From Management
to Leadership

From Management to Leadership

Strategies for Transforming Health Care

Third Edition

Jo Manion

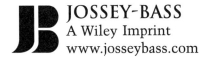

JOSSEY-BASS
A Wiley Imprint
www.josseybass.com

Published by Jossey-Bass
A Wiley Imprint
989 Market Street, San Francisco, CA 94103-1741—www.josseybass.com

Readers should be aware that Internet Web sites offered as citations and/or sources for further information may have changed or disappeared between the time this was written and when it is read.

Limit of Liability/Disclaimer of Warranty: While the publisher and author have used their best efforts in preparing this book, they make no representations or warranties with respect to the accuracy or completeness of the contents of this book and specifically disclaim any implied warranties of merchantability or fitness for a particular purpose. No warranty may be created or extended by sales representatives or written sales materials. The advice and strategies contained herein may not be suitable for your situation. You should consult with a professional where appropriate. Neither the publisher nor author shall be liable for any loss of profit or any other commercial damages, including but not limited to special, incidental, consequential, or other damages.

Jossey-Bass books and products are available through most bookstores. To contact Jossey-Bass directly call our Customer Care Department within the U.S. at 800-956-7739, outside the U.S. at 317-572-3986, or fax 317-572-4002.

Jossey-Bass also publishes its books in a variety of electronic formats. Some content that appears in print may not be available in electronic books.

Library of Congress Cataloging-in-Publication Data

Manion, Jo.
    From management to leadership: strategies for transforming health care / Jo Manion.—3rd ed.
      p. cm.
    Includes bibliographical references and index.
    ISBN 978-0-470-88629-8 (pbk.); 978-1-118-01553-7 (ebk); 978-1-118-01554-4 (ebk);
    978-1-118-01555-1 (ebk)
    1. Health services administration—Psychological aspects.   2. Leadership.   3. Interpersonal
relations. I. Title.
[DNLM: 1. Health Facility Administrators. 2. Efficiency, Organizational. 3. Health Services
Administration. 4. Interpersonal Relations. 5. Leadership. WX 155]
  RA971.M3468 2011
  362.1068—dc22
                                       2010042998

Printed in the United States of America
THIRD EDITION

PB Printing 10 9 8 7 6 5 4 3

CONTENTS

Preface vii

Acknowledgments xv

The Author xvii

1 Leadership: An Elusive Concept 1

2 Cultivating the Leadership Relationship 31

3 Building Commitment: Inspiring Others to Follow 69

4 Communicating with Clarity 115

5 The Art of Effectively Facilitating Processes 179

6 Getting Results 243

7 Coaching and Developing Others 283

8 Going Forward into Our Future 349

References 355

Index 375

To my father . . .
who first set me on my path and instilled in me a
can-do belief with countless repetitions of The Little Engine That Could

To the countless leaders . . .
who have joined me on my journey and inspired me with
their personal insights, stories of wisdom, shared
disappointments, acts of courage, unbridled passion for
their work, and unwavering faith

PREFACE

Welcome to the journey! Whether you are already a transformational leader, an aspiring leader, or simply someone who is interested in a path of continual learning, this book was written for you. Strengthening leadership capacity is a critical challenge facing health care professionals and organizations today. The concepts and principles presented within these pages are essential for those facing the challenge of transforming our health care organizations.

Our world has always been complex; however, in every segment of our lives, the complexity is increasing. Tumultuous change is occurring at break-neck speed and with it comes an overpowering need for individuals who can lead others effectively during these demanding times. Strong and capable leaders are needed who create the direction, remain focused on important priorities amid great distractions, win the commitment of followers and other key stakeholders, and influence others to do what is necessary to achieve a future strategic vision. Unprecedented changes are occurring in executive and managerial health care roles, as well as the manner in which health care organizations function. Health care leaders are assuming nontraditional roles that demand mastery of new and different skills for which they may feel inadequately equipped. The uncertainty of health care reform and the increased presence of government in the health care sector lead to a stressful state of ambiguity. Leaders today face a tremendous challenge in balancing the demands of day-to-day organizational life while learning for the future.

Some organizations meet the challenge of leadership development by recruiting strong leaders from the outside. However, vibrant, dynamic, and flourishing organizations are also committed to developing leaders from within the existing ranks of their managers and employees. Working in partnership with employees to develop their leadership skills is in any organization's best interests. By providing opportunities, active coaching, guidance, and solid experiential learning programs, the organization creates an ever-expanding source of new leaders to navigate amid the turmoil of this decade.

Leadership development is far more than simply an organizational issue, however; it is an intensely personal issue for all health care workers who are being asked to assume increasingly higher levels of responsibility, to be more involved in making decisions about issues that were previously solely the traditional manager's domain, and to serve in leadership roles. Loren Ankario (quoted in "Know How to Lead," 1993) noted that in the first decade of this new millennium, "anyone who is not a leader in his or her own way probably won't have a job." Those words, written almost twenty years ago, have proven to be prophetic. In today's workplace, many employees are seeking—in some instances, demanding—opportunities to serve in roles that influence their work environment even more broadly. In models of shared decision making, organizations consciously develop leaders at all levels.

The concept of leaders at all levels corresponds to societal trends. Overall, the health care workforce is more mature and experienced than ever before in our history. Today's successful health care manager understands that the old command-and-control methodology is no longer appropriate. The work relationship has evolved into a partnership model in which leadership roles are fluid and dynamic, with individuals moving in and out of these roles almost constantly. Facilitating the development of employees' leadership skills makes strategic sense because the entire organization benefits. The organization's foundation is stronger, its structure more resilient, and its future viability more likely in an organization filled with individuals who are leaders or are capable of moving into leadership roles.

To reiterate, this book is written for all health care leaders and aspiring leaders. Seasoned leaders will find that the concepts and skills presented here are essential as they reshape and redefine their roles. The book may also serve as a reference or reminder to which the master leader returns when facing a particular challenge. For new or aspiring leaders, this book can serve as a road map for developing interpersonal skills that enhance the leadership process.

In his book *On Becoming a Leader*, Warren Bennis (1989) notes that leadership courses can teach only skills, not character or vision. He believes character and vision develop in an individual over the course of time, most often as a result of life experiences—learning that occurs beyond traditional course work. However, Peter Drucker believes that all aspects of leadership can and must be learned (Hesselbein, Goldsmith, and Beckhard, 1996). Perhaps it is useful to differentiate between talent and skills, as Buckingham and Coffman (1999) suggest. First, they believe that talent is necessary, and when combined with education and training, determination, and practice, it leads to excellence in practice. In other words, all the determination, education, and training in the world will not help me become a great singer if I do not first have the necessary talent to excel (I am tone deaf and cannot carry a tune). Furthermore, talent cannot be taught; it is there, or it is not.

The presence of the right talent, more than experience, learning, or intelligence, is the prerequisite for excellence as a leader. Skills, however, can be taught and developed. The purpose of this book is to explore the essential interpersonal skills of effective leaders that can be taught and learned: skills that, with study and practice, can increase a leader's effectiveness and strengthen his or her talent base. It is a substantial and in-depth source for the concepts covered. Recent and classic evidence is provided to support the conclusions and writings in this book.

There is an inherent difficulty in writing about leadership. The concepts presented here are most frequently presented in a linear fashion in order to explain them clearly. However, most of these concepts are nonlinear in actual application. Presenting them in a linear fashion can sometimes oversimplify the process and only inadequately give voice to the tremendous complexity that a nonlinear process represents. Only through applying and using these skills does the leader develop them. Yet as learners apply these concepts, they may become frustrated because of the vast number of factors that seem to bear on the outcome. Events and situations rarely unfold in predictable, orderly fashion. The inherent nature of organizations is a state of continual emergence. A particular approach may work well with one individual on a given day, and later the same day factors may have changed enough that the approach needs to be modified. The level of complexity in our environments is almost impossible to comprehend and certainly to describe adequately.

Prior to the publication of the first edition of this book, the American Hospital Association Press and the Center for Health Care Leadership of the American Hospital Association conducted market research on the nature of the leadership gap in health care. Focus groups of more than sixty well-known chief executive officers, board members, physician leaders, consultants, academicians, and community activists revealed five administrative pitfalls driving the emerging paradigm of health care leadership:

- Little or no sense of shared vision and mission within health care organizations

- Ineffective communication skills, especially at the executive level

- Unwillingness to abandon hierarchical control structures, particularly at the executive and board levels

- Refusal to let go of the hospital mentality and traditional modes of service

- Denial of the inevitability of rapid evolution toward capitated reimbursement and managed care

I hope we have made progress in these areas since then. And, indeed, in many organizations, there is vibrancy and passion for the future, and employees work in enthusiastic partnership with executives and managers. Unfortunately, these pitfalls are still present in far too many health care organizations, with tremendous negative consequences as we rapidly move forward to a new future. To offset these weaknesses, leaders will need to take on some nontraditional roles and use innovative approaches for which they may feel unprepared. Mastery of new skills is critical to the successful transition into these roles, and the research shows that these nontraditional skills are clustered into two domains:

- Systems thinking, including skills in collaborative visioning, strategic planning, broad-based decision making, innovative problem solving and process improvement, and stewardship

- Interpersonal abilities, including communication skills, both verbal and nonverbal; coaching; giving constructive feedback; managing conflict; building consensus; delegating responsibility; building teams; and managing change

This book addresses these interpersonal skills, although in a somewhat unusual format. The premise of this book is that leadership exists only within a relationship: if there are no followers, there is no need for a leader. Interpersonal skills in leadership are critical success factors, yet few have written about developing these skills within the leadership context. This book identifies the fundamental interpersonal competencies every transformational leader needs, and it maps out suggestions for improving these skills. It shares examples from health care leaders at all levels to emphasize key points. The concepts in this book are immediately applicable in leadership practice at any level and in any setting where leadership is required and exists.

This third edition contains significantly updated and expanded content. I have added references that reflect current leadership writings and retained classic references and concepts when they are still of value. Some of the most crucial concepts have been around for years, and an older reference date does not necessarily mean the concept is outdated. Learner objectives have been added at the beginning of each chapter at the request of faculty who use this book as a text for their leadership programs. At the end of each chapter are discussion questions with suggested application activities. These can be used for personal reflection or as a basis of conversation with others. In some workplaces, the book is used as a journal selection, with participants reading a chapter and then engaging in dialogue with others about the content. This can serve as a transformational learning tool as it helps move beyond the book knowledge to a more experientially based process.

The first chapter sets the stage by exploring the difference between management and leadership, a concept that even experienced managers and leaders often have trouble grasping concretely. It provides multiple working definitions of *leadership* and identifies key interpersonal requirements.

The chapter examines the reasons that leadership is more crucial today than ever before, as well as several major challenges that contemporary leaders face. Each of the remaining chapters fully examines a key leadership competency.

Chapter Two focuses on establishing the leader-follower relationship, a crucial foundation, for leadership exists only in the context of a relationship. If there are no followers, there is no need for a leader. The chapter addresses the four key elements of this relationship—trust, respect, support, and communication—and includes the nature of collaboration and aspects of forming a partnership. Contemporary leaders will be successful only if they are willing and able to work effectively in partnership with others.

Building commitment among followers is the theme of Chapter Three. A solid base of organizational development theory is presented to increase understanding of the concept of organizational commitment. Executives and managers who inform employees of decisions they have made are seeking compliance or conformance. Most organizational changes occurring today require full commitment from followers to be successful. Commitment is often described as buy-in, a feeling of ownership that goes well beyond mere compliance. Commitment engages the heart and emotions, not just the intellect. What can a leader do to increase the likelihood that key stakeholders—employees, physicians, community members—will commit to the direction the organization takes? The chapter examines both affective and normative organizational commitment. Building a sense of connection and community among all participants and clarifying shared values and a common purpose lead to the possibility of an energizing and inspiring shared vision. Case studies or examples are used to exemplify the power of vision.

Chapter Four deals with the leader's role in communicating effectively, both operationally and strategically. Although seemingly the most simplistic of the interpersonal competencies, communication is central to establishing a healthy leader-follower relationship, and it can be enormously complex. This chapter thoroughly explores verbal and nonverbal communication within the context of contemporary leadership practice. It reexamines long-known principles and concepts in light of today's workplaces and challenges. Several short case examples are shared. It addresses special communication issues such as communicating during times of rapid change, over geographical distances, and with teams.

Many leaders and managers learned their skills in work environments that emphasized outcomes rather than processes. Such organizations often rewarded and promoted the decisive get-it-done individual, whereas they may have seen as slow and plodding the individual who spent the time needed to ensure that the organization followed an appropriate process. Today's leaders must be able to integrate these two approaches and achieve effective outcomes through constructive processes. Key principles of facilitating process are the focus of Chapter Five. The chapter scrutinizes critical processes such as empowering others, resolving conflict, creating effective teams, and leading change and transition. I have separated the critical processes of problem solving and decision making from this chapter and made them the basis of a new chapter focused on getting results. An extension of Chapter Five, the new Chapter Six now includes two alternatives to a traditional problem-solving approach: the action research methodology of appreciative inquiry and a presentation on recognizing polarities and managing them.

The major interpersonal competency, developing others, is the subject of Chapter Seven. Everyone agrees that leaders today must be coaches, and practical, concrete advice is becoming available on how to fill this role. Principles of coaching, teaching, motivating, and encouraging others are this chapter's subject. Effective leaders are continual learners themselves, and they expect others around them to continually grow, develop, learn, and stretch. Good leaders are serious about tapping the potential within each person to expand his or her reach, grow, and increase personal leadership capacity. Systems thinking and collaborative learning are key characteristics of a leader-coach-teacher.

Although mastery of these key competencies does not guarantee immediately successful leadership, it can help those who have innate talents become more effective. Developing and refining leadership skills is a lifelong journey. Circumstances regularly alter, creating the need for new skill sets. I offer this book to stimulate thought and provoke creative action for those on the path to expanding personal leadership capacity. Enjoy the journey!

ACKNOWLEDGMENTS

I gratefully acknowledge the following people who were instrumental in helping to make this book a reality:

- The countless leader colleagues who over the years have shared their experiences and stories with me while on their path
- The colleagues and research participants who willingly and generously gave of their time and wisdom in my pursuit of answers
- Those who have been instrumental in this book's journey over the years: Winnie Schmeling, Richard Hill, and Andy Pasternack and Seth Schwartz at Jossey-Bass
- My husband and lifelong partner, Craig, who has been an unwavering source of support, love, and encouragement

THE AUTHOR

Jo Manion is the president of Manion & Associates, an organizational development consulting practice in Oviedo, Florida. A nationally recognized professional speaker, consultant, and author, she specializes in practical strategies focused on professional and organizational development. Her four decades of health care experience in a variety of organizations and positions have created expertise in the areas of leadership development, the creation of positive work environments, increasing organizational capacity, and the development of effective teams. Her research focuses on the area of the leadership role in creating positive workplaces. A fellow in the American Academy of Nursing, she holds both a master's degree and a doctorate in human and organizational systems from the Fielding Graduate Institute. She is the author of *The Engaged Workforce: Proven Strategies to Build a Positive Health Care Workplace* (2009) and coauthor of *Nature's Wisdom in the Work Place: Managing Energy in Today's Health Care Organization* (2005). She is widely published on a variety of topics.

From Management
to Leadership

1

Leadership

AN ELUSIVE CONCEPT

CHAPTER OBJECTIVES

- Define leadership.
- Differentiate between leadership and management.
- Identify reasons that leadership is especially important today.
- Discuss challenges that health care leaders face today.
- Distinguish between a challenge and an excuse.

Leadership has to take place every day.
It cannot be the responsibility of the few, a rare event,
or a once-in-a-lifetime opportunity.
R. A. HEIFETZ AND D. L. LAURIE, "THE WORK OF LEADERSHIP"

N o other issue is as important in health care today as the development and continual evolution of leaders. "Leadership is the pivotal force behind successful organizations. . . . To create vital and viable organizations, leadership is necessary to help organizations develop a new vision of what they can be, then mobilize the organization to change toward the new vision" (Bennis and Nanus, 1985, p. 12). An organization's success is directly correlated to its leaders' strengths and the depth of internal leadership capacity. The failure of an organization to develop leaders at all levels, relying instead on a few strong leaders at the top, results in dismal outcomes. In the foreword to Gifford and Elizabeth Pinchot's book *The Intelligent Organization* (1996b, p. x), Warren Bennis notes that "traditional bureaucratic organizations have failed and continue to fail, in large part, because they tend to rely exclusively on the intelligence of those at the very top of the pyramid."

In the same way, relying on only formal managers for leadership limits the tremendous possibilities that exist when leaders are acknowledged from within any part or level of the organization. "Solutions . . . reside not in the executive suite but in the collective intelligence of employees at all levels, who need to use one another as resources, often across boundaries, and learn their way to those solutions" (Heifetz and Laurie, 1997, p. 124). Health care is facing a daunting challenge: the development of leaders. "The leadership pool in health care is shrinking in part because companies continue to ruthlessly excise management positions—formerly training grounds for aspiring executives—in the race to become leaner and meaner" (Grossman, 1999, p. 18). And although these tactics may have saved money in the short term, the long-term consequences to health care were significant in the absence of qualified individuals to move into executive and leadership roles. This past decade has seen the further decimation of ranks of managers as older workers are beginning to retire. The tremendous challenges of leadership positions today have resulted in situations in many organizations where the time required to recruit to frontline management positions has extended. The work is less appealing to potential candidates than it was in the past.

Many people fail to understand clearly the distinction between leadership and management; as a result, this narrows the field from which organizational leaders might emerge. In some instances, organizations do not recognize leaders who, without formal positional authority, emerge from the ranks; they sometimes resist them and label them as troublemakers or dissatisfied employees. "It is an illusion to expect that an executive team on its own will find the best way into the future. So you must use leadership to generate more leadership deep in the organization" (Heifetz, Grashow, and Linsky, 2009, p. 68).

This chapter explores the concept of leadership, differentiates it from management, identifies reasons that leadership is so critical in today's health care organizations, and illuminates several major challenges facing health care leaders.

Defining Leadership

Defining leadership is the first step. It is a much more elusive concept than is management. Most authorities on the topic define leadership as influencing others to do what needs to be done, especially those things organizational leadership believes need to be accomplished. The term *transformational leadership* has become repopularized as a result of the Magnet recognition program that identifies organizations with internal cultures strongly supportive of excellence in professional practice. The new model for Magnet has five identified components, one of which is transformational leadership. Leading people where they want to go is easy; in some instances, the biggest challenge is getting out of their way. However, the transformational leader "must lead people to where they *need to be* to meet the demands of the future" (Wolf, Triolo, and Ponte, 2008, p. 202). It's important to note here that the goal of the transformational leader is to transform the organization or department, not necessarily the people within it.

Kouzes and Posner (2002, p. xvii) identify the leadership challenge as "how leaders mobilize others to want to get extraordinary things done in organizations." Max DePree (1989, p. xx) believes the art of leadership is "liberating people to do what is required of them in the most effective and humane way possible." This definition implies that leadership is not something one does to or for the follower but is instead a process of releasing the potential already present within an individual. The leader sets the stage and then steps out of the way to let others perform. True leadership enables followers to realize their full potential—potential that the followers perhaps did not suspect.

Also implied in any definition is that leadership is work. It is about performance: achieving outcomes, getting needed results. Peter Drucker (1992, p. 199) says that "it has little to do with 'leadership qualities' and even less to do with 'charisma.' It is mundane, unromantic, and boring. Its essence is performance." Kouzes and Posner (2002, p. 13) reinforce this message: "Leadership is not at all about personality; it's about practice."

Leadership is mobilizing the interest, energy, and commitment of all people at all levels of the organization. It is a means to an end. "An effective leader knows that the ultimate task of leadership is to create human energies and human vision" (Drucker, 1992, p. 122). Bardwick (1996) clearly states that leadership is not intellectual or cognitive but emotional. She points out that at the emotional level, leaders create followers because they generate "confidence in people who are frightened, certainty in people who were vacillating, action where there was hesitation, strength where there was weakness, expertise where there was floundering, courage where there were cowards, optimism where there was cynicism, and a conviction that the future will be better" (p. 14).

Noted leadership scholar and author Warren Bennis, who has spent four decades studying leaders, describes the leader as "one who manifests direction, integrity, hardiness, and courage in a consistent pattern of behavior that inspires trust, motivation, and responsibility on the part of the followers who in turn become leaders themselves" (Johnson, 1998, p. 293). He concludes that in addition to passion and an intense level of personal commitment, virtually every great leader has four competencies (O'Connell, 2009):

- *The ability to manage others' attention*, through a clear vision of what needs to be accomplished
- *The knack for managing meaning* by communicating well
- *The skill of managing others' trust* through being a person of integrity and good character
- *The self-knowledge* that allows the leader to deploy his or her skills effectively

None of these is easily teachable by the methods often used for leadership development, such as reading widely or attending seminars and formal academic programs. However, all three can be learned or perfected through life's experiences. For most people, the development of leadership capacity is lifelong work—a trial-and-error method of perfecting techniques and approaches and the evolution of personality and individual beliefs. Often the leader is not even aware of exactly how he or she influenced a follower. An opportunity or need to lead appeared, and the leader stepped forward to meet the challenge.

Harry Kraemer (2003, p. 18), chairman and CEO of Baxter Healthcare, believes that the best leaders are "people who have a very delicate balance between self-confidence and humility." They are both self-confident and comfortable expressing their ideas and opinions, but they balance this expression with a healthy dose of humility and an understanding that other people may have better ideas and more insight on any given issue.

And perhaps most telling are the results of research conducted by Jim Collins and his associates (2001). They studied extensively the difference between good companies and compared them to similar companies that had achieved greatness. Although Collins told his research team specifically not to focus on leadership at the top, their final analysis revealed that leadership was a key factor for those companies with extraordinary success. The type of leadership the study revealed was a shocking surprise to the researchers. They found that the characteristics of these successful leaders did not include high-profile personalities and celebrity status but just the opposite: "Self-effacing, quiet, reserved, even shy—these leaders are a paradoxical blend of personal humility and professional will. They are more like Lincoln and Socrates than Patton or Caesar" (p. 12). Their ambition is first and foremost for their organization, not for themselves.

Several years later, Collins (2005) examined leadership in social sector organizations and found a striking difference between the social and business sectors. He described social sector leadership as a "legislative" type of leader. In other words, these leaders do not have the power of decision. Frances Hesselbein, CEO of the Girl Scouts of the USA, was asked how she accomplished her results without the concentrated executive power seen in the business sector. She replied, "Oh, you always have power, if you just know where to find it. There is the power of inclusion, and the power of language, and the power of shared interests, and the power of coalition. Power is all around you to draw upon, but it is rarely raw, rarely visible" (Collins, 2005, p. 10).

The complex and diffuse power structures common in health care organizations means that no executive has enough structural power to make the most important decisions alone. To those from other sectors, the leader may look weak and indecisive when in fact successful leaders in social sector organizations develop incredible skills of persuasion, political currency, and coalition building. Collins (2005) notes that the irony here is that those of us in the social sector "increasingly look to business for leadership models and talent, yet I suspect we will find more true leadership in the social sectors than the business sector" (p. 12). True leadership, says Collins, exists only if people follow when they have the freedom not to.

Distinguishing Between Management and Leadership

How does leadership differ from management? Most would agree that not all managers are good leaders and not all leaders are good managers. However, differentiating between these two concepts concisely and concretely is difficult. A common misconception is that the legitimate authority of a position, such as holding a management job or an elected office, automatically confers leadership skills on the person holding that position. Nothing is further from the truth. In the same way, simply being able to biologically reproduce does not make a person a good parent. Leadership and management are two separate and distinct concepts, although they may exist simultaneously in the same person. In an interview (Flower, 1990), Bennis compares management and leadership on several key points. His viewpoint greatly increases clarity about these two concepts.

Efficiency Versus Effectiveness

The first differentiating point is related to the essential focus of the individual. A manager is concerned with efficiency—getting things done right, better, and faster. Increasing productivity and streamlining current operations are important, and managers often exhort employees to work smarter, not harder. Productivity reports and statistics are crucial for evaluating success. In contrast, a leader is more concerned with effectiveness, asking: "Are we doing the right thing?" The initial question is not, "How can we do this faster?" but, "Should we be doing this at all?" To answer the latter question, a key deciding factor is whether the activity in question directly supports the organization's overall purpose and mission. Is the activity in alignment with the stated values and beliefs of the organization and the people within it? Will it produce desirable outcomes?

A classic example of this difference occurred some years ago in a 480-bed midwestern medical center. As the hospital's volume increased over the years, traffic flow on the elevators became a major problem. Several process improvement teams attacked the problem at various times but came up with no lasting or truly effective solution. After years of frustration, a team assigned to this issue finally came up with a solution: building a new set of elevators for patients only. The intent was to move patients faster and more efficiently, a goal the medical center attempted to accomplish for several hundred thousand dollars.

A couple of years later, the organization went through a major reengineering and work redesign effort. The first questions were: Why are we transporting patients all over the organization? Can we deploy any services to the patient care unit to reduce the distance that patients travel? These are leadership questions; instead of asking how to move patients faster, the project team asked: Should patients be moved at all? How can we reduce movement of patients? This kind of thinking has led to the concept of the universal room: the patient is admitted to a room and remains assigned to that room throughout the entire hospital stay. The level of care may change depending on the patient's needs, but the location of the patient does not.

How Versus What and Why

A second differentiating characteristic is that management is about how, whereas leadership is about what and why. A good manager usually understands the work processes and can demonstrate and explain to an employee how to accomplish the work. Health care, which has a history of promoting people with job or technical expertise to management and supervisory roles, clearly values these characteristics. The highly skilled worker or practitioner becomes a manager, and overall this is the typical pattern regardless of the department or discipline in question. Healthcare workers tend to highly value job expertise in their managers and, in fact, often show disdain for managers who cannot perform at a highly competent level the work of the employees they manage. This is understandable when we examine health care's history. Early hospitals were led and managed by individuals with a high level of technical clinical expertise (physicians and nurses). Only in recent decades have a significant number of executives and managers with nonclinical backgrounds entered health care administration. Some clinical health care workers today still doubt that individuals with nonclinical backgrounds can possibly understand enough to be effective leaders in health care organizations.

Knowing and controlling work processes are essential components of the managerial role—and rightly so. Management's origins were in the factories of the industrial age. The workforce of the late 1800s was very different from today's workforce. Most early factory workers were newly arrived immigrants, women, and children—poorly informed, uneducated, non-English-speaking, and uninvolved employees—working for survival wages. The work was compartmentalized, broken down into small, manageable pieces that one person could easily teach to these early workers. The manager was responsible for ensuring that employees did the work correctly and was often the only person who understood the entire piece of work. The workforce is remarkably different today, where most are considered knowledge workers.

In contrast to a manager, a leader focuses on what needs to be done and why. He or she spends more time explaining the general direction and purpose of the work, and then the leader gets out of the way so that the follower can do it. Someone once characterized a leader as an individual who describes what needs to be done and then says, "It's up to you to impress me with how you do it."

This implies several points. First, the leader knows what needs to be done and can clearly articulate this to others in a way that convinces the followers that it is an appropriate direction. Second, the leader has the patience to share the reasons this course has been chosen and ensures that those reasons are acceptable and valid to the follower. Finally, the leader accepts that the follower may find a new and possibly better way to accomplish the goals. The leader is not wedded to his or her way of performing a task or carrying out a responsibility.

There are many examples of this leadership approach in health care organizations today. When a health care organization is undertaking a major cultural change initiative, executives often present it in a way that first explains the organization's current status, the external environment, and the reasons the board of trustees and executive team believe this initiative is necessary for the organization's future viability. When the case is made well and the reasons are clear, employees in most instances view them as important and valued. When the reasons for the change align with important values and beliefs that frontline employees hold, positive results are much more likely.

Structure Versus People

In contrast, Bennis (Flower, 1990) points out that management is about systems, controls, procedures, and policies—all of which create structure—whereas leadership is about people. Managers spend much of their time dealing with organizational structure. Anyone who has successfully participated in an accreditation visit by an outside agency has a sense of the number of policies and procedures that the average health care institution generates. There is usually a policy or procedure for every aspect of organizational and professional life. Infection control monitoring, risk management reporting, corporate compliance protocols, and patient-complaint resolution are only a few among the multitude of control systems designed to oversee organizational processes. These systems ensure that work is progressing as expected; they are designed to alert the manager to any deviation so that it can be investigated and corrected. Extensive policies and procedures, however, can sometimes be used to substitute for employees' good judgment and initiative in decision making. Relying heavily on the use of written policies and procedures can inadvertently weaken the development of individual decision making in the organization.

Although control is really the essence of management, it shouldn't be construed as a negative. There need to be organizing structures and processes in the most complex organizations. There is continual pressure to reduce variation and increase quality, and this is often accomplished by meeting established standards and expectations. The manager's role is to control processes and structures to ensure that certain outcomes result. "This is managerial control. Managers must have many checks and balances to ensure timely, cost-effective, and high-quality results" (Vestal, 2009c, p. 6).

Leadership is about people and relationships. Leadership exists only within the context of a relationship. If there are no followers, there is no need for leadership, just independent action. Leadership occurs when leader behavior influences someone else to act in a certain manner, and at the core of such a connection between people is trust. Chapter Two explores these concepts in depth. Leadership as primarily a relationship may be disturbing news for managers who have limited people or interpersonal skills, for an individual who has difficulty in working with others will find it virtually impossible to become a transformational leader. A book on policies and procedures cannot replace this key relationship. Fortunately, an aspiring leader can develop and hone people skills, but maintaining them takes more energy if they are not part of the individual's natural talent base.

Status Quo Versus Innovation

Whereas maintaining and managing the status quo are appropriate managerial behaviors (Bennis, 1989), leaders are more concerned with innovation and implementing new processes to create a desired future. This is a difficult area for many health care leaders because most health care organizations have not customarily encouraged or highly valued either creativity or innovation. The words are frequently used and can even appear in the mission statement, but only rarely are health care organizations flexible and fluid enough to encourage true innovation. Most are bureaucratic structures that respond to any deviation from standard practice as something to stamp out, control, or at least limit in some manner.

Punitive responses to mistakes are common, and many managers have learned not to rock the boat or deviate in any significant way. The incident-reporting mechanism is a common example. If an employee reports making a mistake, a familiar response is for the manager to determine what went wrong and how the employee needs to change so that the mistake never occurs again—a return to the status quo. Less frequent is a response that investigates the mistake in partnership with employees to determine why the mistake occurred and what needs to change in the system so that the problem does not occur again. Recent emphasis on patient safety and quality has stimulated a move toward more creative problem solving and resolution without placing blame. Often referred to as a just culture, errors and mistakes are seen as an opportunity for improvement. Investigation is thorough, but responses to these situations are deliberate and based on many factors.

Leaders are always looking for ways to improve the current situation; they are never satisfied with the status quo. A leader's automatic response to a problem or mistake is to consider ways to capitalize on the opportunity that the mistake has created. For this reason, Bennis points out, "bureaucracies tend to suppress real leadership because real leaders disequilibrate systems; they create disorder and instability, even chaos" (Flower, 1990, p. 62).

Because a leader trusts people, he or she knows that the follower can always find a way to improve on the current situation. DePree (1989) describes highly effective leaders as those who are comfortable abandoning themselves to others' strengths and admitting that they themselves cannot know or do everything. This can be frightening to those who are not up to the challenge of continually questioning their own performance or established practices. Fearful individuals may react to this drive for continual improvement as implied criticism: "It was not good enough, and now we have to change it."

Bottom Line Versus Horizon

Managers keep their eyes on the bottom line; leaders focus on the horizon. "With leaders, the future calls to them in a voice they can't drown out. The future is more real than the present; it compels them to act" (Breen, 2005, p. 66). Managers ask: Are we within budget? Are we meeting our goals? What's the deadline? How can we improve our productivity? The manager's emphasis is on counting, recording, and measuring to ensure that everything is on target. It is easy to forget that many things that count—that are important—cannot be counted. By its very nature, leadership and its results are difficult to measure. How do you measure a relationship? What are the concrete, observable outcomes of a healthy working relationship? How do you evaluate the success of an inspiring vision? Good leaders see beyond the bottom line to the horizon, where a vision of a different future for themselves and their followers guides their day-to-day decision making. This vision inspires them as they make difficult decisions on behalf of the organization and the people within it.

A leader with a vision of the future that includes highly engaged and passionate employees who feel ownership of their jobs, make decisions affecting work in their span of control, and work in partnership with the organization's managers knows that in order to attain this vision, the organization will need to continually invest in employee learning and development opportunities. In many organizations today, employees are being asked to contribute more, learn additional skills, and take on more responsibility at the same time that their organizations have severely reduced education departments and learning resources. Leadership decisions to invest in employee education may not look good on the bottom line, but they often are required in order to attain an alternative future. Exemplary leaders recognize that organizations that do not invest in the development of internal staff resources now will have to pay a much higher price in the future.

Another simple example of the difference between focusing on results and paying attention to the future payoff is evident when we observe leaders who become actively involved in coaching their employees for improved performance. If an employee is having difficulty with a key vendor, people in another department, or perhaps a physician, it is relatively easy for a manager to use his or her legitimate authority and step in to solve the problem. Coaching and supporting the employee in solving the problem directly may be more time-consuming and riskier. However, this leadership approach creates stronger, more effective employees, and the payoff is in the future because employees learn how to handle their own problems.

Management and Leadership: A Final Word

That there is a difference between management and leadership is clear. However, it is more of a both-and choice rather than an either-or choice. None of this discussion is to imply that there is not a need for exemplary managers in today's health care organizations, and often the best leaders have strong management skills. Managers will always be needed, and the role is so crucial that everyone in the organization must share managerial responsibilities. Highly efficient employees who understand their work, are able to organize and structure it, and can measure outcomes and take corrective action will always be in high demand. With a greater number of experienced and mature workers in health care today, organizations place higher expectations on employees than ever before. As more employees become self-managing, organizations may reduce the number of formal managers. At the same time, however, there is an increasing need for leaders. According to many scholars, organizations in this country have been overmanaged and underled (Bennis and Nanus, 1985; Kouzes and Posner, 2002; Peters, 1987).

Why Leadership Is in Demand Today

During the 1970s, health care organizations had a burgeoning interest in management development programs. It was recognized that promoting technically competent employees into management positions produced a responsibility on the part of the organization to provide management and supervisory training and education. In the 1990s, there was a shift in all sectors of society to emphasize the importance of leadership skills. The increased number of titles about leadership in a popular bookstore reflects this emphasis. A search on amazon.com produces over sixty-three thousand hits, and when the search is narrowed to health care leadership, there are still 883 titles. Why this focus on leadership? Why is this a compelling issue in today's world? There are at least three major reasons:

- The unrelenting crush of change

- Rapidly shifting paradigms

- Survival

Change

Change has been the byword for over twenty years. Never before has the pace of change been so fast or have the changes altered so deeply the way people live and work. "The change and upheaval of the past years have left us with no place to hide. We need anchors in our lives, something like a trim-tab factor, a guiding purpose. Leaders fill that need" (Bennis, 1989, p. 15). Fundamental changes in health care are occurring so rapidly that it is hard to keep pace. What we all believed to be significant organizational changes in the 1980s—revised job descriptions, new management positions, novel performance appraisal systems—pale by comparison to today's changes, such as new locations for services, innovative business structures, specialty or niche hospitals, distance medicine, virtual patients, health care on the Internet, replacing employees by automation, outsourcing, cross-training of skills, forming partnerships within the community, simultaneously collaborating and competing with the same entity, and merging with other organizations or developing an entirely new system. Annison (1994, p. 1) states the case clearly: "During periods of stability we can be successful by doing more of what we already do; the focus is on management and maintaining the present. During periods of change, the emphasis is on changing what we do and the focus is on leadership."

Shifting Paradigms

Paradigms, or the models through which we view the world, are rapidly shifting. Barker (1992, p. 37) describes it this way: "A paradigm shift, then, is a change to a new game, a new set of rules." This shift creates confusion and unease as well as new possibilities. In some instances, a player in the health care sector changes the paradigm, whereas in other situations, the impetus comes from without. The rules and game plan may suddenly change, leaving those in the game to figure out the new rules.

Competition in health care is a good example of a paradigm that continues to shift. Not so long ago, the major competitor for a hospital was the other hospital in town, just down the road. Today competition comes from everywhere: stand-alone health care facilities, such as ambulatory care centers, specialty hospitals and services, and diagnostic centers in physician offices; hospitals from other communities that set up satellite or full-service facilities outside their originating communities; and even previous customers who decide to become providers on a limited basis. There are now destination health care countries where American citizens can go to receive their care in countries such as India or Thailand, often in hospitals or clinics run by American-educated and -trained individuals. The cost is much less than in the United States.

The lines and boundaries are no longer clear. As the business world has demonstrated, one must sometimes collaborate with close competitors (Annison, 1997). Consumers buying an Apple computer may be purchasing a machine manufactured by Toshiba; MasterCard and Visa collaborate on automatic teller machines and choose to compete on marketing and customer service. Similarly, in health care, two hospitals from competing systems have jointly built a wellness facility in their community, and a major medical center has partnered with a large clinic-based physician practice on several joint projects while competing with it on several others.

Times of great change and rapidly shifting paradigms call for leaders. As Barker (1992, p. 164) points out, "You manage within a paradigm. You lead between paradigms." When times are stable and game rules remain consistent and known, structures, standards, and protocols enhance the manager's ability to optimize the paradigm. In fact, this describes the manager's job exactly. However, during a shift to new paradigms, leadership is required, as Barker explains: "Leaving one paradigm while it is still successful and going to a new paradigm that is as yet unproved looks very risky. But leaders, with their intuitive judgment, assess the seeming risk, determine that shifting paradigms is the correct thing to do, and, because they are leaders, instill the courage in others to follow them" (p. 164).

When paradigms shift and the rules change, everyone involved goes back to zero. Put simply in the words of a colleague, "What got you to the party won't keep you there!" It is time to let go of past successes and look for new ways of doing things. There is no guarantee that the organization, group, or individual who was very good with the old game rules will be as good with the new ones. In fact, the more successful the individual or organization was with the old model, the more difficult it is for him or her to engage in a new way of thinking. A recently observed paradigm shift was seen in 2009 when health care reform was being hotly debated. Business owners and employers were seen as "the bad guy," the ones with a hidden agenda that involved keeping the current system in place. As a result of this political climate, many of these voices were silent when the debate was held, although they certainly represented a tremendous source of knowledge about the system.

When paradigms shift, it is crucial to recognize the change, or your efforts will be fruitless. It is foolish to hold onto the belief that past or current success automatically leads to future success. When we hold to the old paradigm, we may be reluctant to make changes rapidly enough to adapt to the changing external environment. A common behavior is the overreliance on internal expertise and experience, resulting in an aversion to risk taking and a desire to dictate to others how things will be. None of these behaviors will lead to ultimate or enduring success.

The issue of changing paradigms is easy to talk about intellectually but difficult to deal with in its reality. What will it really take to become a fluid and flexible organization, capable of dealing with the enormously tumultuous external environment? How can we provide mobile health care services instead of being limited to an institution and its four walls? How can we shift from the old methods of communicating and move into the tremendous opportunities that new communication technology and the Internet present?

Survival

The final and perhaps most important reason that we need leadership today is survival. Bennis (1989) reported the work of a scientist at the University of Michigan who examined and listed what he considered to be the ten basic dangers to our society, factors that he believed were capable of destroying the human species. The top three are:

- A nuclear war or accident, capable of destroying the human race
- A worldwide epidemic, disease, famine, or financial depression
- The quality of management and leadership in our institutions

There was probably no clearer example of the importance of leadership as during the immediate aftermath of the devastating terrorist attacks on the United States on September 11, 2001. The actions and decisions of our national leaders were crucial. Hasty and reactive actions could have led to even more devastating results. The quality and importance of leaders who emerged was striking.

Leaders are responsible for an organization's effectiveness. As an industry, health care is vulnerable as a result of regulatory changes, technological pressures, globalization, the litigious mind-set, changing demographics, and environmental challenges. Strong leadership is needed to take us into a very uncertain future. Pinchot and Pinchot (1996a, p. 18) eloquently describe the need for leaders: "The more machines take over routine work and the higher the percentage of knowledge workers, the more leaders are needed. The work left for humans involves innovation, seeing things in new ways, and responding to customers by changing the way things are done. We are reaching a time when every employee will take turns leading. Each will find circumstances when they see what must be done and must influence others to make their vision of a better way a reality."

Finally, the role of leaders as it influences organizational integrity is crucial. "There is a pervasive, national concern about the integrity of our institutions. Wall Street was, not long ago, a place where a man's word was his bond. The recent investigations, revelations, and indictments have forced the industry to change the way it conducted business for 150 years. Jim Bakker and Jimmy Swaggart have given a new meaning to the phrase 'children of a lesser God'" (Bennis, 1989, pp. 15–16). Although Bennis wrote those words years ago, they seem prophetic. In the past few years, Americans have become almost inured to corporate scandal and wrongdoing. The collapse of Enron, Arthur Andersen, and WorldCom was just the beginning of what seems to be a never-ending parade of corporate corruption. Many Americans now fully expect that people in positions of power lack personal and professional integrity and can be counted on to lie and cheat. Political corruption and lack of faith in national leaders is at an all-time low.

Health care is not immune to the issue of integrity. Hospital executives indicted for Medicare fraud, home health agencies led by criminals previously convicted of fraud, a cardiovascular surgeon falsifying information and performing hundreds of clearly unnecessary surgeries, a pharmacist diluting chemotherapeutic agents to increase profit, executives at a well-known rehabilitation company indicted for illegal practices, or a community hospital's senior executives convicted of embezzlement: all have made the headlines in recent years. Never before has the need for ethical, exemplary leaders been more crucial as we face the challenges of the next decade.

Challenges Facing Today's Leaders

Today the opportunities and possibilities for leaders are endless, as are the challenges. Difficulties are not all bad. Strong leaders see difficult times as offering tremendous opportunities. Often the times and events that push us the most also have the capability of bringing forth our very best. It's important to notice the difference between a challenge and an excuse. Every one of these challenges presented here can also be used as an excuse in the organization. "I couldn't make a decision when things were so uncertain." "You just can't please everyone. I don't know how you can motivate these young people today!" When we give up on the challenge, we are letting it become an excuse, a reason that we cannot accomplish the results we need. For every one who uses a challenge as an excuse, there is a leader somewhere who uses the same challenge to achieve stunning results.

Demands are different for today's leaders and have ramifications for anyone aspiring to lead others. Recent dramatic upheavals have left no sector untouched. "The financial, political, environmental, and social challenges have affected us all in different ways and, in turn, have impacted our organizations and employees. It leaves us all wondering what will happen next that will change the world we live in and the places we work" (Vestal, 2009a, p. 6). The more a leader understands these issues, the more likely it is that he or she can find the strength and courage to meet the test that these challenges present. A handful of representative challenges include these:

- Accelerating levels of ambiguity and uncertainty
- Workforce issues
- Diversity in the workforce
- Turbulent business and regulatory environments
- The leader's energy drain

Accelerating Levels of Ambiguity and Uncertainty

Probably the most apt description of today's world is uncertainty. Leaders today are dealing with a level of ambiguity and uncertainty almost unparalleled in our memories. Although uncertainty and ambiguity are not measurable, they are palpable in workplaces. Change continues to accelerate at a pace that makes it impossible to predict even the near-term future with any accuracy. And as change begets more change, the challenges become more complex and difficult to meet.

Today's solution rapidly becomes tomorrow's problem that must be dealt with. In no other area is this clearer than in technology. The advent of the electronic medical record (EMR) created visions of a health care environment where workers could be more productive, the electronic processing of medical information making their lives much easier. Nurses would spend more time at the bedside caring for patients. Members of various departments and different disciplines could communicate virtually through real-time computing technology. Errors would be reduced and patient quality increased.

The reality for many people today is quite different from the original vision and the promise implied, if not explicitly made. In many organizations, problems abound with the EMR. Decisions about hardware and software were made with limited or low-quality input from end users, and as a result, they are inadequate to meet practitioners' needs. Organizations invested major portions of their financial resources into technology, only to find it seriously outdated within a few years. Years are spent waiting for upgrades, either because of their lack of availability or lack of resources on the part of the organization. Productivity for many has declined rather than improved. Caregivers navigate multiple screens to access pertinent information. Duplication continues to exist as practitioners are forced to complete screens of information that may not even apply to the individual for whom they are caring, such as a decubitus ulcer assessment on an ambulatory clinic patient. And the quality of patient care? Of course, in many ways it has improved because of the technology capabilities inherent in the EMR. However, the impact of a caregiver or physician sitting with his or her back to the patient busily inputting data into the computer was never considered as a serious consequence of the technology. Relationship-based care, the underlying foundation of an effective relationship between patient and health care worker, can be seriously and negatively affected when caregivers lose the high touch of person-centered care in our high-tech world of today.

Of course, the world is not worse off because of the invention of the computer. And no one would advocate stopping or even slowing the tremendous advances that have been made through technology of all kinds. Nanotechnology holds great hope for treating and curing diseases that have plagued humankind throughout its history. However, these changes often complicate our lives in unforeseen ways. Leaders know that the current change simply brings us closer to the next one.

Living during times of great ambiguity and uncertainty requires tremendous energy, both personal and organizational. Because influencing others positively when we are exhausted is difficult, leaders must take good care of themselves during changing times and manage their energy wisely (Loehr and Schwartz, 2003; Cox, Manion, and Miller, 2005). Not all changes are for the better, and a leader is challenged to remain optimistic and enthusiastic yet truthful. This can be arduous in the face of personal discouragement. Transformational leaders have a high degree of resilience in their ability to demonstrate courage, strength, and flexibility in the face of change and frightening disorder.

Sometimes the challenge for a leader lies in determining which changes to make and which to forgo. It is easy to become swept up in the tide of change and go overboard. Many leaders find change exhilarating and forget that the organization's ability to sustain a certain pace of change may not match the leader's capacity for change. Winston Churchill said, "When it is not necessary to change, it is necessary not to change" (Curtin, 1995, p. 7). This sage advice is easy to forget when all the changes look positive. The knack of looking beyond the initial excitement and potential promise to determine whether the change is necessary and beneficial is a leadership skill worth developing.

Peter Drucker talks about this same issue (Flower, 1991, p. 53), but he refers to it as being effective. He says the leader has to sometimes say no: "The secret of effectiveness is concentration of the very meager resources you have where you can make a difference." Thus, the leader's role is to carefully assess what changes are most important and likely to help achieve the organization's goals and attain its vision while avoiding the energy drain of nonessential change.

The pace of change in the world today results in ambiguity and uncertainty in every arena of our lives. Some of this change will be for the better, but it is likely that at least some will increase the difficulties people experience in both their personal and professional lives. The entire structure of health care is changing. Health care reform will reshape our systems in ways that will create challenges as well as opportunities over the next decade. Other factors at work requiring critical shifts in thinking by health care leaders—for example:

- A shift from current reimbursement structures to pay-for-performance and bundling of costs

- A shift from inpatient acute care to outpatient services, requiring health care leaders to rethink traditional hospital boundaries, investments, and relationships with key stakeholders

- The changing business practices and structures of physicians, moving from independent status to employment

- The continued shift from a discipline-centered production organization to a customer-focused service orientation

- A continuing shift from an illness and disease model to a wellness paradigm with a focus on alternative or complementary medicine

These high levels of uncertainty and ambiguity are to be expected when so many people are in transition. The word *change* means to alter or make something different. Transition is the psychological adaptation to change and is not over until the person can function and find meaning in the new situation (Bridges, 1991). If a transition has occurred, something has been lost, even if it is as simple as loss of comfort with the old way. Thus, stages of transition include stages of grief, which engender some of the most difficult emotions humans face. People often experience and express anger, depression, anxiety, fear, and just plain contrariness. Trying to lead people who are grieving is fraught with difficulties and can tax even the most proficient leader.

These emotions are complex enough to face in an individual, much less when multiplied by hundreds and even thousands in an organization. Understanding where people are in their emotional cycle helps prevent inappropriate or unhelpful responses. The fact that individuals may be in different places at the same time makes the challenge more intense. Adding to the complexity is the fact that the leader may be feeling some of these difficult emotions as well. Chapter Five explores the transition process in more detail.

Workforce Issues

The large number of Baby Boomers nearing retirement age and the declining numbers of younger workers entering health care are rapidly reaching a crisis point. This challenge will be one of the most difficult in this new decade and is likely to remain a paramount concern for many years into the future. A poll of hospital CEOs by the American Hospital Association (2001) found that 72 percent of respondents identified workforce shortages as one of the top three concerns. Demographics alone tell us that workforce shortages are not just a temporary challenge but part of the landscape for many years to come. This has become a major concern of governments and countries throughout the developed world (Manion, 2009a) as they face the unpleasant situation of higher-paid workers exiting the active workforce through retirement and beginning to draw on government pension plans. The result is less tax revenue being collected at a time when entitlement liabilities are increasing. Both organizations and governments are seeking ways to delay retirement age through legislation and making the workplace more attractive for older workers.

In the not-so-recent past, one of the biggest issues in the arena of workforce management was the recruitment and placement of qualified people. "Never before have organizations paid more attention to talent . . . keeping it. Stealing it. Developing it. Engaging it. Talent is no longer just a numbers game; it's about survival" (Kaye and Jordan-Evans, 2002, p. 32). Workforce shortage issues were not limited to one discipline or one job category in organizations but cut across all boundaries. Although the literature often focuses on the cost of turnover of higher-paid professionals such as pharmacists, nurses, and physical therapists, a significant cost is also associated with the turnover and vacancy of workers in positions such as housekeepers, dietary aides, and nursing assistants. This cost may be lower per individual, but the sheer number of these workers employed in the average health care organization makes the cost almost prohibitive. A study of long-term care organizations reported turnover rates of nurse aides near 100 percent annually. This represents a tremendous cost to the organization, one that far exceeds the financial impact.

In the more recent past, the tremendous economic downturn has changed the landscape considerably. There are now fewer vacant positions. In many instances there are many more applicants for a position than will be hired. The unemployment rate has skyrocketed, and the official statistics likely underreport the true situation because they don't take into account those who are unemployed and have given up looking for work. In health care organizations, many part-time workers have converted to full-time positions or opted for more work hours when they are able to get them. Temporary staff members working in agencies are seeking a job where there is more stability in their work hours. Close-to-retirement workers are delaying their exit from the workforce in order to replenish personal retirement accounts depleted during the downturn. The result is that our organizations have fewer vacancies. However, many of these people made these decisions not by free choice, but because of a perceived need to do so. The new workforce challenge in health care organizations has become how to attain high engagement levels of employees when they are there from a lack of choice. Chapter Three addresses this issue more fully.

The stability and quality of the workforce is directly linked to better outcomes and higher-quality services in our organizations (Aiken, Clarke, and Stone, 2002; American Hospital Association, 2001; Gelinas and Bohlen, 2002; Unruh, 2004). The quality of the workplace has become even more important when the external environment is so uncertain. The challenge for today's health care leader is to create positive work environments that not only attract high-quality candidates but retain them (Jazwiec, 2009; Manion, 2009b). And although people seldom join an organization today with the intent of remaining in its employment throughout their career, simply extending the length of tenure of high-quality employees by several years can have a positive impact on vacancy and turnover rates.

Diversity in the Workforce

When frontline health care leaders are asked what their greatest challenges are today, increasing diversity in the workplace is almost always near the top of the list. As a leader in a recent program noted, "In our organization, there are sixty-five different languages spoken." Globalization has certainly made an impact in the workplace in terms of the cultures and ethnic groups of the people who work together. However, this is not the only diversity creating increased challenges for leaders. Never before has there been such diversity in workers' ages. For the first time in history, four generations are actively working side-by-side in our workplaces.

Although we have always been aware that the generations differ in attitudes and beliefs, focusing primarily on the differences can increase friction among members of these age cohorts. While it may actually be less of a problem between coworkers, juggling the different needs and desires of such a variety of people can be a daunting challenge for leaders. Generational cohorts are defined as a group of individuals who experienced similar major events during their formative years. However, with the pace of change accelerating so wildly, the time required to produce significant differences between age groups may be compressing; whereas our grandparents were markedly different from our parents and from us, now there are significant differences between three siblings ages twenty-one, seventeen, and twelve (Maun, 2004). All of this adds to the tremendous complexity for leaders.

The challenge for health care leaders can feel overwhelming at times. How can one person lead such a diverse group of employees who are providing service and care to an even more widely diverse group of patients and families? How can we benefit from the creativity and opportunity that such diversity represents while respecting the many differences and not allowing relationships to degenerate into unmanageable conflict and confusion?

Turbulent Business and Regulatory Environment

The business environment within which health care organizations exist is tumultuous and unpredictable. Declining levels of reimbursement, increasing costs of products and materials, new business models, government-managed health care reform, the availability of Internet-based health care, the litigious mind-set, the appearance of watchdog groups focused on patient outcomes and safety, escalating workforce issues and worker demands, increasing competition from physicians, and the demands of increasing regulation: all serve to foster uncertainty in the health care marketplace. These create tremendous challenges as well as opportunities for leaders. Struggling to stay one step ahead requires leaders to spend tremendous energy and renew their commitment day to day and sometimes even hour to hour.

A story illustrates this challenge perfectly. In Africa each day, a lion wakes up. He knows he will need to outrun the fastest gazelle if he is to eat that day. Each day in Africa, a gazelle wakes up and knows he will need to outrun the fastest lion if he is to stay alive that day. The moral: it does not matter if you are a lion or a gazelle, as long as you wake up running. This translates to health care as, "Every leader must wake up and be ready to face the challenges every single day or be left behind.

Our appreciation of the rapidity with which the business environment can change began in the late 1990s. One home health agency lost over 60 percent of its reimbursed business overnight with a change in the reimbursement of phlebotomy. Hospitals with healthy bottom lines experienced severe reversals in their financial picture within months due to unanticipated reimbursement changes. Previously stable organizations have found that their financial situation can radically change within a few months. The recent economic downturn has had an impact on organizations with major investment portfolios just as significantly as it has had for individual citizens. The financial health of today's health care organizations can best be described as highly volatile.

The Leader's Energy Drain

In light of these challenges, or perhaps as a result of these issues, health care leaders face the personal challenge of maintaining and expanding their own energy capacity. This is likely the ultimate leadership challenge of this decade. In the face of increasing demands and escalating complexity in our environment and work, how do leaders locate and protect their sources of personal energy? And perhaps more important, how do they increase their capacity to deal with these multiple challenges?

Health care leaders not only have permission to care for themselves, they have a responsibility to do so (Collins, 1992). When you think of the tremendous national resource our outstanding leaders and managers represent, they are indeed a precious asset. Often these leaders come from the ranks of people who started their career in service to others or as caregivers. Self-care may not come naturally to those who have spent their life in service to others. As Collins (p. 5) writes, "Caring for others is a hazardous occupation . . . those of us who care for others have trouble caring for ourselves."

Everything we do consumes energy. Understanding the flow of energy within a system, whether the organization or the self, is a way to increase our proficiency at managing energy and ultimately, increasing our capacity (Cox, Manion, and Miller, 2005). Loehr and Schwartz (2003) believe that managing energy, not becoming increasingly proficient at managing time, is the key to high performance and personal self-renewal. "Once people understand how their supply of available energy is influenced by the choices they make, they can learn new strategies that increase the fuel in their tanks and boost their productivity" (Schwartz, 2010, p. 65). The most effective strategies are rituals that help replenish stores of physical, emotional, mental, and spiritual energy. A ritual can be as simple as shutting down e-mail for a couple of hours a day or taking a midafternoon walk to get a mental breather.

We know that most people in leadership roles fully expect to work well beyond a forty-hour week. According to a survey reported in the *Harvard Business Review* (Perlow and Porter, 2009), of one thousand professionals, 94 percent said they put in more than fifty hours a week, with nearly half that group turning in more than sixty-five hours a week. And that doesn't include the hours at home monitoring their BlackBerry and e-mail. Too many managers and leaders today report spending their last day of vacation at home going through e-mails that have accumulated so they don't have to deal with all of them on their first day back on the job. Perlow and Porter (2009) found that designating periods of time off, called predictable time, increased people's effectiveness. The biggest problem was getting these people to take the time off. It meant not checking e-mail and voice mail. The result was happier, more engaged workers and increased productivity and effectiveness. Finding and keeping a reasonable balance of work, family, and personal worlds is a remarkable yet crucial feat for today's organizational leader (Friedman, 2008; Bowcutt, 2004; Fields and Zwisler, 2004; Larson and William, 2004; Kemp, 2009; Ulreich, 2004; Van Allen, 2004).

A less frequently considered source of energy drain is the depletion many leaders experience in the spiritual domain when they face ethical and moral issues in the workplace that they feel unable to influence. This can create high moral distress, which has been defined as "the inability to translate moral choices into moral action" (Coles, 2010, p. 28). It occurs when a person knows ethically the right course to take but feels or is unable to act on it. The result is a perception that personal values or core ethical obligations are being violated. When this occurs, there is a tremendous depletion of personal energy, and it spirals out into the organization in negative ways. Moral distress happens at every level in organizations from the caregiver in the intensive care unit who is forced to participate in what is perceived as futile care to the highest-ranking executive who feels unable to be honest and transparent with board members for fear of losing his or her job. During an assessment in one organization, staff nurses admitted to entering false information in the EMR because it "forced them to do so" in order to move on and complete their work. These issues are rarely addressed openly in organizations because they are difficult to talk about. Truly excellent leaders are willing to do things for others and take the moral high road without regard to what's in it for them (Kaplan, 2008). Being a leader means being willing to speak up, even when you're expressing an unpopular view.

These are only a few of the major challenges that health care leaders face today. The increased complexity of our world today demands intense passion, courageous action, and unwavering belief and faith from its leaders. Challenges can help us focus and force us to reaffirm our commitment on an ongoing basis.

Conclusion

Developing leaders and increasing internal leadership capacity is one of the most important issues facing health care organizations. In defining leadership, it is important to distinguish between leadership and management. The growing need for strong leadership is directly related to the unrelenting crush of change we experience today, which in the health care world is reflected in the rapid shifting of paradigms and concern for survival into the future. The many challenges for leaders are closely intertwined and interdependent:

accelerating uncertainty and ambiguity, workforce issues, increasing diversity in the workplace, the tumultuous business and regulatory environment, and the need for managing one's own energy capacity. These factors have resulted in a tremendous sense of urgency in health care organizations and have made clear the need for the identification and development of internal leaders, as well as the mastery of new, nontraditional skills for these leaders.

DISCUSSION QUESTIONS

1. Think about people who have been effective leaders who influenced your life in a positive way. Why did you follow them? How were you influenced by them? What were the leadership behaviors they exhibited that you observed or remember?

2. What does your organization emphasize: leadership or management? Consider carefully both the verbal and the behavioral messages from established organizational leaders.

3. Think about your own skills and competencies. Where do your strengths fall? Are you a stronger leader or a stronger manager? Where do you have opportunities for increasing your capacity?

4. Reflect on the activities of your day. What do you spend most of your time doing? Are they managerial or leadership activities? Do you need to change your mix of activities? What would you gain from increasing your activities in a particular area? What are the barriers that keep you from doing so?

5. Think about the person to whom you report. Where do that person's strongest skills lie: in management or leadership? Why did you select one or the other? What kind of impact does this have on you?

6. Think about a time when you were at your very best: you were passionate about what you were doing, highly engaged and committed, and getting results that were important to you. As you think back about this situation, were you demonstrating any leadership or management characteristics?

7. What are your biggest challenges as a leader today? If you are not currently functioning as a leader, what are the biggest challenges that leaders in your organization, religious organization, community, or our country face today?

2

Cultivating the Leadership Relationship

CHAPTER OBJECTIVES

- Define the key concepts of emotional intelligence.
- Relate the four elements of a healthy relationship.
- Define a working concept of trust.
- Identify three steps for repairing broken trust.
- Identify examples of conditional and unconditional respect in the workplace.
- Explain the importance of both negative and positive event support.
- Describe the ratio of positive to negative interactions and its impact on the quality of the relationship.

The only definition of a leader is someone who has followers.
Some people are thinkers. Some are prophets. Both roles are
important and badly needed. But without
followers, there can be no leaders.

PETER DRUCKER, *MANAGING FOR THE FUTURE*

Leadership exists only within the context of a relationship. It is an intensely personal experience, a process of relating to another person, who, if influenced, becomes a follower. All definitions of leadership include the ability to influence others to do what needs to be done. It is a dynamic interaction between leader and follower, changing each irrevocably.

Emotional Intelligence

The emphasis on the importance of the relationship between the leader and the follower has become evident in recent years. Research in the area of emotional intelligence clearly demonstrates that the emotions of the leader directly affect the atmosphere and quality of the leader's relationships with others (Goleman, 1994; Goleman, Boyatzis, and McKee, 2002). The emotionally intelligent leader is one who is able "to generate excitement, optimism, and passion for the job ahead, as well as to cultivate an atmosphere of cooperation and trust" (Goleman, Boyatzis, and McKee, 2002, p. 29). These leaders need competencies in four domains: self-awareness, self-management, social awareness, and relationship management. Figure 2.1 presents these domains, as well as the competencies that exist within them. Closely intertwined, these competencies form the basis of leadership effectiveness in the workplace.

An early definition of emotional intelligence was "the ability to perceive and express emotion, assimilate emotion in thought, understand and reason with emotion, and regulate emotion in the self and others" (Mayer, Salovey, and Caruso, 2000, p. 396). This means that the leader has a high degree of self-awareness and is able to recognize his or her own emotion accurately. Not only is this self-awareness accurate, but the individual is able to regulate a response to the emotion. Here's a clear example. Several employees were very

Figure 2.1 Emotional Intelligence Competencies

	Self (Personal competence)	Other (Social competence)
Recognition	Self-Awareness Emotional self-awareness Accurate self-assessment Self-confidence	Social Awareness Empathy Service orientation Organizational awareness
Regulation	Self-Management Emotional self-control Trustworthiness Conscientiousness Adaptability Achievement drive Initiative	Relationship Management Developing others Influence Communication Conflict management Visionary leadership Catalyzing change Building bonds Teamwork and collaboration

Source: The Emotionally Intelligent Workplace © 2001. Reprinted with permission of John Wiley & Sons, Inc., Hoboken, NJ.

angry about a recent administrative decision and confronted their manager by saying, "We're surprised you aren't angry about this. What's the matter with you?" The leader took them by surprise when she replied, "Oh, do not mistake me, I am very angry about this. But I don't need to let that anger erupt all over everyone here. I can control it." Those brief words gave the employees a beautiful role model of an emotionally intelligent leader capable of regulating her emotions.

Emotional intelligence is not limited to the individual domain. The leader also is competent in relationships with others, resulting in social awareness as well as effective relationship management. These build on the personal competencies of recognition (emotional self-awareness, accurate self-assessment, and self-confidence) as well as self-regulation (emotional self-control, trustworthiness, conscientiousness, adaptability, achievement drive, and initiative). The social competencies related to social awareness include empathy, a service orientation, and an organizational awareness (Cherniss and Goleman, 2001). Other authors and scholars have identified the importance of these competencies as well. "The caring part of empathy, especially for the people with whom you work, is what inspires people to stay with a leader when the going gets rough. The mere fact that someone cares is more often than not rewarded with loyalty" (Champy, 2003, p. 135).

Social Intelligence

Further research from the emerging field of social neuroscience—the study of what happens in the brain while people interact—provides scientific basis for three elements long believed to influence the effectiveness of a leader: empathy, intuition, and rapport, all of which increase the quality of relationships and social interactions. One of the most important discoveries is that certain things leaders do, "specifically, exhibit empathy and become attuned to others' moods—literally affect both their own brain chemistry and that of their followers" (Goleman and Boyatzis, 2008, p. 76). This has led to the appreciation that effective leadership is about having powerful social circuits in the brain and has prompted an expansion of the concept of emotional intelligence. Awareness of this latest research allows a leader to identify practical, socially intelligent behaviors that can reinforce the neural links between the leader and his or her followers. It requires an understanding of mirror neurons, spindle cells, and oscillators.

A stunning recent discovery in behavioral neuroscience is the identification of mirror neurons in widely dispersed areas of the brain. These neurons reproduce the emotions of others as we detect them through their actions. As a result, working collectively, these neurons create an instant of shared experience. Specifically, a leader's emotions and actions prompt followers to mirror those feelings and deeds. Leaders who are tightly controlled and humorless rarely engage the mirror neurons of their followers. One who laughs and sets an easygoing tone taps into the potential of a follower's mirror neurons and often triggers spontaneous good humor and connections with others. "Top-performing leaders elicited laughter from their subordinates three times as often, on average, as did midperforming leaders. Being in a good mood . . . helps people take in information effectively and respond nimbly and creatively" (Goleman and Boyatzis, 2008, p. 77). This explains the process by which emotions are so contagious.

Intuition is linked to the functioning of spindle cells, a specific class of neurons with a body size about four times that of other brain cells and an extra-long branch to make attaching to other cells easier and transmitting thoughts and feelings to them quicker. It is now believed that these spindle cells account for intuition or having good instincts. This is the talent to recognize patterns and is usually based on extensive experience.

The third class of specialized neuron is the oscillator, which has been found to account for the establishment of rapport, sometimes referred to as resonance, between people. These neurons coordinate people physically by regulating how and when their bodies move together.

Certainly some individuals are far more socially intelligent than others. And intentionally taking on these behaviors may appear contrived and artificial to others. However, it is possible to work on developing social intelligence. Suggestions include:

- Listen attentively, and think about how others feel.
- Attune yourself to the moods of others.
- Seek to understand what motivates other people, especially those from different backgrounds.
- Make an effort to be sensitive to other people's needs.

These deliberate behaviors can contribute to the strength and connections of these specialized neurons.

The Leadership Relationship

The quality of the leader and follower's relationship directly affects the leader's effectiveness. Without the foundation for a healthy relationship, aspiring leaders cannot attain extraordinary outcomes. Although troubled leaders seldom return to the basic components of a healthy relationship when they are frustrated by followers who do not follow, the answer to their difficulties often lies within this basic concept. This chapter outlines the essential elements of a healthy leader-follower relationship and examines briefly the concepts of collaboration and partnerships, both of which depend on a willingness to relate at an interdependent level, probably the most complex of relationship forms.

Essential Elements of a Healthy Relationship

Leaders who relate comfortably to others often take for granted their talent for forming relationships. Their relationships have a naturalness and a spontaneity that result in mutually beneficial outcomes. When a particular leader-follower situation is not going well, the relationship-centered leader often reflects first on the connection with the supporter to determine the issues. And because the leader is already skillful in this area, the assessment process is not likely to produce undue anxiety. But if the leader is not naturally talented at forming strong relationships, this affects both the accuracy and ease of the assessment process. However, it is possible to increase interpersonal competency in this area.

Established effective leaders often intuitively understand the essential elements of a healthy relationship. And when something is wrong, intuitive signals alert the leader. A successful leader-follower relationship has at least four essential elements (Figure 2.2):

- Trust
- Mutual respect
- Support
- Communication

These elements are essential because the absence of any one can damage the relationship. In fact, without any one of these elements, a relationship would not be considered healthy and flourishing. Each is explored here.

Figure 2.2 Essential Elements of a Healthy Relationship

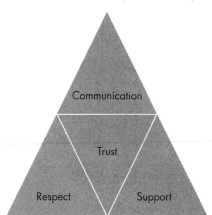

Trust

Trust is a crucial first component in any relationship. It is a necessary condition for closeness to occur so that appropriate social interactions can take place. Closeness implies that sense of connection with another human being that is so important in a leader-follower relationship. But how do people decide whether to trust another person? Recent research (Zak, 2008) has revealed the neurobiology of trust. In his review of animal and human research, Zak found that the cues, in the form of positive social signals and interactions, given off by one person stimulate the release of a neurotransmitter and hormone in the brain that stimulates others to trust him or her. And furthermore, a person who is trusted tends to be more trustworthy. Further research revealed evidence of a negative or opposing side of this trust-forming mechanism. A person who feels distrusted is likely to have a negative reaction; for some, it is simply a negative emotion, while for others it can actually increase aggression.

According to *Webster's Encyclopedic Unabridged Dictionary*, *trust* means you can rely on the "integrity, strength or ability of a person or thing. Confidence implies conscious trust because of good reasons, definite evidence or past experience." Without trust or confidence in the person attempting to influence them, people will not follow that person's direction or lead.

Confidence is a reliance and dependence on the person we trust to attain the results needed to benefit everyone. Vestal (2005) defines confidence as having an expectation of a good outcome. Piper (2010) refers to trust as the sublime duty in health care leadership. In an organization, when the individual attempting to lead relies primarily on the legitimate authority of his or her position, the relative health of the relationship can be deceptive. People may do what that leader wants not because they agree or believe in the direction the leader sets or the request he or she makes, but because they believe they must comply or suffer painful or undesirable consequences.

Kramer (2009) distinguishes between tempered trust and presumptive trust. The second, presumptive trust, describes situations when we have no suspicions. We approach these with trust that everything is as it appears and that things will work out. We treat others as trustworthy, and in the large majority of instances, they act in a trustworthy manner. Morse (2005) suggests a possible downside to this type of trust in a team or work relationship. He points out that when levels of trust are high, there may be less tendency to monitor outcomes as closely. To overcome this potential issue, he suggests that deliberate monitoring of outcomes is helpful and should be established openly so others don't interpret these actions as a sign of mistrust.

Tempered trust is a little more difficult. Kramer (2009) acknowledges that to survive as individuals in the organizational context, we must learn to trust wisely and well. If we put our trust in the wrong person, the consequences can be disastrous. His first suggestion is to begin with honest self-awareness. If you tend to trust the wrong people, ask yourself what cues you have been missing. If you are good at recognizing cues accurately but have difficulty forging trusting relationships, work to expand your repertoire of trust-building skills. For instance, start with small acts of trust of the other person that will foster reciprocity. Develop clearly articulated expectations and clauses for disengagement. When these are clear, it is easier to trust.

Understanding the concept of trust is imperative for anyone aspiring to lead others. Warren Bennis (Flower, 1990) offers a concrete, applicable framework for understanding trust within the context of a leadership role. He defines three essential ingredients for trust: competence, congruence, and constancy. Examining these three components provides a guide for any leader who is seeking to more fully understand his or her personal effectiveness (see Figure 2.3).

Figure 2.3 Essential Elements of Trust

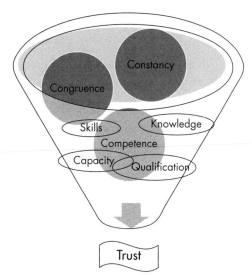

Competence

Webster's defines *competence* as the "possession of required skill, knowledge, qualification or capacity." The application of this definition in a leadership context is clear. Supporters must believe that the leader has the skill and knowledge to do what is required. "Whenever we step in front of the crowd and say, 'Follow me,' the implication is that we know where we're going and what we want to achieve and that we're committed to giving our very best efforts" (Melrose, 1996, p. 20). Confidence in a leader develops from working with that person and from seeing evidence of the leader's past performance demonstrating competence. Both skill and knowledge are included in this definition. Knowledge alone is insufficient. The leader may know that followers need accurate information and clear communication, but an unskilled leader who is unable to articulate clearly will be greatly hampered. And the reverse is true as well: an individual may be a charismatic, powerfully effective communicator, but if he or she is unable to back up the rhetoric with performance and outcomes, trust is weakened, if not severed entirely.

This explains, at least partially, why changing key leaders in organizations can result in a troublesome situation. Establishing trust and confidence in new leaders takes time. Nevertheless, many health care organizations embarking on major change choose to alter the managerial and executive structure and working relationships, eliminating or combining positions. Entire departments find themselves in a new reporting relationship. Leaders in these new positions are then expected to lead their followers through the changes, yet they are severely disadvantaged because they must first form a trusting relationship. Although this sequence of events may be appropriate, organizations should carefully consider the sequence's impact on the time required to create change. In one midwestern hospital, the CEO routinely changes reporting relationships every couple of years because he likes to keep people off balance—in his words, "to shake things up a bit." What he fails to see is the effect on productivity and the cost in terms of relationships. Careful evaluation of outcomes can determine the long-term impact on organizational relationships. Do the long-term consequences outweigh the disruptive environment in the short term?

Qualification   Qualification is an interesting factor in competence. The field of health care has a notable emphasis on expertise as a necessary qualification. Some people simply do not follow an individual unless the person has a particular qualification they believe to be important, such as a clinical discipline background or a certain academic degree. Whether the qualification actually prepares or enables the leader to function competently is a moot point; to a potential follower, it can become a critical issue with significant repercussions. Organizations that have consolidated departments and replaced two or three managers with one often encounter significant obstacles when the manager no longer shares the background or expertise of the department's employees. Although this is not an insurmountable obstacle, it can take longer for the new manager to establish a trust relationship with employees because of a need to prove competence in the face of what appears to be a significant qualification issue.

Capacity   Capacity issues influence the level of trust in the leader. If others see a leader as having too much to do, too many responsibilities, juggling too many balls, a question of trust may arise. Can this leader handle the current situation? Will it be too much? What if it pushes the leader over the edge? A leader who appears frazzled and out of control creates uneasy followers. Personal endurance and a phenomenal capacity for work often go hand in hand with effective leadership. "Never let them see you sweat" may be an appropriate motto but should not imply that a good leader never lets followers see the reality of a difficult situation.

In one West Coast hospital undergoing significant organizational consolidation of leadership roles, a newly appointed executive had a personality style characterized by spontaneity, impulsiveness, and a high degree of self-disclosure. As the initiative progressed, this leader was given more and more responsibility because she was very capable. She quickly reached the point of overload and began manifesting counterproductive behaviors such as volatility, extreme distractibility, and pure panic. Her communication patterns became dysfunctional as a result of her intense anxiety. Her erratic behavior with her followers clearly transmitted her anxiety, and she began to lose their trust. In this situation, skill, knowledge, and qualification were not at issue. Instead, her followers feared that she could not handle the heavy load. Adequate capacity was the issue. Figure 2.4 summarizes these factors related to competence.

Figure 2.4 Factors Related to Competence

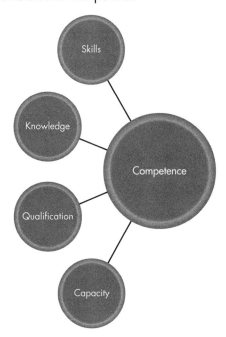

Congruence

The second key element of trust in this context is congruence, meaning consistency or agreement between verbal (or written) messages and the leader's behavior (Lorimer and Manion, 1996). When what a leader says is highly congruent with what he or she does, the followers perceive the leader as honest and trustworthy. If the leader says one thing but does another, the result is an enormous credibility gap with followers. Most would agree that leaders must walk the talk. The leader's integrity and character are important. Followers need to believe that leaders act in accordance with their personal beliefs and are honest not only with themselves but with followers. This is more important than the followers' agreeing with the leader's beliefs. "Effective leadership . . . is not based on being clever; it is based primarily on being consistent" (Drucker, 1992, p. 122).

Common Discrepancies   Examples of discrepancies are common in any work setting. One department leader in the hospital maintenance department established employee work teams and assured team members that they would have responsibility for decisions that affect their work. After almost a year of working together as a team, two new team members that no one on the team had expected joined them. Their manager had hired these additional members without including the team in any way in the decision. The team members felt betrayed by the manager, and the ensuing breach of trust was difficult to repair. They wondered what other decisions the manager had made without their ideas or input.

One of the most serious problems with congruence is that inconsistent messages are often inadvertent. The leader usually does not purposely engage in behavior that is contrary to previous messages he or she has sent but instead, without realizing it, acts in direct contradiction to the oral and written messages delivered. This happened in one organization that stated that competence was a key organizational value. Yet when attempting to determine which employees to lay off during an economic downturn, tenure was the key selection criteria. Tenure and competence are not the same thing, and many employees were offended and angered by what appeared to be a decision-making criterion inconsistent with a stated, and often-touted, organization value. When employees questioned this, the senior executive leading the initiative became defensive and angry but eventually listened to the feedback and changed the decision-making criteria. The organization then used tenure as a final determining factor only if the employee in question first met the criterion of competence.

Another hospital handled a similar situation differently. When confronted with the incongruity between the stated organization value of competence and use of tenure as a selection criterion, the administration of this community hospital retained tenure as the deciding criterion. They reasoned that this was not the appropriate time to correct problems with employee competence that managers had not dealt with previously. Although it may sound reasonable, their choice created a major credibility issue. By saying that managers had never dealt properly with unacceptable or poor employee performance, they were basically admitting that they had never held true to the organization's stated value of competence.

Avoiding Discrepancies   A leader must scrupulously examine and be aware of behavior that others might interpret as incongruent, although avoiding all discrepancies is virtually impossible. Thus, it is especially important for a leader to promote openness and honest feedback from followers. An executive team in one northeastern medical center worked diligently to establish such an open environment, making certain that employees knew their leaders wanted feedback if their behaviors appeared incongruent. These leaders knew that their initial reaction to feedback would determine the amount and usefulness of future feedback that employees would give and were very careful to listen fully and react nondefensively when employees brought discordant messages to their attention. In some instances, leaders changed behavior deemed incongruent to their message. In other cases, communication was unclear, and the parties resolved the problem by sharing additional information. This openness did not occur overnight. Many employees were—and some still are—hesitant to provide feedback because they feared reprisals. This fear is a common obstacle when the leader holds a hierarchical position and has legitimate power over employees.

Giving the leader feedback on incongruent behavior is much more difficult than it may appear. The majority of employees are unwilling to say anything, even if they see that the leader is about to make a mistake. If their feedback is discounted by verbal or body language, they become unwilling to speak up in the future. Some of this reluctance to speak freely and honestly is related to early socialization messages. Chaleff (1996) explains that people learn from an early age to obey authority, to say, "Yes, sir" and "Yes, ma'am," and that this conditioning runs deep. Overcoming these deep internal messages takes work. "We are afraid that if we question authority we will be viewed as a nuisance, pushed out of the loop, overlooked for promotion, even fired. We fear the consequences of speaking up far more than we are afraid of the more serious consequences of not speaking up" (p. 16).

Detert and Edmondson (2007) set out to systematically identify factors that cause employees to either bring ideas to their manager or withhold them. Although these employees had multiple mechanisms through which to present their ideas as well as repeated encouragement from the organizational hierarchy to do so, "half the employee respondents . . . revealed that they felt it was *not* 'safe to speak up' or challenge the traditional ways of doing things" (2007, para. 2).

Multiple reasons for not speaking up were uncovered. Self-preservation, or the innate protective desire, is so powerful that it even inhibited speech that clearly would have been intended to help the organization. The researchers found that the perceived risks of speaking up felt very personal and immediate to employees, whereas any future benefit to the organization from sharing their ideas was too uncertain and too distant to have an impact. In some instances, employees feared speaking up because of previous hostile or otherwise uncomfortable reactions from the manager. Seemingly untested assumptions also led to silence. Employees sometimes withhold information or comments because they perceive that the manager is the champion or owner of the project, process, or idea.

Gentile (2010) spent four years studying the moments when people decide whether to speak up about an ethical issue and what they say when they do. She has identified further rationalizations for the decision to remain silent. The first is the belief that the particular behavior is standard practice and it isn't going to change. A second is that this is "no big deal." An example of this thinking occurs when a problem or issue is uncovered, and the reaction is, "Well, no one has complained about it yet, so why bother to fix it?" Other common reasons include telling ourselves that it isn't our responsibility and the belief that loyalty means not saying anything.

Transformational leaders can create a climate that encourages employees to speak up and speak out on issues. The first step is to set the expectation and clearly communicate what is desired behavior. When people do speak up, their willingness to do so must be positively reinforced, even if they say something the leader doesn't necessarily want to hear. The behavior can be acknowledged and appreciated visibly to others in the organization. Certainly the leader must respond in a nondefensive and positive manner. The basic leadership strategy is to make it a more positive experience for the follower to speak up than to remain silent.

Another way to view congruence involves congruity between what leaders do in their personal and public lives. People who do not live up to commitments to their family or who cheat their neighbors often hide behind the belief that what happens in their personal lives should not affect their leadership roles. Like it or not, if followers see untrustworthy personal behavior, this affects the level of trust they place in their leaders.

Constancy

Constancy is the third and final ingredient of trust that Bennis identified (Flower, 1990). It implies that the leader is reliable, dependable, and consistent. A good leader keeps commitments and follows through on promises made. If it becomes clear that a promise or commitment cannot be met, the leader communicates openly and honestly with followers to inform them of the changed circumstances—ideally before the followers confront the leader.

Availability and Accessibility   To many followers, availability and accessibility are part of constancy. For leaders to be most effective, they must be accessible to followers and not just at prescheduled, formal times. Some of the best dialogues occur spontaneously. When the leader is also a manager or executive, the role's formal trappings may distance the leader from followers. Common examples are isolated office locations or the presence of secretaries who see their role as protecting or buffering the leader from others. Although being completely available twenty-four hours a day is not possible, neither should the leader be inaccessible to followers. The leader must find a balance, for the perception that the leader is available is potent in developing a collegial relationship with followers.

One key way that leaders create a positive work environment is by being visible (Manion, 2004b). Peters and Austin (1985) coined the term *management by walking around* (MBWA). This suggests that the closer a leader is physically to followers, the more this establishes a sense of connection and understanding. And it is true that the leader who sees a situation with his or her own eyes is certainly better informed than one hearing about it from a third, potentially biased party. As time pressures increase, a leader often sacrifices visibility and availability. Whatever constraints may exist, they are never as serious as the threat to a leader's effectiveness from followers who do not feel a sense of connection and as a result do not follow. And the presence of the leader is not limited to physical presence. We are much more linked electronically than ever before in our history. Although a leader's prompt and effective response to e-mail or telephone contacts is not as powerful as physical presence, it can still be reassuring and supportive.

These ideas seem like common sense or intuitive knowledge that is self-evident. However, availability and accessibility are difficult to achieve in these demanding times. The massive amount of change creates an environment filled with uncertainty, and followers have many questions. They may not perceive all changes as positive and may be unhappy, even angry, about the organization's current direction or decisions with which they disagree. Every leader today knows how daunting it is to face a crowd of antagonistic followers, and avoiding these situations and withdrawing from contact with followers is a natural tendency. Herein lies one major difference between the transformational leader and the not-so-effective leader: the transformational leader stays more visible and involved, more accessible and available to followers during these times. As in a sporting event in which a team finds inspiration from cheerleaders when it falls behind and is losing the game, the excellent leader knows the importance of being present during significant unrest. This leader understands that his or her mere presence is a message of support to uncertain followers.

Being able to count on the leader's presence is important to followers, although some leaders feel uncomfortable if they do not have answers to complex or difficult questions that followers raise. Many of today's leaders are managers, or were managers in the past, who have been socialized to believe that the manager's job is to have answers. A good leader understands and accepts, however, that having all of the answers is impossible. It takes phenomenal courage on the part of the leader to stay present with others when they are looking for answers that he or she does not have. Yet followers respect leaders who are not afraid to admit that they do not have the answers. They are encouraged when a leader communicates the belief that they will find the answers by working together. This presence during trying times is a tremendous gift the leader gives to others.

Behavior   Constancy also refers to stability of personal characteristics. The leader who experiences extreme fluctuations in mood, is quick to anger, or responds with knee-jerk reactions has more trust problems with followers. Take the leader who is excessively positive about ideas, unrealistically optimistic about the chances for a project's success, and effusive with praise on one day but scornful the next day. Followers are left with an uncomfortable feeling of uncertainty, which impairs trust. Although it is next to impossible for a leader to be completely balanced and thoroughly predictable, the degree to which the leader avoids these surprises contributes to followers' trust in the relationship. Consistency of behavior is important. (See Figure 2.5 for the factors related to constancy.)

Figure 2.5 Factors Related to Constancy

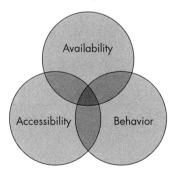

The Presence of Credibility

When these three elements of trust are present—competence, congruence, and constancy—followers can place credibility in the leader and his or her actions. Kouzes and Posner (1993a, 1993b) have studied credibility extensively. They believe credibility relates to how a leader earns the trust and confidence of his or her constituency. They have found that "people want leaders who hold to an ethic of service and are genuinely respectful of the intelligence and contributions of their constituents. They want leaders who will put principles ahead of politics and other people before self-interests" (1993b, p. xvii). Credibility is a way of maintaining or regaining people's faith in their institutions and the individuals who lead them.

Repairing Broken Trust

The three key ingredients of competence, congruence, and constancy must all be present for a healthy relationship. If mistrust is present, examining these three areas can help to sort out the probable causes. When mistrust is apparent in potential followers, one possible approach to the solution is for the leader to ask the followers: What has happened to damage trust? Leaders with the courage to ask this question are often rewarded with insight. Unless the leader asks the question sincerely, however, followers may be reluctant to discuss situations in which they believe the leader let them down. Bennis (1989) points out that good leaders encourage respectful dissent so that they can know the truth about a situation, even if it is not what the leader would like to hear. In fact, good leaders need people around who have contrary views and serve as devil's advocates. These are very difficult conversations to have. O'Toole and Bennis (2009) suggest rewarding contrarians by listening to their ideas, using their views to challenge your own assumptions, and recognizing and thanking them for their contributions.

Nevertheless, there will be times when trust is damaged. Rogers (1994) identifies three steps to repairing broken trust:

1. Acknowledging

2. Apologizing

3. Making amends

Acknowledging   Acknowledging broken trust is tough for many leaders. Few leaders purposefully set out to destroy trust, and admitting that something has happened to damage it in this relationship is difficult. In fact, some people find it almost impossible to talk directly about issues of trust. It seems they prefer to call it something else, anything else, rather than accept it as distrust. Perhaps acknowledging a lack of trust implies a personal fault of some kind, and this belief makes honestly examining these situations especially onerous.

Susan is a senior vice president in a community hospital in Texas. The hierarchy in her organization is very rigid, and rules and policies are plentiful. All employees, including managers and executives, are required to use a time card. For years employees were required to have the individual to whom they reported sign their time cards, but managers and executives did not follow this rule. Problems developed with one manager, including questionable entries and inaccuracies in recording sick or absent time. As a result, Susan began to require that all managers and executives have their time cards signed. The reaction was predictable: people felt they were no longer trusted. Susan was adamant that her requirement for the double-check on the time cards was just policy, but her assurances did nothing to assuage their feelings. When pushed, she finally admitted that she wanted to enforce the policy because of performance problems with one individual. Even when confronted directly, she continued to deny that there were any trust issues. It was clearly a lack of trust (albeit well deserved) in the one individual who had been found altering and falsifying time cards.

Acknowledging is not just about recognizing a break in trust; it also means accepting ownership for behavior. It may mean publicly acknowledging that a mistake in judgment was made or that a particular decision did not bring about the required outcomes. This can be particularly difficult for leaders who may feel that they ought not talk about their mistakes because it can weaken the trust with their followers. However, refusal to acknowledge errors and poor judgment calls often results in followers' questioning the leader's level of accountability. Admitting that a mistake has been made disarms critics and makes employees more likely to own up to their own mistakes (O'Toole and Bennis, 2009).

Apologizing   Apologizing for a breach of trust is difficult for many leaders. This does not mean accepting fault for something that is not the leader's
responsibility. If it is the leader's responsibility, the apology may sound like
this: "I made a mistake, and I am sorry," or "I am sorry that my decision has
caused these difficulties for you." If the leader is not culpable, the apology
may sound different: "I am sorry to hear you feel this way; the decision was
right for this situation," or "I am sorry that is what you heard. Let me try
explaining this again." Another possibility is simply to say, "I am sorry that
happened." This is often described as a blameless apology.

Apologies are very difficult for some people because they believe that apologizing diminishes their stature or damages the other person's respect for them.
Many managers and executives have been socialized in a hierarchical system in
which formal leaders do not admit mistakes to employees, perhaps because they
believe it may weaken their authority. The problem with this attitude is that
what one most hopes to avoid is exactly what occurs: people lose respect for
individuals who cannot admit they were wrong or made a mistake.

In one community hospital undergoing a major work redesign initiative
in the late 1990s, employees showed significant distrust of administration.
Five years before, a layoff had occurred, and executives had made several
highly visible and devastating mistakes in the way they handled the process.
While the executives talked about these mistakes behind closed doors,
employees talked about them openly. The executives closed ranks and never
talked with employees about these mistakes. The pervasive organizational climate was antagonistic, fueled by a workforce that did not trust the executives
to manage this new challenge because employees did not believe the executives had learned anything from the layoff. How different the environment
might have been if the executives and employees held an open dialogue and
shared ideas about what they had learned during and since the layoff.

Making Amends   The last step in repairing broken trust is to make
amends. If something can be corrected or if a behavior is not repeated, these
are ways of making amends. Sometimes the easiest thing to do is to ask,
"How can I make this right? How can I make amends?" In many instances,
an apology is enough. However, if there is behavior to be changed and one

makes the commitment to do so, the leader must follow through on this commitment. Reestablishing trust may take longer than expected. People will be watching closely to determine whether they can believe the leader's promises. Nothing is worse than an insincere apology offered with no real intent to change or rectify the situation. These apologies leave others feeling manipulated and more distrustful than before.

Making amends also implies some reciprocal behavior from the follower. If the leader changes his or her behavior and acts in trustworthy ways, followers at some point need to let go of past wrongs. A leader in one organization found that his early behavior when first appointed to his position resulted in a reputation that still haunts him ten years later. He needs to address this lack of trust from followers and should perhaps ask for their trust.

Mutual Respect

The second essential element in forming a healthy relationship is mutual respect between leader and follower, which means having esteem for or valuing the other person or his or her skills or characteristics. In a leader-follower relationship, the leader can offer respect in two ways. In the first, the leader offers respect unconditionally to followers. This respect is not contingent on superficial attributes such as position, education, or socioeconomic status but recognizes the contributions, actual and potential, of the individual. This does not mean that the leader would withhold respect for an individual's achievements in education or position; instead, he or she would *not* withhold respect from an individual because this person does not have a particular level of education or position of authority.

In health care, because we extend unconditional respect to patients and families regardless of their situation, we often assume that this same respect exists among health care workers. All too often, however, people offer respect merely because of the status or authority inherent in a title. Just as a person leaving a position often becomes a nonentity because that person no longer has a title, management may not recognize certain employees as leaders because these staff have no formal title. Some believe that individuals with particular educational qualifications are most capable or are the only ones with the ability to solve certain problems. These are all examples of respect based on superficial attributes. A leader understands fully that another situation may cause a reversal of positions, placing the leader in a follower position.

The respect a leader extends to followers is a result of a sincere belief that followers are partners who have ideas, abilities, solutions, and a keen interest in the situation. Max DePree (1989) says that the excellent leader begins with understanding the diversity and breadth of people's gifts, talents, and skills. "Understanding and accepting diversity enables us to see that each of us is needed. It also enables us to begin to think about being abandoned to the strengths of others, of admitting that we cannot know or do everything" (p. 9). Relating to followers as colleagues is a characteristic of a transformational leader (Burns, 1978). Extending respect to others includes seeking input, soliciting opinions and ideas, and then using these in making decisions. It also means providing freedom within the relationship, allowing give-and-take to occur.

The second way a leader can offer respect is based on performance. In other words, we observe a person's skills or abilities and see that he or she obtains desirable outcomes. This type of respect may be differential: we do not guarantee the same level of respect to all people but base it on their individual performance. In this case, we withdraw respect if the individual does not achieve appropriate or desirable outcomes. In other words, the individual who makes repeated mistakes and does not learn from them may experience the consequences of losing others' respect and even being removed from a position.

Unless respect is clearly defined by the people who work together, there can be behaviors that inadvertently demonstrate a lack of trust of people. Less important is the dictionary definition and more important is how coworkers define respect. For many people, respect is shown by behaviors such as asking others for their opinion; including them in decisions that affect their work; using their ideas and opinions when the other makes a decision; letting them finish their thoughts before responding; and understanding what they do and its importance. In a recent assessment in a midsize hospital, respect was identified as one of the driving tenets of the culture. Yet employees reported a pervasive sense of lack of respect for them and their work. In the words of one of the nurses, "I've never been in an organization where nurses are less respected." The results of the assessment came as a shock to the executive team, who felt they did respect the caregivers. However, the climate was one of extreme scarcity and toxicity: failing equipment, inadequate supplies, inadequate staffing, unresolved long-standing problems, and abusive physician behavior toward the nurses that no one ever addressed. The nurses reported their issues and problems over and over again, to no avail. Because they endured multiple disruptions in their workday trying to track down missing equipment or find supplies or equipment, their conclusion was that they and their work were not respected. The failure to address disruptive physician behavior was perceived as a lack of respect for the nurses.

Support

The third element that characterizes a healthy relationship is support. To support is to nurture or to provide sustenance, a two-way street going from followers to leaders and from leaders to followers.

Recent research sheds light on the concept of support. Social support in the face of negative events has been reported and long accepted to be crucial for recovery and healing from difficult situations or losses. Individuals with a strong social network are found to deal with difficulties more easily because of support provided. Recent research by Maisel and Gable (2009) examined positive event support and found that others' reactions to a person's good news dramatically influence the level of support that the individual perceives.

Positive Event Support

In most people's lives, positive events occur three to five times more often than negative events. Sharing these with others capitalizes on the positive occurrences, and positive emotion increases in the relationship. It has been found that when these events are shared, a person experiences less loneliness, greater connectivity to others, and greater life satisfaction (Maisel and Gable, 2009). Who these positive events are shared with is likely contingent on how the other person responds. There are four possible responses based on how active or passive the response is and whether it is primarily constructive or destructive (see Figure 2.6).

Figure 2.6 Responses to Positive Events

	CONSTRUCTIVE	DESTRUCTIVE
ACTIVE	"That is so great! I am so proud of you. You'll really make a difference! Tell me more about it!" (Good nonverbals)	"Are you kidding me? Those committees never really do anything. How do you think you're going to have the time to do this?"
PASSIVE	"You have good ideas and I'm sure you'll do great." (Warmth but no active emotional expression)	"Yah, like that's going to get you anywhere!" (Roll your eyes and snort with disbelief)

Say that Jane, one of your strongest employees, has just been asked to serve on a systemwide committee to focus on creating a positive culture in the workplace. She is elated and bursting with pride at this recognition. An actively positive response to her news is to respond with enthusiasm and encouragement. You ask questions that demonstrate your interest in this new project she is taking on and express your pride that others see some of the same strengths in Jane that you do. You tell her this will reflect on and affect your department in a positive manner. Jane cannot help but feel supported by your warm and genuine regard.

There are three other possible reactions. The first is an actively destructive response: you respond with dismay at having to provide her time off her schedule so she can attend regular meetings. You are quick to point out that these committees are often created to pay lip-service to their purpose, but they quickly disband without achieving any lasting results. You hope she won't be surprised or upset when this happens! Your cynicism is expressed not only through your verbal response but through your skeptical body language as well.

The second destructive response is more passive but still clearly communicates your feelings. You roll your eyes, snort with disbelief that she would be so gullible to think this is a great opportunity, and then brush off her enthusiasm with your disinterest. Clearly these two responses will not communicate support.

The third possibility is somewhat paradoxical: a positive but passive response to Jane's enthusiasm. You might respond with a brief but warm comment such as, "You always have good ideas, and I'm sure you'll do great on this committee." However, you then move quickly onto the business at hand and somewhat brush aside her enthusiasm and desire to talk more about this request. Maisel and Gable (2009) found that this third response, although positive, was a let-down for the person sharing the good news. In some ways, it felt more diminishing than an actual negative response would have.

This research found that a person is better off to have a day when nothing positive happens than a day when something really positive occurs but they've shared the event with others and had only less than actively positive responses. The cue for the leader is to respond to these situations with just a bit more emotion than the person sharing the event is expressing. Positive event responding in an active constructive manner is important for relationship building.

Negative Event Support

Consistency of support is critical; without it, trust wavers. If a leader offers support only when everything is going smoothly and then withdraws it during vulnerable times, it is of virtually no value because the followers cannot count on it. The net result in the relationship is uneasiness and uncertainty about whether this time the support will be there. Ironically followers most need support when leaders most frequently withdraw it: when mistakes occur or when someone makes a poor decision or an error in judgment. In a healthy relationship, the giver freely offers consistent and visible support to the receiver.

A leader's response to mistakes or errors is often the clue followers have as to the consistency of support that the leader extends. If punitive consequences are the norm, people do not feel supported. Punitive consequences to mistakes can occur in the form of shaming, blaming, humiliating followers, or reducing their future opportunities. Simply stepping in and taking over a situation or project, and thereby relieving the follower of responsibility for correcting the consequences that resulted, can appear as a lack of support.

Interestingly, if others observe the leader engaging in negative, punitive behavior with any follower, the action is enough to damage trust even with followers who were not directly involved. This is not to imply that there should not be appropriate consequences for a person making the same mistakes repeatedly.

Communication

The final essential element of healthy relationships is open, honest, and positive communication. No leader is effective without the ability to communicate with others. This requires excellent communication skills and a willingness to talk through issues. A leader may be highly skilled but unwilling to do the time-consuming work of communicating. (Because of the scope and importance of this element, Chapter Four is devoted to communication skills.)

There is, however, one aspect of communication that has less to do with skill and more to do with self-awareness and deliberate intention. Recent research from the field of positive psychology has determined that the ratio of positive-to-negative interactions is a key indicator of a healthy relationship. In corroborating research, both Fredrickson (2009) and Losada and Heaphy (2004) discovered that a ratio of at least three-to-one positive-to-negative interactions must exist for the relationship to be described as flourishing. Losada, with a passion for mathematical modeling of group behavior, conducted research on work groups and tracked three dimensions of their group behavior when engaged in strategic planning sessions: whether team member's statements were (1) positive or negative, (2) self-focused or other-focused, and (3) based on inquiry (asking questions) or advocacy (defending a point of view).

The high-performing teams in Losada's research had higher connectivity and a balance on these three different dimensions. For example, they asked questions as much as they advocated for their own positions. And there was a balance of inward- and outward-focused behaviors. He found that the high-performing teams had a positive-to-negative ratio of at least six-to-one. Low-performance teams had ratios below one-to-one, and mixed-performance teams were around two-to-one. The mixed-performance teams were interesting because of the low resiliency they demonstrated. In other words, they might start out positively and seem to be making progress, but if they encountered extreme negativity, they descended into self-absorbed advocacy. Negativity (which destroys the positive-to-negative ratio) caused the mixed-performance teams to lose their good humor, as well as their flexibility and ability or willingness to question. They ended up languishing in a cycle where each "fought their own corner" and became critical of everything else that might be suggested.

Low-performance teams began where the mixed-performance teams ended up. They were caught in a negative downward spiral, a doom-and-gloom loop. Members did not listen to each other and were unwilling to consider new or different ideas because they were mired in advocating their own positions. Forward progress becomes almost impossible in this state.

The high positive-to-negative ratio describing flourishing relationships demonstrates two core principles that have tremendous application for the leadership relationship. The first is that positivity opens and expands us and provides the energy for us to consider new and different ideas and approaches. Second, it broadens and builds our capacity and resources. In this case, it builds our social resources. The connectivity we feel with each other expands and leads to better outcomes. The teams with higher positivity were more flexible and resilient and experienced demonstrably better outcomes.

What are the ramifications for contemporary leaders? It means that there is a crucial tipping point that must be attained for a relationship to be healthy and serve us well. That ratio is between three-to-one and eleven-to-one. There are always negatives that we must deal with. No life is filled with 100 percent positive events and emotions. If someone fails to meet a commitment he or she made to you, feeling hurt is an appropriate reaction. If a coworker or employee behaves in a purposelessly hurtful way to another, anger is justified. If you lose a valued team member, grieving that loss is appropriate. So the idea here is not to totally eliminate all negative comments, feelings, events, or experiences. The challenge is to increase the positive so that when the negative situations occur, they don't overwhelm the positive. This means we must be on the lookout for what's going right and monitor our comments and reactions so that they are predominantly positive. Focusing on what is going right releases energy to deal with problems.

As a leader, another extremely important ramification is that we need to set the expectation and coach our employees to focus on the positive. When the team begins to fall within the three-to-one up to eleven-to-one positive-to-negative ratio, a tremendous momentum builds within the group. And it is not just the leader who provides this. It stems from the partnership of everyone working together.

Creating a Trust-Based Organizational Climate

Healthy relationships are the foundation of a trust-based organizational climate. Effective leaders continually scan their environment and the reactions of organizational members to assess levels of trust. We are becoming increasingly aware of the direct correlation between a positive, trust-based work environment and the competitive advantage of the organization. "We are a society in search of trust. The less we find it, the more precious it becomes. An organization in which people earn one another's trust, and that commands trust from the public, has a competitive advantage. It can draw the best people, inspire customer loyalty, reach out successfully to new markets, and provide more innovative products and services" (Ciancutti and Steding, 2001, p. ix).

This message echoes the earlier work of Reina and Reina (1999), who examined closely the issues of trust and betrayal in workplaces. They write, "Unmet expectations, disappointments, broken trust, and betrayals aren't restricted to big events like restructurings and downsizings. They crop up every day on the job. Leaders are beginning to realize that people's trust and commitment to the organization affect their performance" (p. ix). Reina and Reina offer a model for understanding the complex and emotional issue of trust and betrayal in organizations today. They believe it is possible to create an organizational climate in which transformative trust exists. Four core characteristics that produce transformative trust are conviction, courage, compassion, and community.

As important as trust is, it is not as prevalent in organizations as we would hope. In March 2007, Leadership IQ (Murphy, 2007) surveyed 7,209 executives, managers, and employees to assess trust in the workplace. The findings were startling. The first verified that trust levels significantly predict employee loyalty and commitment to the organization. Approximately 32 percent of an employee's desire to stay or leave the organization is the result of feeling, or not feeling, trust toward the person to whom he or she reports. While trust was found to be a significant driver of employee loyalty, there's room for improvement in many organizations. Only 20 percent of the respondents strongly trusted their organization's top leadership. Another 36 percent moderately trusted this group, and the remaining 44 percent ranged from not trusting to strongly distrusting their top leaders.

So the question becomes: How do we build a culture of trust in the organization? O'Toole and Bennis (2009) believe that organizations will be unable to build such a culture until leaders learn how and communicate honestly. It is not enough to talk about candor and transparency; people must believe their leaders are honest. In an organizational context, transparency means being frank, free from pretense or deceit, and being clear, obvious, and readily understood. These certainly have implications for a leader's communication skills and philosophy. If this culture is set by the leaders, staff will be encouraged to speak up and speak out with honesty about their concerns and without fear of reprisal. They also suggest that contrarians be rewarded by being listened to and thanked for their ideas.

The Leadership IQ study (Murphy, 2007, p. 5) identified five aspects of trust that were the best predictor of employee loyalty. They all validate the previous content on trust. In order of importance, they are:

1. If I shared my work problems with my direct boss, I know that he/she would respond constructively.

2. My direct boss makes smart decisions.

3. My direct boss is honest and truthful.

4. My direct boss helps me grow and develop professionally.

5. I receive consistent direction from my direct boss.

In *Built on Trust* (2001), Ciancutti and Steding talk about intentionally creating trust in the organization. They offer a model for deliberately and systematically establishing and maintaining high levels of trust in these ways:

- Obtain closure with all communication. This means coming to a specific agreement about who will do what and by when.

- Make a commitment: a positive intention to complete what the parties agreed to with no conditions. If you are unable to follow through or fulfill the commitment as agreed to for any reason, let the other person know immediately.

- Ensure that communication is direct, open, and honest, which eliminates dysfunctional forms such as talking behind people's backs, withholding information, and gossiping.

- Insist on speedy resolution of difficulties, which refers to clearing up unresolved issues as soon as they become apparent and as soon as possible.

Ciancutti and Steding (2001) include other principles as well, such as being responsive to each other, telling the truth, agreeing to a no-surprise practice, handling issues at the lowest possible level in the organization, and relying on managers who serve as daily role models in each of these aspects.

The Nature of the Leadership Relationship

Establishing and cultivating a healthy relationship with followers is an initial step in developing the ability to influence others. This can be accomplished by ensuring that the four elements of a healthy relationship—trust, mutual respect, support, and communication—are in place. Understanding the concepts of collaboration and partnership is also important because these describe the nature of effective leader-follower relationships.

Collaboration and partnering are terms similar in meaning. Collaboration refers to work or labor accomplished together, and partner is derived from the word partake, meaning "to share." The essence of a successful leader's relationship with followers and key stakeholders is a combination of collaboration and partnership. Collaboration has become a buzzword, found in many journal articles and workshop titles. But like most other buzzwords, it is one that people overuse and misuse without a true understanding of the concept. A good leader may not need to know the actual definition but certainly needs to live the concept in relation with followers and colleagues.

Collaboration

Collaboration has multiple meanings, but the most useful is that of working together, especially in a joint intellectual effort. Leader-follower collaboration means that interactions between leader and follower enable the knowledge and skills of both to synergistically influence the decision the two are making or the work they are accomplishing (Manion, 1989). Synergy is a biochemical term meaning that the whole is greater than the sum of its parts. In the leadership context, it means that when the leader and follower work together, they are likely to generate more and better solutions and alternatives than either would by working alone. Dictionary definitions rarely bring a concept fully to life. To more completely understand collaboration, examining the relationship between coordination, cooperation, and sharing mutual work is helpful (Baggs and Schmitt, 1988). These three ingredients compose the whole of collaboration (see Figure 2.7).

Coordination

Coordination is the summary of individual ideas. It occurs when two or more people come together and share their points of view and experiences to ensure a harmonious combination or interaction. One executive team meets regularly on Monday mornings for a short time, sharing plans for the week, discussing major issues, and briefly reviewing its members' calendars. Their intent is to coordinate efforts. Another example is a patient conference in a patient care department that is often held for a similar purpose. Individuals from different disciplines and shifts come together to compare their assessments of patients and coordinate their efforts. Coordination is based on sharing information.

Figure 2.7 Elements of Collaboration

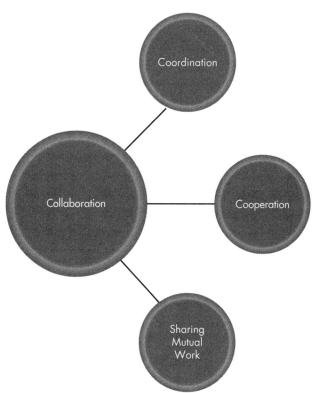

Cooperation

Cooperation implies planning and working together in an actively helpful manner; it is thus more than being passively cooperative or simply accommodating. Cooperation as it relates to collaboration means meeting the other person's needs yet being assertive in meeting one's own needs; being aggressive and uncooperative, in contrast, is being competitive.

Sharing Mutual Work

Sharing mutual work in collaboration means sharing goals, planning, problem solving, decision making, and responsibility. Contrast this with consultation, in which sharing occurs during the planning phase but allows the individual to proceed alone in implementation.

True collaboration requires all three elements in healthy amounts: coordination, cooperation, and mutual work. Too often a leader makes a decision and then expects others to coordinate and cooperate in its implementation. The leader may honestly feel that he or she is being collaborative because there is a general feeling of cooperation. However, unless involved parties made the decision mutually, it is not collaboration in the true sense of the word. The very basis of any partnering relationship is collaboration.

Partnership

Successful relationships of the future will be characterized as partnerships, which form at all levels in our society. Communities are forming partnerships with businesses and industries. Former competitors such as Apple and IBM are creating business partnerships. In a community in the Midwest, two hospitals of competing systems are considering building together a third facility needed in their area. Strategic partnerships are appearing with more regularity in health care, between health care systems as well as individual organizations (Blouin and Brent, 1997). Managerial partnerships are found at the executive and managerial levels (Manion, Sieg, and Watson, 1998; Heenan and Bennis, 1999). Tomorrow's leaders need to work in partnership with others. It is the very essence of the leader-follower relationship. As Heenan and Bennis (p. 5) write: "In a world of increasing interdependence and ceaseless technological change, even the greatest of Great Men or Women simply can't get the job done alone. As a result, we need to rethink our most basic concepts of leadership."

The philosophy and approach of "every man for himself" in organization life is gradually going by the wayside. In the past, organizations often rewarded managers for the size of their turf. The larger their budget and the more direct reports and greater number of personnel in their departments, the greater their status was. Organizational environments were competitive and predominantly unhealthy. If the organization was to meet one manager's request, it would deny another's. Today the manager who is a leader understands the importance of forming alliances and partnering with colleagues to accomplish results. The effective leader of tomorrow will be able to form collaborative associations with others to achieve the organization's mission. This is much more complex than it first appears because an individual, group, or organization may at one time be a competitor, a partner, a distributor, or a supplier. Balancing these complex relationships takes a high level of maturity and skill.

Although successful leaders are those who are able and willing to partner with others, not everyone is suited to being a partner. Partnering may well be the highest level of interpersonal development. Stephen Covey, author of *The Seven Habits of Highly Effective People* (1989), identifies stages of development and their ramifications in the professional world. As healthy individuals mature and develop, they progress from a state of dependence to independence and then to interdependence. Each of these stages of development represents significant and substantial evolution. In the stage of dependence, the individual relies on others. In the stage of independence, reliance on the self increases; the individual has taken responsibility for behavior and ownership of feelings and accomplishments. At this point, the individual is capable of moving to the higher interdependence level of development to work effectively with others and share responsibility and recognition (see Figure 2.8).

Covey (1989) points out that only independent people can make the choice to become interdependent. So highly dependent people have difficulty moving into true interdependence. Independent people may choose not to

Figure 2.8 The Development Continuum

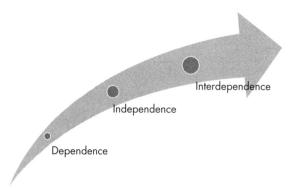

become interdependent and in fact may see relinquishing control to others or sharing decision making as a weakness. Executives in health care systems across the country are learning to balance the mixture of independence and interdependence as they partner with colleagues to lead in a variety of ways.

This development continuum, as illustrated in Figure 2.8, is significant to understanding the leadership relationship. Both Bennis (1989) and DePree (1989) describe leaders as seasoned, mature people who have recognized the need for—and have consciously chosen—interdependence with their followers. The excellent leader does not go it alone but derives energy and ideas from follower colleagues. A healthy leader-follower relationship has true synergy: the two achieve more together than either could achieve alone. Neither leader nor follower exists in a vacuum; they function in a reciprocal relationship.

Interestingly, the concept of partnership has been with us since the earliest of times. In *The Chalice and the Blade*, Eisler (1987) describes the shift from a partnership societal model in the earliest human history to a dominator model. It is clear from her research that "war and the 'war of the sexes' are neither divinely nor biologically ordained" (p. xv). Based on her understanding and interpretation of historical artifacts and findings, the earliest human societies existed in which "difference [was] not necessarily equated with inferiority or superiority" (p. xvii) and neither gender was subjugated to the other. This concept is relevant to today's organizations. Many people are involved in organizations that are "working to create more mutual relationships, democratic institutions, and equitable societies . . . they want personal and social power to be used with and for others, not over or against them. They believe that conflict can be resolved collaboratively and peacefully" (Eisler and Loye, 1998, p. viii).

Collective Responsibility and Accountability

In any partnership, the members must retain a sense of personal responsibility and accountability. But a new dimension is added in the leader-follower relationship: the sharing of collective responsibility and accountability. For the relationship to thrive and continue to flourish, all elements of a healthy relationship discussed in this chapter must exist on both sides of the partnering agreement. The leader must be trustworthy, as must be the followers. Respect is mutual, support is consistent, and communication two-way and predominantly positive in nature. Without these things, the partnership withers and dies, its potential never fully realized.

Conclusion

The quality of the leader-follower relationship directly correlates to the effectiveness of the leader and the ability of all involved to achieve necessary outcomes. Emotional intelligence and a relationship based on trust and confidence, mutual respect, support, and honest communication create a vital association. The nature of the relationship is one of collaboration and partnership. Neither is easy to attain but is worth every ounce of effort it takes. The benefits of these relationships go well beyond the personal level to the level of organizational trust. "Employees demonstrate more cooperative, helpful, and tolerant behaviors and thus reach their goals more effectively when they trust in their coworkers, managers, and institutions" (Altuntas and Baykal, 2010, p. 191).

Although many people discount the need to deal with such basic relationship principles, they are the foundation for a leader's effectiveness. They are anything but simplistic. Relationships in today's world are "parallel and simultaneous, connected, murky, multiple, and interdependent" (Bennis, 1989, p. 101). Forming healthy relationships is complex, ever changing, and always challenging for transformational leaders.

DISCUSSION QUESTIONS

1. List or categorize all the types of relationships that apply to your work group—for example, coworker to coworker; shift to shift; job categories (the pharmacist and pharmacy tech; the physical therapist and physical therapist assistant; registered nurses, licensed practical nurses, nursing assistants, or techs; manager and staff; supervisor and staff; department to department; and so on. Use the four essential ingredients of a healthy relationship presented here (trust, respect, support,

and communication) to assess the quality of these work relationships. What opportunities exist for improving relationships?

2. Are there any current or lingering issues of trust between people in your department or work group? In your organization? What steps could you take to begin to address these issues?

3. As a leader, what behaviors on your part demonstrate your trust of other people? What are the behaviors you see within your department or work group that show people trust each other? What behaviors do you see or engage in that demonstrate distrust of others?

4. What examples of presumptive trust and tempered trust do you see or experience?

5. Have you ever broken trust with anyone? Have you apologized?

6. Think of a time you felt betrayed by someone or something that happened in your workplace. How did you react? Do you carry the sense of betrayal with you, or were you able to resolve it? How has this affected your level of trust in others?

7. Go to www.PositivityRatio.com and complete the Positivity Self Test. Track your scores over time (for example, biweekly for several months). How do your scores affect your leadership practice? What can you do to increase your positive-to-negative ratio with your followers?

8. What are the ways you demonstrate conditional and unconditional respect for others? Are there some people you respect more than others? Is that respect based on superficial characteristics, such as title, age, tenure, or is it based on performance?

3

Building Commitment

INSPIRING OTHERS TO FOLLOW

CHAPTER OBJECTIVES

- Distinguish between compliance and commitment.
- Define the concept of commitment.
- Compare the three forms of organizational commitment.
- Identify strategies for building affective organizational commitment.
- Outline a process for building normative commitment.
- Write a leadership or personal mission statement.
- Develop a personal or work-related vision for the future.

Compliance is a matter of the mind;
commitment engages the heart.
JO MANION, *FROM MANAGEMENT TO LEADERSHIP*

L eadership is more than influencing others to follow a specific direction; it is creating a desire in the followers to do so. "It is relatively easy to lead people where they want to go; the transformational leader must lead people to where they *need to* be to meet the demands of the future" (Wolf, Triolo, and Ponte, 2008, p. 202). With a healthy leader-follower relationship, followers are more likely to choose the path the leader indicates. A healthy relationship, however, is only the beginning. The leader will be more effective if he or she differentiates the concepts of personal and organizational commitment and also understands the difference between commitment and compliance. Leaders who understand the various forms of organizational commitment, as well as the stages of commitment formation and key factors that result in commitment, can consciously choose behaviors to support this process. The current emphasis on employee engagement and its relationship to a positive work environment (Manion, 2009b) requires leaders to fully understand these concepts in order to avoid unnecessary frustration and the expense of the shotgun approach, in which they try everything in the hope that something works.

High levels of employee commitment are crucial for organizational success. As a concept, commitment is almost synonymous with engagement. Certainly both imply a high level of emotional involvement and passion on the part of the employee. Martin and Schmidt say engagement is "the level of personal connection and commitment the employee feels toward the firm [organization] and its mission" (2010, p. 58). The tremendous impact on

Note: This chapter is adapted from Jo Manion, "Strengthening Organizational Commitment," in *The Health Care Manager*, © 2004. Used by permission of the publisher: Lippincott Williams & Wilkins, Baltimore, Md.

service quality and financial viability has been demonstrated through multiple sources. Employee engagement has been found to be a leading indicator of financial performance. Employee discretionary effort, defined as the willingness to go above and beyond, was found to be as much as 50 percent lower among highly disengaged employees than their coworkers with average engagement (Martin and Schmidt, 2010). High levels of employee commitment and engagement also help debunk the belief that loyalty in organizations is a thing of the past. It should be noted that commitment goes both ways. Organizational leaders must create environments conducive to high levels of employee commitment. And employees also owe the organization a certain loyalty whereby they demonstrate good intentions and positive engagement in their work (Spitzer, 2007).

Although teaching people how to build commitment through reading and classroom work is difficult, if not impossible, an academic and theoretical understanding of the concept can serve to influence a leader's behavior in ways that increase the follower's level of commitment. Peter Senge (1996, p. 10) describes the importance of commitment that leaders and followers share when he writes about leading learning organizations: "We have seen no examples where significant progress has been made without leadership from local line managers, and many examples where sincerely committed CEOs have failed to generate any significant momentum." In other words, no leader accomplishes a major change or program initiative alone; it requires a vital partnership with followers, all working in concert to carry out the plan.

Compliance

In the past, when formal managers were considered the primary source of leadership in the organization and the old command-and-control methodology was still acceptable, compliance seemed fairly easy to attain. Followers were simply told what to do, and they were expected to conform or acquiesce regardless of their own opinions or ideas. Two factors today make mere compliance inadequate. The first is the nature of the workforce. A clear majority of the members of today's health care organizations are older, more mature, and experienced, and they feel more involved in their work than ever before.

Second, the changes occurring are no longer mere tweaks to the system but instead fundamental, complex alterations to the very way we deliver service. The success of this deep level of change requires more than mere compliance on the part of those individuals who will implement these changes. Compliance means conformance: people do what they have been directed or asked to do. There may be very little personal involvement. Commitment is a personal pledge to a position or issue. It is a matter of giving oneself in trust to the issue or solution. Compliance is a matter of the mind; commitment engages the heart.

Commitment

Understanding the underpinnings of personal and organizational commitment is crucial for health care leaders in today's business environment. Accelerating change, increasing organizational challenges and crises, workforce shortages, and mounting external environmental pressures make the need for committed and fully engaged employees more important than ever before.

The Concept

Commitment is the act of pledging or engaging oneself. To commit is to bind or obligate oneself, as in committing to a promise, a certain course of action, or even another person. A review of the classic organization development literature sheds further light on the concept. Brickman, Wortman, and Sorrentino (1987, p. 2) studied commitment extensively and say it is "a force that stabilizes individual behavior under circumstances where the individual would otherwise be tempted to change that behavior. . . . Commitment is whatever it is that makes a person engage or continue in a course of action when difficulties or positive alternatives influence the person to abandon the effort."

We see commitment in the workplace daily when people remain at work despite unpleasant or rapidly deteriorating conditions. All of us can remember days when everything seemed to go wrong and we would rather have been somewhere, anywhere, else. It was our commitment that kept us at work.

The early work of Rosabeth Moss Kanter (1972) included a study of thirty U.S. utopian communities to determine whether their commitment practices were related to their chances of success. Contrary to a prevalent notion at the time that utopian communities exist for people who want the freedom to do whatever they want, Kanter found a general tendency for the most stable and successful communes to spend more time and effort instilling commitment in their members. In other words, they made an effort to ensure that their members acted in ways beneficial to the community.

Commitment contains a directional element (Trigg, 1973). An individual can never be just committed; one must be committed to something or someone. Commitments are not free-floating but instead are attached to a person or a thing. Commitment also implies a strong evaluative element: people must believe in the truth and inherent value of that to which they commit. Commitment indicates a belief that an organization or job is a good one, worth supporting, and important in some way. People do not commit to organizations that they believe are trivial, deceitful, or potentially corrupt. They make a judgment about an organization or job in light of their own values.

Presupposing certain beliefs, commitment involves a personal dedication to the actions those beliefs imply. So commitment is more than belief; it is a strong enough belief that compels action. To illustrate this observation, consider the example of membership in a professional association. Members obviously reflect differing levels of commitment. One may believe that the association advances the profession, which is of value, but choose not to join and support the association. There is no action, thus no commitment, even though the individual may recognize the association's value. Or one may join and pay dues but not participate in committees, task forces, or local membership meetings. One's actions show some commitment to the association. Or one may be an active member of the association, involved and participating, contributing in numerous ways. This shows a higher level of commitment.

The essence of commitment is in the "relationship between the 'want to' and 'have to.' . . . Commitment involves three elements: a positive element, a negative element, and a bond between the two" (Brickman, Wortman, and Sorrentino, 1987, p. 6). This makes commitment a distinctive and compelling psychological process. The connection between the two elements, not merely their joint presence, is critical for commitment. Furthermore, the nature of this connection and bonding determines the nature of the commitment.

Even the most absorbing of commitments has negative elements. Examples include the spouse who nurses a partner through a devastating and lengthy terminal illness; the manager who spends inordinate amounts of time at work, often at the expense of personal relationships; the highly skilled surgeon who has made heavy sacrifices to learn those skills and runs risks daily in exercising these skills. And even the most alienated commitment contains a positive element. "People who stay with a job or marriage after the life has gone out of it may no longer have the reason that initially drew them, but they still have reasons, they still have something of value that they do not wish to lose. . . . Thus the pension the person derives from the job, or the reputation and security from the marriage, become more valuable" (Brickman, Wortman, and Sorrentino, 1987, p. 7). In other words, the investment the individual made in the commitment has become more important than the original reason for the commitment.

> People experience commitment in at least two different ways. If the negative element is salient, persistence is the manifestation. If the positive element is stronger, enthusiasm is manifest. Persistence characterizes behavior that people continue to enact despite their sense that it calls for them to make sacrifices and resist temptations—they may have to work hard and resist the pleasure of quitting. Enthusiasm characterizes behavior that people enact without ambivalence about what the behavior costs, out of a sense that the behavior itself is meaningful. Persistence in commitment reflects the call of duty; enthusiasm goes beyond the call of duty [Brickman, Wortman, and Sorrentino, 1987, p. 10].

This is an important cue for leaders in the workplace. If people seem to have lost their enthusiasm, this does not necessarily mean that they will leave the organization, but it may mean that the negative aspects of the job have overtaken the positive. Logically, when persistence is all that is keeping the person in the job, the individual is likely closer to the next step, severing the commitment.

Interestingly, adversity plays an important role in the formation of commitment (Lydon and Zanna, 1990). Without the negative element or adversity and the existence of alternatives that the individual must sacrifice, that person has not made a true choice. Adversity can serve as a catalyst in the development of commitment. It can strengthen and affirm a commitment. Researchers have most commonly studied this in the realm of romantic commitment, finding that romantic love develops more strongly in the face of opposition. This chapter addresses ramifications in the workplace more fully in a later section.

Stages of Commitment

Commitment has five stages, and these help us understand the process and issues related to each stage (Brickman, Wortman, and Sorrentino, 1987). Briefly described here, these stages also give insight into the breaking as well as the making of commitments. See Figure 3.1.

Figure 3.1 Stages of Commitment Formation

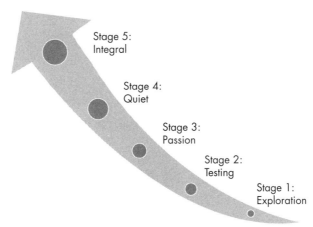

Stage 5:
Integral

Stage 4:
Quiet

Stage 3:
Passion

Stage 2:
Testing

Stage 1:
Exploration

Stage One: Exploration

Commitments in stage one are exploratory. During this stage we explore a potential activity or relationship with concern only for the positive elements that might make further exploration worthwhile. These are pre-commitments because they often involve a positive orientation toward the potential object of commitment and significant reflection has not yet occurred. Beginning commitments are often positive and somewhat superficial. Recall your early stages of a job search or your exploration of a possible promotion.

Stage Two: Testing

Commitments in stage two can be best described as testing. By this point, we have encountered some negative elements or events, and we are assessing our willingness and ability to accommodate these. We may have been involved in testing the environment, for example, to determine the manager or coworker's willingness to make concessions and contribute in some meaningful way to the employment relationship. Or we test ourselves to determine our ability to solve the problem or accomplish a task or activity. This stage also involves a search for information, but the focus is on negative and troubling aspects rather than the positive attributes inherent in stage one. The focus at this point is external, and the crisis is one of encountering unfamiliar and perhaps unexpected events. We discover that the honeymoon is over. The new job or organization has failed in some way to meet our expectations.

Stage Three: Passion

Passionate describes the commitments of stage three. This stage is characterized by the first major synthesis of positive and negative elements as well as recognition of the entire process as a commitment. Commitments at this stage are fiercely positive, with denial of any negative features, and such commitments are highly self-conscious and deliberate (Brickman, Wortman, and Sorrentino, 1987). The individual at this stage is sometimes fanatical, acting in ways that are rigid and without regard to costs. It is almost as if we need a more rigid, positive view in order to remain committed once we have a more realistic view of negative elements in the situation.

Stage Four: Quiet

The commitments of stage four are quiet. This stage emerges more slowly as the energy we need to maintain the passion of stage three fades, along with the ambiguity of the previous stage. This leads to the crisis of this stage, which occurs because we have attained the object of the commitment and now must focus energy on retaining and sustaining the commitment. Familiarity and comfort, characteristic of this stage, can undermine the effort required to sustain it. As Maxwell (2003) says, "Commitment is the will of the mind to finish what the heart has begun long after the emotion in which the promise was made has passed" (p. 8).

The orientation of this stage is intrinsic, with the threat coming from inside the person. Boredom is the crisis. Many who reach this stage in their work commitments begin looking around within the job at this time, seeking new opportunities or new ways to experience challenge again.

Stage Five: Integration

Stage five commitments are integral. These commitments represent a higher level of integration of both positive and negative elements, with the integration being more flexible and complex than earlier bonding. The structure that exists allows awareness of both the positive and negative elements and the entire commitment flows in and out of consciousness. During stage five, "individuals have the capacity to treat their commitments in a cognitively simple or mindless way, simply acting out of habit or following a well-known script" (Brickman, Wortman, and Sorrentino, 1987, p. 179).

These five stages are helpful for understanding how we establish commitments and the process we go through when making commitments. They provide increased clarity about the reactions to expect, and this can be reassuring for people who may be feeling confused by the differing dynamics of the various stages.

Perhaps one of the most important reasons to understand the stages of forming a commitment is that such understanding increases our appreciation that forming a commitment is a process. Therefore, commitments are dynamic rather than static, changing in their characteristics as they become deeper and more strongly affirmed.

Organizational Commitment

Researchers have studied commitment in a myriad of contexts, but the focus here is commitment in the work setting. There are many definitions of *organizational commitment,* with the simplest being an employee's expressed intent to stay. Wiener (1982) points out that behaviors resulting in organizational commitment possess the following characteristics: (1) they reflect some personal sacrifice made for the sake of the organization, (2) they show persistence, and (3) the commitments indicate a personal preoccupation with the organization, such as devoting a great deal of time to organization-related activities. These characteristics vary in degree depending on the strength of the commitment.

Other elements of organizational commitment that scholars have identified include a strong belief and acceptance of the organization's goals, a willingness to exert effort on the organization's behalf, a strong desire to maintain membership in the organization, and group cohesiveness (Kanter, 1972; Makin, Cooper, and Cox, 1996). Group cohesiveness is the "ability of people to 'stick together,' to develop the mutual attraction and collective strength to withstand threats to the group's existence" (Kanter, 1972, p. 67).

Types of Organizational Commitment

Extensive research has revealed at least three specific types of organizational commitment. Understanding these enables leaders to influence the level of employees' commitment more significantly.

Continuance Commitment

This form of commitment is based on the fact that the employee recognizes the benefits to be gained for aligning with the system as well as sacrifices to be made or costs to be paid. This is a cognitive process. The balance between costs and rewards must tip in the direction of rewards in order for an employee to remain in the system. Early research on commitment focused on side bets (Becker, 1960). In the organizational context of employment, the term *side bet* can refer to anything of value that the individual has invested, including money, ego, time, and effort that the employee would lose or might deem worthless if he or she were to leave the organization. Such investments might include contributions to nonvested pension plans, the development of organization-specific skills or status, or any specific organizational benefits that no other organization can duplicate. Thus, the threat of a loss binds the person to the organization.

Employees committed to the organization primarily for financial reasons such as pay and benefits are not as likely to be committed to the organization's values (Mayer and Schoorman, 1998). In fact, they may actually become a liability to the organization because they may have higher-than-normal levels of dissatisfaction and lower levels of job performance (Meyer and others, 1989).

Affective Commitment

Affective commitment occurs as a result of events and occurrences that increase an emotional connection with the employee's work group and lead to increased group cohesiveness (Kanter, 1972; Iverson and Buttigieg, 1999). Over the years, we have seen that lower rates of turnover have been related to strong emotional and affiliative ties with the work group. When the commitment to relationships within the workplace is strong, the ties of emotion bind group members to each other as well as to the community they form.

Today a sense of community within the workplace has become increasingly important for many people because it may be the only source of community in which they participate. Decreasing involvement in family, religious institutions, and neighborhood activities; increased geographical distances from family members and childhood communities; and harried and full work lives have all combined to escalate a general feeling of isolation and disconnectedness from the typical communities of the past (Manion and Bartholomew, 2004).

Affective commitment is based on the strength of positive feelings that increase the emotional bond. It also explains why turnover has costs beyond monetary impact. Turnover ruptures relationships and threatens the work group's cohesiveness (Barney, 2002; Manion, 2000a, 2000b, 2004a, 2009b).

Normative Commitment

The final form of organizational commitment comes from the recognition that one's personal values and beliefs fit with the organization. "Commitment to uphold norms, obey the authority of the group, and support its values, involves primarily a person's evaluative orientations. When demands made by the system are evaluated as right, moral, just, or expressing one's own values, obedience to these demands is regarded as appropriate" (Makin, Cooper, and Cox, 1996, p. 69). This is known as moral commitment or normative commitment, and there is less deviance and challenge to authority when it exists.

This explains at least partially why congruence between an organization and a leader's stated values and behavior is so critical. A breach in moral commitment occurs when employees perceive the organization or leader acting in ways inconsistent with stated beliefs or in ways significantly different from the employee's values. We have all seen the effects of this at one time or other. For example, one midsize community hospital in the Midwest states clearly that its most important value is quality patient care. Yet employees openly and disdainfully argue that the organization's true value is quality *physician* care, because in numerous and highly visible examples over the years, executive behavior has not supported the organization's slogan, "Patients first." Instead, what the physician wants rather than what the patient needs has guided decisions and action. What started as a catchy phrase meant to exemplify the organization's values has become a liability in building employee commitment.

Although these different types of commitments may lead to stronger organizational support and affiliation, the nature of each of these links to employees is quite different. "Employees with a strong affective commitment remain with the organization because they want to, whereas those with strong continuance commitment remain because they need to" (Meyer and Allen, 1984, p. 152). As a result, the daily performance and behavior of these employees are different. Those who value and want to remain part of the organization are likely to exert considerable effort on the organization's behalf, whereas those who feel compelled to stay to avoid financial or other costs may do little more than the minimum required to retain their employment.

This also explains the current reality of workforce issues. With the significant national economic downturn beginning in 2008, the issues within our workforce have changed dramatically. Prior to 2008, finding and recruiting the right person for the job was a major issue. There was a strong emphasis on retention of employees. Today employee turnover rates have plummeted, and position vacancies have declined. With the high national unemployment rate, most people have been affected directly or indirectly. Part-time employees have converted to full-time status or increased their hours if possible. Those near retirement age are delaying retirement plans. Per diem and temporary staff members are seeking jobs where they are more assured of a certain number of work hours. Unfortunately many of these people fall into the category of continuance commitment. They may be in the workforce not by choice but because of need. The primary issue is no longer retention, but engagement of the hearts and minds of people who would rather be there less or someplace else entirely.

As in the past, health care organizations also contain many employees who "stayed but left," that is, they resigned psychologically a long time before. Coworkers can easily identify these people because they rarely behave in a manner that exhibits any affective commitment. In fact, studies have found that employees with continuance commitment evidenced lower job performance and less promotability (Meyer and Allen, 1984). More recent research has found that affective and normative commitment led to positive organizational outcomes (such as lower absenteeism and intention to leave as well as a higher acceptance of change), whereas continuance commitment led to greater inflexibility. In terms of rewards and benefits, merely introducing higher wages increases the person's "perception of low alternatives but has no effect on improving the alignment of employee goals with the organization" (Iverson and Buttigieg, 1999, p. 327).

Normative commitment is especially important to consider for those seeking to understand generational differences in our workforce. Millennials (born between 1981 and 2000) and Baby Boomers (born between 1946 and 1964) share "a heightened sense of obligation to make a positive contribution to society and to the health of the planet. Respectively, 86% and 85%

say it's important that their work involve 'giving back'" (Hewlett, Sherbin, and Sumberg, 2009, p. 73). That's not as true for Generation Xers (born between 1965 and 1980), who are 10 percent less likely to find this important. When these people are in an organization that shares their important values, engagement is stronger.

Leadership Interventions

When a leader understands the essentials among the three types of organizational commitment, it becomes clear that efforts focusing on strengthening affective and normative commitment bring longer-term benefit. Makin, Cooper, and Cox (1996, p. 81) sum it up nicely: "In simple terms . . . people stay with the organization because they want to (affective), because they need to (continuance), or because they feel they ought to (normative)." The more a leader understands about the process of commitment, the more consciously he or she can select leadership behavior that encourages employees to form a commitment.

Recognizing the commitments and understanding the dynamics in severing or dissolving commitments is also crucial. Otherwise actions can inadvertently lead employees to further psychological disengagement from the organization. For example, dissolving a team, ending a service, or closing a department may be a wise business decision, but if the organization does not provide emotional support to employees in a way that recognizes the value of their commitment and helps them through this transition, their attachment to the organization as a whole may suffer irreparably.

Organizations most often emphasize continuance commitment during times of workforce shortages, using strategies such as adding recruitment incentives, increasing salaries, and improving benefits. Yet this form of commitment is the weakest and can actually be harmful. Organizations can more likely attain positive outcomes by focusing on and strengthening affective and normative commitment. These two types of commitment are closely related and more likely to develop personal and organizational commitment.

Approaches for Building Affective Commitment

Affective commitment is based on the emotional and social connections the employee has with and within the organization. Studies have shown that a person's experiences during the initial months of employment are perhaps the most crucial in developing affective commitment. Focusing efforts to ensure that the organization meets the employee's expectations of it is important. During times of significant change, such as the early days of an employee's employment, there is a need to continually clarify roles and pay attention to the formation of healthy relationships with new employees.

The nature and quality of an employee's work experience during his or her tenure in an organization influence commitment. The work experience is a major socializing force, and it significantly influences the extent to which employees form affective attachments with the organization. Experiences found to influence commitment included the work group's attitudes toward the organization, organizational dependability and trust, and perception of one's importance. In addition, efforts that support the development of healthy working relationships in work groups are a crucial beginning for the formation of this strong commitment. Peer relationships are important, but so is the relationship of the individual with organizational leaders and others with whom interaction is common such as patients and families, people in other departments, and physicians. Healthy relationships, as defined in Chapter Two, are based on trust, mutual respect, consistent support, and good communication. The formation of healthy relationships is at the heart of affective commitment and has been addressed in detail earlier.

Approaches for Building Normative Commitment

Three components to building normative commitment are essential (Figure 3.2):

• Shared values

• A common mission or purpose

• A shared vision

Figure 3.2 Steps for Building Normative Commitment

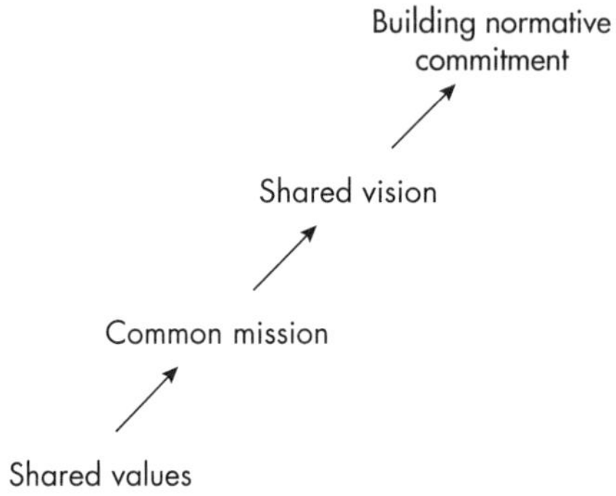

Identifying and working from shared values, a common sense of mission, and a mutually developed and held clear vision are three concrete ways a leader builds normative commitment among followers. The more fully these exist and the degree to which each has meaning for the followers, the greater the level of commitment. In recent years, these concepts have become popularized and common in the organizational language.

These concepts, though simple in meaning, are rarely easy to attain. Implied in each is that the leader first has extraordinary insight into what is personally and organizationally important in his or her leadership practice and can comfortably and clearly articulate it to others. Then the concept is more likely to become personally relevant to the followers, who deem it important enough to commit wholeheartedly to the effort and help the group attain results.

Deeply held values, a clear sense of mission, and a shared vision are often leadership attributes rather than specific skills. Guided activities may help a leader clarify his or her beliefs in each area but cannot develop them if they are not already present. Usually forged by life's experiences and the development of one's character, personality, and beliefs, these elements reveal themselves over time. For optimum leadership effectiveness, these are not only present but are vibrant and vital within the leader's day-to-day practice.

Shared Values

Employee engagement has been linked to the alignment and fit between organizational and individual values (Morgan, 2005). Alignment of values shared between leaders and followers and between individuals and the organization is necessary for the development of organizational commitment. Values are pervasive, deep-seated standards that affect all aspects of life. They are beliefs that one holds to be of worth, such as the value of kindness, freedom, or teamwork. There are group and individual values, all of which may exist simultaneously for a person. Societal values are beliefs that most members of a society hold, such as independence, personal freedom, and choice. Organization values are beliefs common to most people in an establishment, such as service to others, competence, and quality. Family values, although sometimes construed as a political statement in today's world, are simply beliefs about what's important within the family unit (however it is defined), such as commitment, support, honoring each other, and caring. Personal values are beliefs that the individual holds, such as integrity, honesty, challenge, and achievement. In addition to these categories, an individual may hold work values; in the case of a leader, these often become the person's leadership values. These are the beliefs they hold for this aspect of their lives. Respect for others, integrity, honesty, and competence are examples of what a leader's values might be.

Aligned Values

In an individual who experiences a high level of congruence among the different aspects of his or her life, these values overlap and are in sync with one another. High levels of energy and enthusiasm for life are the result. Each arena of life supports and reinforces the others. Personal power and effectiveness are at a peak. Contradiction among values in these different areas creates dissonance, resulting in disturbance for an individual. Three choices exist at this point. The individual may take steps to reduce the dissonance, perhaps by redefining the value to make it fit the situation. Another option is to suppress the uncomfortable and possibly painful feelings that arise and deny that there is any discomfort. This happens when we turn away and pretend not to see a situation that offends one of our values. The third alternative for a person of integrity is to take steps to change the aspect of life that holds unacceptable contradictions in values. We can do this by addressing and bringing forth concerns about the situation or even removing ourselves from the dissonant situation permanently.

Gilbert, in *Strengthening Ethical Wisdom: Tools for Transforming Your Health Care Organization* (2007), examines the concept of ethical erosion in an organization. "Research shows that it is in the small steps and small decisions that lead ever well-meaning individuals and their organizations into ethical conflicts—a slippery slope that can ultimately undermine the organization's viability" (p. xiii). Conflicts in values that are ignored or swept under the rug can create a dangerous situation in the organization. For example, an employee sees questionable physician behavior (abusive language, unacceptable performance, or unethical practices) and brings it forward to administration, only to be told that nothing can be done about it. The patients, employees, and the organization itself are at increased risk. Ignoring the behavior not only condones the practice, but it also may actually escalate its occurrence over the years, potentially leading to a poor practice environment, a direct effect on the quality of patient care and potential legal action.

Prioritizing Values

Life is about choices. An individual with integrity is continually aware of the values that serve as a foundation for his or her life and recognizes the choices that must be made. However, we do not always see or experience choices with great clarity. In any of the arenas of society, organization, family, or work, our stated values may not correspond to the values we truly hold. Rhetoric can easily drown out the truth. A society may say and believe it values personal independence but then inadvertently institute policies and programs that encourage dependence among some citizens. A health care organization may say that it values service and community when in truth its primary focus is on the bottom line: profits and reputation. The earlier example of one organization's slogan of "Patients first" became a source of great dissonance and dissatisfaction for employees as they observed decision after decision that clearly valued physicians first. The credibility gap grew wider with each new decision and subsequent assurance of "Patients first."

Examining one's feelings of discomfort takes courage, for intuition may be the only thing that is saying something is wrong. An individual with much invested in the current system may find it difficult to admit that his or her values are not in alignment with those of the organization.

A person of integrity acts in accordance with his or her beliefs. If the values of the organization or group do not match, the individual first assesses the situation to determine whether change is possible. Action follows, based on a belief and hope that the individual can influence the situation. Perhaps leaders in the organization haven't recognized the incongruent messages their decisions are sending. Honest feedback and open dialogue about a perceived mismatch between a stated value and observed behavior need to occur. If nothing changes, the individual's choice becomes clear: stay or leave. "In the work setting, a lack of congruency between personal and organizational values decreases job satisfaction and work productivity and ultimately may lead to job burnout and turnover" (McNeese-Smith and Crook, 2003, p. 260).

In some instances, an individual's assessment of the situation results in a decision to stay so that the individual may meet another highly held personal value. For example, individuals who highly value security and providing for their family's needs may choose to remain in an organization even though other values are not congruent. Such an individual may hope that this is a temporary situation, and it is healthier if the individual is able to see clearly the choice that he or she has made. Too many times an individual remains in a dissonant situation and suppresses feelings of rebellion against the differing values. Over the long term, one may even lose sight of or change one's values, telling oneself that these values are not worth leaving for.

Courage to choose a different path can be just as difficult when the conflict is between beneficial values. Which is most important? Which choice will be most true to the beliefs that the individual holds dear? Jane, a leader in a health care agency, discovered the difficulty inherent in choosing between two seemingly good values. She strongly valued security and stability and had spent most of her professional career in positions that aligned with these values. Fortunately, these positions also provided her opportunities to meet other values that she held dear: challenge and achievement. In fact, these differing values were very compatible for most of her years in health care. With every challenge she met, every goal she achieved, the higher were the rewards and the greater the financial security and sense of stability she attained. As a vice president at the corporate level in a home health agency, she most enjoyed the new projects and service development aspect of her work.

But the company appointed a new CEO, and within six months, Jane became aware that the company's philosophy had changed significantly. Her position became responsible for monitoring and ensuring regulatory compliance and advocating with state legislators. Although Jane was highly skilled in these areas, she now missed the challenge and sense of achievement she had previously enjoyed. She tried to negotiate a role change so that she would be challenged and excited about work again but was unsuccessful. To make matters more difficult, the new CEO significantly increased her salary, and Jane's sense of security was stronger than ever before. Her choice was difficult: Would she stay and be true to her value of security and stability, or would she seek another position full of challenge and the opportunity to grow again? After much soul searching, she resigned and became an entrepreneur, starting her own business, which over the years became more successful than she originally dreamed was possible. Challenge and achievement were more important to her than security and stability.

Jane's story illustrates the importance of values. They guide daily decision making and give a sense of direction in day-to-day existence. Holding the values of security and achievement simultaneously can lead to a crisis point in a career when situations force an individual to choose between remaining in a seemingly secure, well-paying job and seeking a new job with greater challenge. When actions are in accordance with the values one holds, events flow more smoothly.

The Result of Shared Values

When people share values, the result is a tremendous feeling of connection and synergy. Of course, this requires that leaders and followers can clearly define their values. They know what beliefs are most important in their lives. However, if they never discussed their values, anyone may make a false assumption—either that values are in agreement or that they differ. Open dialogue about beliefs benefits both leaders and followers, because people who share values feel united.

The ramifications for a leader who is trying to build commitment to a certain idea are clear. The leader must be absolutely sure about his or her values and how this decision supports these values. If there is incongruity, the leader experiences feelings of dissonance that he or she reflects in subtle ways to followers. When the path chosen is consistent with the leader's values and followers share them, commitment blossoms. The ability to articulate and communicate clearly is critical for this process to succeed. Not only are the technical skills of communication important, the leader also needs the courage to speak from the heart and share his or her deeply held beliefs regardless of the feelings of vulnerability this may create. "The challenge we all face is to find ways to use the workplace as a forum in which to express and embody our deepest values. We can derive a sense of purpose, for example, from mentoring others, or being part of a cohesive team, or simply from a commitment to treating others with respect and care and from communicating positive energy. The real measure of our lives may ultimately be in the small choices we make in each and every moment" (Loehr and Schwartz, 2003, p. 140).

Mission

A vivid, vibrant sense of mission that provides a focus for both individual leaders as well as organizations is the second step of forming normative commitment. Clarity of mission provides focus in a world that can feel fragmented and out of control at times. Organizations and individuals who define and understand their primary purpose are much less likely to be distracted by all of the other choices that fight for their attention. Gilbert (2008, p. 1) believes that having a noble purpose is one of the disciplines of daily practice that strengthens organizational integrity and makes likely the delivery of ethical health care: "Noble purpose is the calling of healthcare expressed in the vision, mission, and values of an organization and those who work in it. It is a powerful, unifying force. A focus on it brings together different parts of the healthcare community who might otherwise find themselves in conflict. It diminishes their differences and mobilizes powerful collaborations for change."

During these turbulent times, remaining focused on the organization's primary mission helps reduce the expenditure of unnecessary energy. Peter Drucker, whose contributions to the leadership and management field, spanned over fifty-four years, preached about steadfastness and clarity of long-term vision: "He recognized that leading in turbulent times requires foresight about where things are heading as well as judgment about what not to change. He would remind us that the best preparation for a smooth journey, even as we steer across troubled waters or leap across chasms, is a clear sense of meaningful purpose" (Kanter, 2009, p. 70).

The power of a clear purpose can be seen in a broader context as well. Kanter (2008, p. 44) analyzed some of the world's largest companies and found that clarity of mission and values serves as a guidance system for these global giants: "Employees once acted mainly according to rules and decisions handed down to them, but they now draw heavily on their shared understanding of mission . . . they more readily think about the meaning of what they do in terms of the wider world." She also found that clarity of values turned out to be another ingredient in the most successful of these organizations. Holding common values and standards and having clarity of mission allowed people on the front lines to make decisions consistent with these even under pressure.

"The first responsibility of the leader is to define reality" (DePree, 1989, p. 11). In an organizational context, leaders have the task and responsibility of determining both the purpose and the future of their organizations. Beckhard and Pritchard (1992) note that the white-knuckle turbulence of rapid change is forcing most leaders to reexamine the very essence of the organization along with its basic purpose, its identity, and its relationships with customers (internal and external), competitors, and all other key stakeholders. Mycek (1998, p. 26) asks: "What is the true business of healthcare? Is it the 'high-tech, high-touch' blend of dedicated caregivers and state-of-the-art technology that was prophesied in the late 1980s? Or is healthcare purely a commodity—products and services that are bought and sold at the lowest price, on the spot market?" The questions today are becoming more and more difficult. In addition to defining the organization's mission, leaders also need a clear sense of their own mission or purpose.

Strong leaders have a clear sense of mission; they know why they are here and are clear about their purpose. Mission is a reason for existence—of the individual, the project, the team, or the organization. A clear mission defines the purpose and gives direction and focus. It enables an individual to decline opportunities that detract from this true purpose. "It's easy to say 'no' when there is a deeper 'yes' burning inside" (Covey, Merrill, and Merrill, 1994, p. 103).

Over time a person's mission in life evolves. A person grows into a leadership role by fully experiencing life and learning from its many lessons through extensive reading, dialogue with others, travel, trial and error, and observation. People in leadership roles are continual learners, always seeking the lesson in a situation, even when it is difficult or painful. Reflective practice is growing in popularity today (Taylor, 2004). Reflection is a powerful tool that individuals can use to better understand what motivated actions and behaviors, what reactions came of certain situations, how outcomes were attained, and what is really important.

Leadership Mission Statement

Every leader needs a personal mission statement, which may or may not include a leadership mission statement. For some people, these are two different but compatible statements. A leader needs to distinguish between his or her purpose as an individual and as a leader. Writing these statements takes "deep introspection, careful analysis, thoughtful expression, and often many rewrites to produce it in final form" (Covey, 1989, p. 129). It means sorting through a great deal of extraneous material to reach the core reason for one's existence and the way one is to achieve that purpose. The leadership mission statement usually includes the leader's values and often the means by which he or she will achieve the mission.

A strong sense of connection between leaders and followers results from leaders' being open and sharing their personal or leadership mission statements. They may initially feel vulnerable and embarrassed because this statement is very personal. But if the leader is sincere and humble rather than arrogant and egotistical, this is a powerful way of disclosing more of himself or herself to followers. Even if a supporter does not totally agree with or fully value a leader's mission statement, understanding between the two still increases.

An individual without a sense of purpose is like a rudderless ship—buffeted about by every strong wind that happens along. People without purpose do not make good leaders. It is difficult, if not impossible, for an individual to lead if he or she has no inner sense of direction or understanding of purpose. And in our tumultuous, rapidly changing times, simply adopting someone else's purpose because doing so is politically savvy or expedient is not enough. There must be a strong inner sense of knowing and a connection to this identified purpose, or it does not serve during stressful times.

Aligning Missions

This clarity of personal purpose enables leaders to determine whether there is a match with their organization. If the organization's purpose or mission is diametrically opposed to a leader's purpose, he or she may feel that carrying out his or her mission is not possible. If encouraging and nurturing followers to function independently and interdependently is part of a leader's mission statement but the leader is in a bureaucratic, heavily hierarchical organization within which there is no intention of empowering employees, this leader would have difficulty feeling successful. Or if a leader sees his or her primary purpose as developing others but recent expansions in scope of responsibility have made it difficult, if not impossible, to serve as a coach for others in the workplace, this role may no longer meet the leader's primary purpose.

Clarity of mission also helps the leader keep a perspective on his or her day-to-day work. If there isn't a clear link between a person's purpose and his or her daily activities, work can easily become drudgery. Mackoff and Triolo (2008a, 2008b, 2008c) report on a study of nurse manager engagement. They found that a manager's "ability to maintain [this] clear line of sight emerged as the crucible in longevity, vitality, and excellence" (2008a, p. 21). They describe this notion of line of sight as the ability of individuals to understand how their daily activities contribute to the organization's purpose and goals, as well as to their own purpose and goals. For health care managers, this means creating "a meaningful, ongoing link between their daily management activities and the goals of patient care" (2008a, p. 21).

Exemplary health care leaders today demonstrate an abiding sense of personal and organizational purpose. Many see themselves as stewards for health care in their communities. Chawla and Renesch (1995) describe this as a willingness for leaders and managers within health care organizations to be accountable for the well-being of the larger community by operating in service to colleagues, patients, families, and other stakeholders. This enduring sense of operating for the benefit of others and for something bigger than any individual helps create committed partnerships with followers. Robert Greenleaf describes it this way in the collection of his private writings, *On Becoming a Servant-Leader* (Frick and Spears, 1996, p. 2):

> The servant-leader is servant first. . . . It begins with the natural feeling that one wants to serve, to serve first. Then conscious choice brings one to aspire to lead. . . . The difference manifests itself in the care taken by the servant—first to make sure that other people's highest-priority needs are being served. The best test, and the most difficult to administer, is: Do those served grow as persons? Do they, while being served, become healthier, wiser, freer, more autonomous, more likely themselves to become servants? And, what is the effect on the least privileged in society; will they benefit or, at least, not be further deprived?

Alignment of purpose between individuals and organizations creates a tremendous sense of synergy and unleashes passion for the work. The values, mission, vision, and strategies must represent the highest aspirations of the organization and those who choose to work within it. "The calling to care for and enrich the quality of life for patients, to support their families in times of stress, and to lift the wellness of communities served by the organization, is implicitly or explicitly stated in the vision, mission, and value statements. This calling is the heart of what draws many to healthcare" (Gilbert, 2008, p. 3). Simply ensuring that health care professionals can lead and deliver on their noble purpose increases organizational commitment (O'Brien, 2011; Ott and Abrams, 2008). Both the organization and every individual within it must have the intention and unwavering commitment to do the right thing, to act with integrity and ethical behavior in every situation.

Vision

The third step for building normative commitment among followers is through development of a shared vision. In recent years, *vision* has become a byword in management and leadership circles. Everywhere managers and leaders are exhorted to have a vision. We see example after example of governments, organizations, and people for whom vision made a difference. And all are impressive. Joel Barker in *The Power of Vision* (1990) raises the question: Does vision come first, or does the success of an individual, organization, or government lead to a vision? In each instance he examined, the vision came first, leading him to conclude that "vision has the power to change our lives."

All leaders understand vision because of its presence in their lives. Vision may not be a concept that is easy to explain, but leaders relate to this idea because they have experienced it. They see the future differently than other people do: leaders see what is possible and dream, while others merely predict. Vision is really hope for the future and is based in optimism. It is the ability to rise out of the current daily turmoil and see something different for the days and years ahead.

The leader's vision is not necessarily accurate, but it is almost always desirable and positive. Leaders who inspire others with a future vision follow these three crucial steps:

1. Define and describe the vision.

2. Engage in dialogue about the vision.

3. Create a structure to enable the vision.

The first involves describing the vision, the second is talking about it with others who must help create the new future, and the final step is putting a structure in place to ensure realization of the vision.

Step One: Define and Describe the Vision

A future vision is a picture the leader has of the horizon. The power of vision is in its expectancy; it's a picture of a preferred future rather than a forecast of a predicted future. Peter Drucker has been credited with saying, "The best way to predict the future is to invent it" (Cooper, 1999). Rather than what might be anticipated, it is a desirable future to be sought. It is an illumination of tomorrow based on what the leader believes is possible. Vision takes imagination and optimism. "It is the ability to see beyond our present reality, to create, to invent what does not yet exist, to become what we are not yet. It gives us capacity to live out of our imagination instead of our memory" (Covey, Merrill, and Merrill, 1994, pp. 103–104).

Some leaders seek or rise to a leadership position because they have a vision of what the future could be—a vision that drives and inspires them to lead. When the leader is armed with the vision, the work of putting structures in place to achieve the desired future becomes simple. Sometimes the position comes first, whether it is a formal leadership position in an organization, appointment to chair a committee or task force, or election to an office. The individual discovers that he or she has the responsibility and obligation to take the lead in a situation. Perhaps there is a clear mission but only a general vision of the outcomes.

The first step is to develop the vision, but this may be more difficult than it sounds. Like the process of creativity, using a deliberate intuitive process is valuable. The intuitive process starts with preparation by coming to understand as much as possible through reading everything related to the situation, talking with people, and drawing on experience. The second step is to let all information and ideas incubate until a spark occurs, leading to illumination, the third step. As the vision becomes clear, it is important to create as much detail as possible. Concrete, specific descriptions of a preferred future help others see the vision as well. John F. Kennedy, when speaking of the U.S. space program in his 1961 State of the Union Address, did not say: "We will be the world leaders in space exploration." Instead, he said that before the end of the decade, the United States would have a man on the moon and return him safely to earth. His vision was explicit and definite.

To be inspiring, the preferred future must be a stretch, a far reach from the present. Martin Luther King Jr. said, "I have a dream that one day this nation will rise up and live out the true meaning of this creed—we hold these truths to be self-evident: that all men are created equal" (Anderson, 1990, p. 11). At the time, in segregated America, this was a tremendous stretch from the reality. Peter Senge (1990) says that once a vision is identified, the greater the distance it is from the current reality, the more creative tension exists. Creative tension is the pull between the vision and the present. This tension acts like a giant rubber band, pulling toward a new future. During the growth toward a new future, if the new future seems impossible, it is just too distant; Senge says it is better to extend time frames than to compromise the vision. Settling for less is the first step toward mediocrity.

Step Two: Engage in Dialogue About the Vision

A leader alone cannot achieve the vision. New realities are created when everyone the vision affects works together. A successful organization or association encourages multiple leaders and in the same way recognizes the need for multiple visions. These visions are more influential if they are in alignment, forming a cascade of visions in the organization, as illustrated in Figure 3.3. Everyone has his or her own vision of the future, and a shared vision is created when people engage in dialogue about the vision. They discuss, explore, and modify their visions based on what they learn from each other. A shared vision occurs when two or more people have a similar picture for the future and are each committed to having the vision.

Figure 3.3 A Cascade of Visions

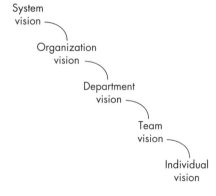

Senge (1990, p. 206) wrote, "Today, 'vision' is a familiar concept in corporate leadership. But when you look carefully you find that most 'visions' are one person's (or group's) vision imposed on an organization. Such visions, at best, command compliance—not commitment. A shared vision is a vision that many people are truly committed to, because it reflects their own personal vision." When the shared vision reflects these personal visions, there is a deep sense of caring about reaching the future. Senge describes this shared vision: "A shared vision is not an idea. It is not even an important idea such as freedom. It is, rather, a force in people's hearts, a force of impressive power. It may be inspired by an idea, but once it goes further—if it is compelling enough to acquire the support of more than one person—then it is no longer an abstraction. It is palpable. People begin to see it as if it exists. Few, if any, forces in human affairs are as powerful as shared vision" (p. 206).

Shared visions do not happen unless there is plenty of dialogue about the future. There needs to be open give-and-take, honest questioning, and stimulating conversation about the vision. Abraham Lincoln is a wonderful example of a leader who understood and applied this concept. "Throughout the war Lincoln continued to visit his generals and troops. . . . He always had a kind word for them, frequently telling them his vision of America and how important they were in achieving victory in the cause for which they were fighting" (Phillips, 1992, p. 19).

Step Three: Create a Structure for the Vision

Although Martin Luther King Jr. said, "I have a dream," and not, "I have a plan," it is not enough to have a dream without a structure in place to ensure the new reality is achieved. In a piece of folk wisdom, the Noah principle is described as: "No more prizes for predicting rain; prizes only for building arks!" The ark in this case is the structure that enables attainment of the desired vision. Some people are great dreamers but unskilled when it comes to implementing those dreams. Leaders need both skills: "Leaders not only have a vision, they work unusually hard to execute it well. Leaders are implementers, not just strategists; doers, not just dreamers" (Berry, 1992, pp. 2–3). Structure includes the steps to be taken to create the future. A person can dream of winning the lottery, but if he or she never purchases a ticket, the dream can never come true.

Bennis and Nanus (1985) describe vision as the management of attention, and in this simple statement, they capture the power of vision. With a clearly articulated vision and followers who believe in it, the vision itself focuses the attention of the vision community. It keeps people looking to the future, hopeful and expectant about its possibilities. "A leader envisions the destination their followers want, they have the superior skill to guide the journey, and they have the belief to drive the group forward in the face of adversity" (Fagiano, 1994, p. 4).

Shared values, a common purpose or mission, and a shared vision together produce the ability to influence others. An individual leader's personal and deeply held values influence the direction or mission chosen. And a strong sense of mission creates the possibility of commanding visions powerful enough to forge a new future. When you examine major accomplishments, no matter the scope, these principles are at the heart of the success. The vision may be one a new manager holds of converting a negative, toxic work environment to a positive, healthy department with high levels of mutual trust and respect, open communication, and powerful collaboration. Or as in one organization, there was a desire to develop a labor management partnership to replace the current contentious labor-management relationship that exists. Perhaps it is an innovative new business structure the leader sees as a possible alternative to the way things are being accomplished now. No matter the scope, a clear, positive vision is a guiding light.

Three case studies are offered here to illustrate the importance and power of a compelling vision. The first is the story of an organization attempting a major culture shift and attainment of Magnet status designation. The second is a more local example, a department director with a vision for a new form of service delivery. The final example describes a failed vision in a large tertiary medical center.

CASE EXAMPLE 1
MAGNET DESIGNATION OF A HOSPITAL SYSTEM

The journey started with the dream of one person, Carolyn Johnson, vice president of patient care services at Wolfson Children's Hospital in Jacksonville, Florida, who knew of the Magnet designation for hospitals and believed it was a process for strengthening the internal culture of an organization based on practice excellence. Magnet designation is awarded only to organizations with strong internal cultures that support the practice of professional nursing. In truth, however, it reflects an environment conducive to professional practice throughout the organization. She saw the potential of reaching this designation as a way to advocate for the professional practice of nursing within her facility, with the outcome being a high quality of patient service delivered. And as with all other great achievements, this one began with one person's passion. During a meeting of the organization's workforce development senior leadership impact team, headed by Diane Raines, system senior vice president for organizational effectiveness, Johnson put the idea forward as a way to recruit high-potential employees and retain them through high levels of engagement. The team's purpose was to look ahead to the future and determine strategies to prepare for workforce issues. They agreed to research and evaluate her suggestion, and the process began.

Team members reviewed the literature, conducted telephone interviews, and completed an on-site visit to another Magnet-designated hospital in Florida. With the review of all of the information, others became convinced that this was the right path. It has often been said that the greatest of journeys begin with just one step. For Baptist Health, this was the first step. Instead of being overwhelmed by the need to convince everyone in the system, Johnson began by convincing ten people that this was the right thing to do. Each of these ten convinced ten others, and the journey toward Magnet designation for the entire system was under way.

Baptist Health, a five-hospital faith-based system, is headquartered in Jacksonville. Of its over eight thousand employees, three thousand are nursing employees. The five hospitals are geographically separate and represent 1,018 in-patient beds. Baptist Home Health also provides in-home care to an average of 650 patients daily. This massive system was already doing many things right. A high-level gap analysis clearly found that several of the standards were already being met; however, it also revealed intriguing possibilities for improvement.

The Preparation

A stretch vision ignites passion, and there was ample excitement as the possibilities were considered. Raines described the first crucial strategic question that had to be answered: Would each hospital engage on its separate journey, or should the medical center with all of its entities seek designation as an entire system? These two options were weighed carefully and rationally because the decision could be important to success. In considering whether to go as individual hospitals, the advantages were that this approach would allow focused effort and honor individual hospital cultures and processes. Implementation could be staged more deliberately and would have been easier to achieve. However, there would be difficult decisions to make, for example, who would go first and who would be last. Also, enthusiasm would need to be maintained over a much longer period of time.

Engaging on this process as a systemwide initiative also had many perceived advantages. It would, they believed, unite the hospitals and accelerate the development of a system culture. Because it would require the development of system infrastructure, including shared policies and a shared governance structure, it was more complex. Intense focus would be required at both the individual hospital and collective levels. The process would be much harder and at the time was not recommended by the American Nurses Credentialing Center (ANCC, the body that confers Magnet designation). Designation as a system is more complex because each entity within it (the hospitals), as well as the system, must meet the standards.

Raines says, in retrospect, that the final decision shifted toward seeking Magnet as a system because of factors in the organization's recent history. Three years before, Baptist had separated from another system in Jacksonville. There existed a strong desire and often frequently expressed strategic need of the system's executive leadership "to recreate the Baptist system." Pursuing Magnet designation was seen as a potential vehicle for strengthening their identity and reality as a true system.

Another early conversation was focused on considering the question: Is Magnet for nurses or all staff? Overwhelmingly the answer was that this designation would change the culture throughout the system; rather than focus exclusively on nursing, it would include the relationships and practice of everyone within the system, from frontline employees through executive and board leadership. The success of this was reflected in the final report by the ANCC appraisers, which said: "Collaboration in this highly complex, matrixed organizational structure is commendable." "Relationship-based, interdisciplinary collaboration work is evident." And "There is a commitment to supporting *all* staff in career development and mobility within the system."

The first year of the journey involved communicating with all key stakeholders and refining the vision. Messages were crafted for each key constituency: the governing board, executive leadership, nursing staff, medical staff, and employees from all other disciplines and functions within the system. The overlying message was that Magnet equals excellence, but this message needed to be translated for the different audiences because excellence can mean different things to different people. Through dialogue with these stakeholders, the overall vision was continually tweaked and strengthened. This resulted in a vision statement that was concrete and clear enough that all members of the vision community could see it as well. It truly became a shared vision, dynamic and inspiring enough to create momentum toward change.

The vision illuminated the stretch that would be required to achieve it. Analysis began of what it would take to reach Magnet designation. Estimates were made of needed resources and decisions made about where these would be obtained. It became clear that infrastructure needed to put in place and changes made that would support attainment of the vision. Raines became the first system chief nursing officer. She was new to this executive role, which itself was new to the system. She credits the Magnet overlay as being instrumental in helping the system adopt and adapt to this new role.

Communication

Getting eight thousand people to move in the same direction is no minor feat. Communication was one of the biggest challenges. The foundation for nursing excellence at Baptist Health is caring relationships with patients and their families, the entire health care team, and the community. This model, developed by nurses at Baptist, describes the aspects of nursing most important to them. A systemwide communication strategy to explain the Magnet journey was developed based on this foundation. At the beginning, there was little use of the intranet for communication, and systemwide communication was accomplished through an employee newsletter. A great deal of work needed to be accomplished in this area.

As the gaps in communication were analyzed, numerous opportunities appeared. A detailed communication structure was laid out that included designated individuals responsible for communicating details and ideas to others throughout the structure. This communication team, ultimately led by the vice president for marketing and communications, was instrumental to the success of the project. This communication structure resulted in increased informal and formal communication about the process and achievements to date. Everyone was targeted, but with special emphasis where there were significant gaps in knowledge and understanding; two examples included the medical staff and colleagues in departments other than nursing.

Multiple formal channels of communication included the development of monthly posters that reported on progress of each of the forces of Magnet. These were shared on "Magnet Mondays" at an information booth in the lobbies of each hospital where new posters were introduced every month. Magnet rounds were instituted, occurring on all shifts, providing opportunities for questions and answers as well as direct feedback from first-line employees. The employee newsletter was used in a special edition to introduce the Magnet journey, and updates have been highlighted in every subsequent issue.

One of the key communication strategies was to make the journey personal for every employee. This included recognizing practices and stories that exemplified the desired behaviors. These were shared actively using the intranet. Stories were posted for everyone to read and appreciate. Rewards and recognition were given in the form of a variety of celebratory activities. Ice cream parties, pizza, cupcakes, and candy were always enjoyable. Fun, interactive games that focused on Magnet made everyone feel like a winner. One particularly creative and successful activity was making a quilt at each hospital to represent the Magnet journey. Each department was furnished with materials and asked to make a square that represented their contributions to the Magnet journey. These squares were made into a quilt for each facility. They were such a hit with staff that a traveling show of quilts was undertaken so they could be shared with each hospital. Today they are prominently displayed in the lobby of the hospital each represents.

The employee intranet evolved into a vital communication hub called Magnet Central. What began as a place to post Magnet Council meeting minutes and photos of members became the place to go to for news and information for everyone in the organization. It was accessible to employees from their work stations and their own computers. It has been used to deliver an interactive survey instrument, share departmental information, and provide links to the Medical Library and Joint Commission, and it includes reading lists for those interested. However, it has become more than merely a source of the latest information on Magnet; it is also a source of inspiration. Videos are posted, posters are shared, contest winners are congratulated, and stories are celebrated.

Magnet designation was awarded four years after the journey began with Carolyn Johnson sharing her vision with her colleagues. The journey was rough at times, and many barriers and challenges had to be overcome. However, Baptist's story is one of how one person's vision can become a shared vision and then a reality in even the most complex of systems.

Lessons Learned
At many times, the journey seemed too hard and impossible to attain. Raines said that if they had realized just how difficult it would be to achieve this vision as a system, their original decision might have been different. Many times during the process, a point would be reached when people wanted to throw up their hands and toss in the towel. It just seemed too hard. Letting people whine a bit and complain at times gave them the space to let off steam. This energy was turned around by asking people to remember why the decision was made to undertake this initiative.

"We've set three thousand and more people on this path. Do we really want to stop now?" The answer was, "Of course not." So how do we overcome the current obstacle? There was such an overall commitment to the vision that no one wanted to be the person, the hospital, or the department that kept the system from achieving this designated status. The overall vision continually recalled people to the purpose of their efforts and gave voice to their belief that the momentary discomfort and difficulty would be worth it in the end.

A second major lesson learned is that no matter how well you estimate the resources, time, and energy a change such as this will take, the cost will always be more. A major change initiative takes a massive amount of time and attention from those involved. In the beginning, it is almost incomprehensible. Perhaps this is why leadership optimism is such a defining characteristic of success. Belief is necessary. Martin Luther King Jr. said: "Faith is taking the first step even when you don't see the whole staircase."

Recognizing and celebrating incremental progress was an important strategy for building and keeping the momentum going. Finding the bright spot, the one example where it works, and then understanding that one example fully leads to greater learning. Sharing examples widely throughout the organization increased the adaptability of the entire system.

At the time of Baptist's designation of Magnet, it was the first and largest system in Florida to attain this status. Other systems have done it one hospital at a time, and in the future, other systems will exceed this achievement. Nothing, however, will take away the tremendous pride and sense of accomplishment inherent in making a vision of this magnitude a reality.

CASE EXAMPLE 2
IMPROVING THE DELIVERY OF CARE:
A DEPARTMENT LEADER'S VISION

The scope of this case example is more limited than the development of an integrated health care system but no less significant in terms of its impact on the people being served. It involved Joan, a director of women and children's services in a five-hundred–bed community hospital in a western state. (She prefers to remain anonymous.)

Her areas of responsibility encompassed six patient care departments: labor and delivery, postpartum, newborn nursery, neonatal intensive care, and two pediatric units. When Joan was recruited to this organization, these departments were managed in a traditional fashion and were gradually declining in market share because their obstetrical services were basically unresponsive to customers' requests.

Joan had been in her position for three years and was well respected throughout the organization for her innovative leadership style. During those three years, she had established good relationships with employees in the various departments and had gradually hired new managers who more closely shared her values of employee empowerment and participatory leadership, as well as family-centered maternity care. In spite of a traditional medical staff and administration who preferred to maintain the status quo, Joan held a vision of a women's service in which care was organized around the family unit instead of segregated into four different departments.

As Joan and her new managers began implementing innovative programs and services, the hospital's market share for obstetrics began slowly regaining ground. After three years, the service was bursting at the seams, requiring more postpartum beds and bassinet space. The closest patient care area available was a rehabilitation department in the next wing of the hospital. An expansion was planned for an additional ten postpartum beds and a small nursery for newborns to be added to the new unit. However, this new patient care unit was so small that staffing would be a significant problem unless employees were cross-trained to care for either mother or baby. Suddenly, Joan's long-held vision for a mother-and-baby unit was possible. Commitment to this vision began with frequent discussions with all stakeholders. Employees, managers, and physicians were all involved in planning discussions. Major educational sessions were offered to introduce the concept to key stakeholders.

In several instances, commitment was difficult to gain because the people involved held values that differed from Joan's belief in maintaining the integrity of the family unit. In addition, this change represented a major impact on postpartum and newborn nursery employees, many of whom believed they would not be able to learn the new skills needed to care for both mothers and babies.

A planning committee of employees and physicians worked out details for the expansion unit. Employees volunteered and were then selected and trained. The implementation process proceeded smoothly, and within months, the new department had a waiting list of expectant parents. Demand for this service was so intense that the hospital converted the original postpartum unit to mother-and-baby care two years later.

What had started with one individual's vision became possible only when those within the vision community shared the vision. Together they created a powerful new reality that improved health care in the area.

CASE EXAMPLE 3
VISION FAILED

Successfully attaining a vision creates tremendous feelings of pride and accomplishment for the individuals involved. There is optimism for the future, and people see the direction in which they are headed. In this final example, however, the outcomes were not positive: individuals made errors in judgment, and the results actually damaged the organization's viability.

This is the story of a large community hospital. The CEO had been reading about vision and believed his organization needed a clear vision. He assigned two interested and capable individuals within the organization as internal consultants to develop a vision statement. They interviewed the CEO and one or two other key executives to gather ideas and concepts, then developed a positive stretch vision from these ideas. The first draft of the vision statement was beautifully worded and certainly far reaching, and it seemed to be the direction in which the organization was already heading. The two consultants met with the executive leadership group to share this vision and engage in dialogue about it. This step was only moderately successful because the discussion was somewhat stilted and limited. Nevertheless, the group identified strategies for sharing the vision with employees, with the next step to include holding focus group discussions.

Based on input from these focus groups, the consultants made minor changes in the vision. But most important was the concern that managers and employees alike raised relating skepticism and doubt about executive commitment to this vision.

This response and concern fell on deaf ears. The CEO disregarded the advice of the two consultants. The internal consultants then prepared the final draft and presented it at a department managers' meeting, with overheads and fine rhetoric. Healthy working relationships and a positive work environment formed the foundation of the vision. The consultants concretely presented the terms with many strong examples. However, there was limited buy-in from anyone in the organization.

Four years later, the organization had undergone repeated crises, internal conflicts, a successful union-organizing effort, and the stressful effects of a rapidly changing external environment. Where other organizations' vision of a new future had guided them through turbulent times, this organization emerged weaker and more disorganized than it was before the development of the vision. What was the problem? At least three factors prevented the attainment of the vision. The first was the CEO's mistakenly held but strong belief that the organization should have only one vision. Over the years, he and members of his executive group had discouraged the development of additional, congruent visions by individuals and teams, preferring that the only vision in use be the organization's vision statement. The organization actively discouraged departments and work groups from developing their own vision to fit within the organization's vision. The end result was a preponderance of individuals and teams who saw the organization's vision statement as administrative rhetoric that did not directly apply to them or their team.

A second factor was the executives' unwillingness to consistently model their behavior on the very behavior they expected from employees. Highly visible examples of the old command-and-control approach to management continued to occur in spite of the language in the vision statement about valuing employee empowerment. And the executives never got around to holding themselves accountable for the relationship behaviors they expected from others. The final nail in the coffin was the internal managers' lack of commitment to the vision. Most of the communication about the vision came from the internal consultants rather than the CEO. Although the vision sounded inspiring, the managers were cynical about ever attaining it. Over time the employees who were initially committed to the vision felt betrayed, which caused cynicism that became quite virulent about what they felt was a bogus vision statement.

Common Pitfalls

Leadership interventions for strengthening employee organizational commitment seem relatively straightforward. However, as with any other issue dealing with human behavior and interactions, there are often hidden pitfalls and challenges to consider. Several of the most common issues are addressed here.

Mistaking Compliance for Commitment

Effective leaders grasp the difference between commitment and compliance and do not mistake one for the other. Leadership is more than influencing others to follow a specific direction; it is creating a desire within the followers to do so. Because many leaders also have the legitimate authority of a position, they may be tempted to rely on giving others direction about the needed actions and behaviors.

At first glance, it may seem easier to seek compliance than invest in the preparation time required to build commitment. Simply telling people what to do and expecting conformance takes less time. The time it takes to gain commitment is illustrated in Figure 3.4. The arrow indicates a project, decision, or action that must be implemented. The preparation time for gaining compliance appears to be relatively short, whereas gaining commitment requires a long, intense preparatory period of lengthy conversations, exploration of shared values, dialogue about purpose, open sharing of information, and collaborative development of the vision and plan. All of these steps lead to the internal shift within the followers that indicates a deep

---

Figure 3.4 Comparing Compliance and Commitment in Terms
            of Time Investment

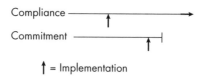

level of commitment to the outcome (illustrated by the longer line before implementation).

The paradox, of course, is that if leaders provide thorough preparation and treat stakeholders as partners on the journey, they can attain the desired outcome much faster. When organizations seek mere compliance, leaders find they have created an open-ended process with no closure because there are always some who do not comply (the open-ended compliance line in Figure 3.4). They simply have not bought in to the concept and do not support it. Unfortunately, it does not take many of these people within a group to sabotage and undermine a vision. And in too many cases, the resistant behavior may be covert and not readily apparent. In either of these situations, full compliance and closure is never attained. A strong leader understands the difference between compliance and commitment and consciously decides when commitment is needed and when mere compliance is enough. This requires a high level of judgment on the part of the leader.

Failing to Offer Choice in the Work Environment

When leaders understand commitment, the importance of choice in making a commitment is clear. Brickman, Wortman, and Sorrentino's construct of commitment (1987) indicates that commitment comprises a positive element, a negative element, and a bond between the two. This implies that there are alternatives to be considered and evaluated. If there is no choice, there is really no commitment because there are not two elements between which a bond is formed. Thus, choice is essential to the concept of commitment. The opportunity of choice is an important construct in American culture: "For Americans . . . making a choice provides an opportunity to display one's preferences and, consequently, to express one's internal attributes, to assert one's autonomy, and to fulfill the goal of being unique" (Iyengar and Lepper, 1999, p. 350).

"Choice is crucial to commitment" (Waterman, 1987, p. 299). Employees choose whether to commit and follow the path they chose. Commitment cannot be forced, and this means that a leader must face the possibility that people may choose not to follow. Waterman writes: "If the most competent and trusted people won't commit, the leader should take another look at the cause itself. It may be ill-conceived or stated in a misleading way" (p. 299). And forcing a choice prematurely is risky. Leaders must be comfortable with employees' making their own choices in their own time about the commitments they make because once they have made a choice, research has demonstrated that they are less open to new information (Brickman, Wortman, and Sorrentino, 1987). People need more information in order to change a decision than to make one. Demanding compliance on a course of action that requires employees' full engagement and support is hazardous because it may preclude the possibility of ever achieving true commitment.

Probably the most important ramification in providing choice has to do with understanding why emphasizing continuance commitment is so damaging. If salary and benefits levels are high, the employee perceives fewer alternatives because leaving the organization costs too much. An employee who feels trapped, even by positive circumstances, is less likely to be positively engaged. So although competitive compensation packages are desirable, other rewards, such as job variety, promotion opportunities, increased autonomy, and coworker support, are probably more effective (Iverson and Buttigieg, 1999).

Insufficient Communication

Recognizing that making a commitment is a rational decision-making process underscores the critical importance of communication. Information is crucial in any decision-making process, for it forms the basis for decisions. This relates back to the recommendation that there be an open flow of information about the leader's and employee's individual values and mission, as well as the organization's values and mission. Involving employees in developing a shared vision of what this venture will look like in the future helps create enthusiasm and commitment. Honest and sincere dialogue between a leader and followers helps further shape and enhance the direction. As Senge (1990) pointed out, only when the vision is shared is true commitment to and engagement with it possible.

How do we get from thought to action? The choices may seem overwhelming. Rational decision making requires accurate information. What are the alternatives? What are the consequences of choosing different alternatives? "The essential conflict between rational thought and functional behavior can be put very simply. Rational thought requires consideration of all available alternatives. Effective action requires the pursuit of one alternative, not necessarily the best one, and the ignoring or suppressing of the others" (Brickman, Wortman, and Sorrentino, 1987, p. 51). Decisions must be made and action taken even if compelling arguments exist on both sides of the issue. Being rational means that an individual chooses the best alternative. Thus, a key issue in rationality is whether the individual is aware of the alternatives and his or her reasons for choosing one above the other.

The influence of a commitment needs to be respected. "To whatever extent people are rational, they are less so following commitment" (Brickman, Wortman, and Sorrentino, 1987, p. 35). When circumstances result in the dissolution of commitments, especially those we have asked people to make, we cannot expect a rapid resolution to the emotions involved. A recent example illustrates this. In a small Georgia community, two hospitals with a long history of fierce competition were set on a course to merge. The CEOs in each facility worked diligently to gain the commitment of employees, physicians, and community. Their strongest argument was that this course of action was the only hope for the survival of both facilities. People were convinced and became quite committed to the merger. Imagine the difficulties when the merger fell through.

Missing the Possibility of Escalating Commitment

Another key aspect that effective leaders understand is the concept of escalating commitment. This social psychology concept is related to our need for self-justification. "Escalation is self-perpetuating. Once a small commitment is made, it sets the stage for ever-increasing commitments. The behavior needs to be justified, so attitudes are changed; this change in attitudes influences future decisions and behaviors" (Aronson, 1995, p. 192). This is why many savvy telemarketers begin by asking a question to which the person answering the telephone can respond only positively. It sets the respondent up for a positive second response. Similarly, if a leader can get even a small commitment first, it sets the stage for more significant commitments later.

Conclusion

Compliance from followers is not enough during these difficult and demanding times. Exemplary leaders build among followers commitment to a certain course of action. Such leaders also understand the different forms of organizational commitment and know how to capitalize on these to create a positive work environment. They focus their efforts predominantly on building affective and normative organizational commitment. Shared values, a mission common and relevant to all, and a shared vision are three specific ways in which a leader can build normative commitment among followers. Jim Collins (2008) has found that deep abiding values and a clear purpose are two key factors found in organizations that survive tumultuous challenges and thrive over time.

Affective organizational commitment occurs when healthy relationships and a strong sense of connection exist among people in the workplace. When these two forms of commitment are present, employees do more than just comply with directions set by those leaders; they want to follow the path. Together these things inspire passion and provide the energy and courage to create a new reality. Sometimes we have to believe in something before we can visualize it. And we won't see it until we believe it.

DISCUSSION QUESTIONS

1. Think of something to which you are committed. How did your commitment begin? What has kept it strong over time? Which is the positive element, and which is the negative element, of your commitment? Did you go through the five stages of commitment formation? For this example, what stage of commitment are you currently in?

2. Which form of organizational commitment (continuance, affective, normative) do you think is the strongest in your organization or work group? What examples do you see of each of these forms of commitment?

3. What are your most important work-related values? Ask yourself: "What do I stand for? How do I treat my coworkers or colleagues? What do I mean by ethical behavior? How do I want to be known by others?"

4. Once you have a list of your important values, identify the specific day-to-day behaviors you engage in that demonstrate you live by these values. Are there gaps between what you say you value and how you live your life? What values do you say you hold but find you don't express frequently enough? What values are you more likely to neglect during periods of high stress?

5. Think of an example when your values were in conflict with each other and you had to decide between competing values. How did you decide which values were more important? What was the situation, and how did you resolve it? In retrospect, did you make the right decision? Would you change that decision today?

6. Are you living up to your values on a daily basis? If not, what is a first step you can take now to ensure that you are living by your most important values each day?

7. Do the people with whom you work know what your most important values are? What can you do to emphasize values in your leadership practice? How can you talk with employees or peers about your values or those of the department or organization?

8. What are your personal mission and your leadership mission? Why are you here? What do you do, and for whom do you do it? Take some time to reflect, and then write a personal and a leadership mission statement.

9. What is your future vision? Where do you see yourself in five years? What will you be doing? How will you get there?

10. What is your vision for your area of responsibility three years from now? Have you shared and engaged coworkers or employees with this vision? Is it a stretch vision?

11. Consider your organization's values, mission, and vision statement. Are your own values, mission, and vision congruent with those of your department, service, or

organization? Are any of your important values in conflict with the organization's values or behaviors?

12. Find someone whose vision has made a difference in his or her life. Ask him or her to share this story.

13. Sit down with at least three other people and talk with them about your leadership values, mission and vision. What was it like to do this? What kind of reaction did you get?

4

Communicating
with Clarity

CHAPTER OBJECTIVES

- Identify the impact of communication philosophy on the organizational or department culture.

- Describe a linear model of communication.

- Discuss the principles of effective listening.

- Differentiate among the various levels of listening.

- Identify basic principles for effective questioning.

- Discuss examples of common nonverbal messages communicated through the use of time, touch, space, appearance, body posture, voice tone, and eye behavior.

- Identify basic principles of e-mail etiquette.

*The greatest problem of communication
is the illusion that it has been accomplished.*
GEORGE BERNARD SHAW

No other skill set is more directly linked to the effectiveness of a leader than the ability to communicate clearly. Efforts to establish a leadership relationship, build commitment, manage processes, and develop others are futile without superior communication skills. Although some people believe that simply being articulate is enough, there is far more to proficient communication. Good leaders cultivate openness in their communication; they believe followers desire and deserve information pertaining to their work. Exceptional leaders have a high degree of emotional and social intelligence competencies, one of the most important being the ability to communicate not just information but emotion. They clearly recognize that through their communication, they establish connections with others (Kowalski and Yoder-Wise, 2003).

And as important as it is to skillfully communicate, the leader's philosophy and attitude toward communication precede the development of this competency. If the leader holds a bias toward open sharing of information and true transparency in his or her interactions and behaviors, information between people in the workplace will flow freely. Relationships will be strengthened through the establishment of trust, and employees will feel supported and valued. This requires the courage to be frank and direct about concerns and issues, as well as the willingness to extend trust that information shared will be used in a helpful and positive manner. It also requires the highest level of integrity on the part of the leader. A person may have the gift of articulate communication, but if this is used to self-promote and distort truth, the level of betrayal that followers will feel is deep and difficult to repair.

This chapter tackles the issue of sharing information openly and explores several communication techniques for leadership effectiveness. It presents special issues in leadership communication. Many people overestimate the ease of meeting this competency because it appears to be simple, and almost everyone has attended some kind of communication course or seminar. Managers and leaders today spend more of their time communicating than ever before, yet the most common complaints from followers concern communication: "We don't get enough information"; "Nobody is telling us anything"; "Communication here is rotten."

Exacerbating the problem are those individuals who overestimate their effectiveness at communicating. "A few individuals may exhibit exceptional interpersonal skills, a great many others may demonstrate weak, negative, or virtually nonexistent interpersonal skills. Such considerable difficulty as we know exists . . . because most individuals do not believe there is anything wrong with the way they communicate face-to-face. . . . Most persons inherently believe they are better communicators than they actually are" (McConnell, 2004, p. 177). These people believe that if they open their mouths and words flow out or they have sent an e-mail or posted a memo, they have communicated something. This leads to a false sense of security and sometimes an attitude of arrogance: "I've communicated; if they didn't get it, that's their problem." Perhaps nothing destroys the leader's effectiveness as quickly as a lack of information and miscommunication. Distrust rapidly grows, and the leader's credibility shrinks.

Communication is a necessary component of emotional competency. The effectiveness of our relationship skills hinges on our ability not only to attune ourselves to or influence another person's emotions but also to take this knowledge into account when we communicate. Emotionally intelligent leaders who exhibit communication competency "are effective in the give-and-take of emotional information, deal with difficult issues straightforwardly, listen well and welcome sharing information fully, foster open communication and stay receptive to bad news as well as good" (Cherniss and Goleman, 2001, p. 37). A healthy and open dialogue depends on the leader's staying attuned to others' emotional states and controlling his or her own impulses to respond in ways that might impair or restrict open communication.

Defining Communication

Communication is the act of interchanging or imparting thoughts, opinions, ideas, emotions, or information by verbal speech, writing, or other methods. It has been described as the flow of information from a sender to a receiver by way of a channel (Figure 4.1). The channel might be verbal, the written

Figure 4.1 The Communication Loop Model

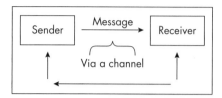

or spoken word, or nonverbal, such as body language or the environment. When the receiver gets the message and experiences the same meaning as the sender, communication is complete. The sender may either perceive a change in the receiver's behavior or hear that the receiver has received the message, and this feedback closes the communication loop.

This description of communication is, of course, overly simplistic. It depicts the process as completely linear, when in fact it is likely better described as a nonlinear process. A multitude of factors interact simultaneously and affect the quality of the communication. In any communication, for example, all parties come to the situation with assumptions, prejudgments, experience, and emotions that affect what is happening in the existing moment. Often these are unacknowledged and sometimes locked in the subconscious mind. Although they may not be overt, they can significantly influence our perception of the situation. External conditions can also dramatically affect the communication effectiveness and flow of information. Standing in a line at the airport and making a light-hearted remark about explosives on the airplane would likely have been ignored before the terrorist attacks of September 11, 2001.

The linear nature of this diagram also creates a false sense of simplicity about what is a complex process. A socially and emotionally savvy leader who is communicating with others is continually assessing his or her own emotions as well as reading the complex signals the other person is sending. This is a significant disadvantage of communicating electronically: it is impossible to read the cues the other person is sending you if you cannot see his or her face or body. This highlights the importance of using good judgment in determining the selection of channel for communication. Tough conversations, where it is important to evaluate the other's reactions, should be reserved for face-to-face communications.

Common Problems

As simple as it may seem, this linear communication loop model highlights several problematic areas. A skilled communicator understands these potential problems and takes steps to avert them when possible.

Noise

Noise anywhere in the system can reduce the likelihood of transferring a message accurately. Noise is more than loud or distracting sounds that impair the ability to hear. It can be anything that hampers the ability to receive the message accurately, including the state of the receiver's body or mind (the presence of tension, anxiety, or any intense emotion), elements that cloud the message (jargon, words with multiple meanings, assumptions, and biases), and attitudes of the receiver toward the message (perhaps the message is something the receiver does not want to hear or has prejudged).

Choice of Channel

Another potential problem area is the choice of channel. Announcing major organization changes by e-mail rather than face-to-face communication may send the wrong message. Cultural differences influence this as well. In Japan, if the manager does not communicate a major change individually with each employee, the employees feel insulted. American managers, in contrast, assume that a general announcement will suffice. Differences in expectations can lead to misread situations. Not long ago, a director in a small community hospital was in the process of selecting a new manager for a department. She had included employees in the interview process and had reviewed and used what she had learned from them in making the final decision. On the day the decision was to be announced, her plan was to simply go to the department, make the announcement, and then send out an e-mail to all employees. She discovered that many of the employees who were not working that day expected a personal telephone call from her with the results of her decision. Although most of us might feel this is unreasonable, nevertheless, the mode of communicating the final decision had never been discussed and it obviously created unrealistic expectations and hurt feelings.

Changing channels unexpectedly can affect the clarity of the message. If the usual channel between the sender and the receiver is the face-to-face spoken word, switching to a formal written memo can add unintended emphasis. If the message is negative, the change in channel may so accentuate its tone that it raises exaggerated emotions in the receiver, making a correct interpretation of that message difficult.

John, the manager of environmental services, and Mary, the manager of a patient care department, found themselves in this kind of situation. They communicated frequently, mostly talking face-to-face, about issues and problems related to the environmental services function in the patient care area. The previous year, there had been repeated problems because of the increased responsibilities assigned to the environmental service workers as a result of work consolidation efforts. Mary, frustrated after a particularly bad day, sent John an e-mail outlining unresolved problems. Because she was irritated, she also sent a copy to John's supervisor, as well as to her own.

John felt blasted by the e-mail as well as betrayed because Mary also sent it to his supervisor, as well as up her chain of command. The e-mail contained nothing that they hadn't talked about before, but the channel selection accentuated the message dramatically and almost destroyed John's willingness to cooperate further with Mary. Although most leaders are aware of these basic principles, it is still easy to get caught up in a situation and make a poor judgment. Leaders need patience to persevere in the face of these challenges.

Judgment needs to be used in selecting the appropriate channel. Delivering negative messages or criticisms electronically is fraught with difficulty. It is too easy to misinterpret the message or read into it more than was there. The words may read much harsher than they were intended, and if the sender is unable to see the reaction of the receiver, it is difficult to undo the harm that may have been caused. Furthermore, it is simply too easy to send an e-mail in the heat of anger. Thomas (2004) has done extensive research on how staff members handle their anger and reports that one of the most disturbing aspects is the vehemence of employees' anger directed at each other. This anger comes out in bickering, backbiting, needling, snapping, and cutting remarks directed at each other. In her research, she found that these employees "were constantly writing each other up," which included nasty notes on locker room doors, as well as reporting each other to supervisors. "Today," she writes, "hostile messages from coworkers can be transmitted even faster in workplaces with networked computers—in those snippy e-mails with a little zinger at the end" (p. 116).

Responsibility

The issue of ownership is another potential problem. Although the receiver has some responsibility to respond to the message received, the sender retains full responsibility for the message until the feedback loop is closed. If the sender gets feedback that the message was not received clearly, the sender's responsibility is to resend the message, perhaps modifying it in a way that increases the likelihood of understanding or choosing an alternative channel for the communication. If no feedback is forthcoming, the sender seeks a response that is appropriate to the situation—for example: What did you understand me to say? Have you acted on the information I sent you? What action have you taken? Communication is a covenant between sender and receiver, and too often the sender believes that his or her responsibility ends once the message has gone out.

Feedback

On concrete, tangible issues, feedback may result from observing the receiver's reaction or behavior after receiving the message. Perhaps the worst mistake the sender can make, however, is to assume that because the message was sent, the responsibility has shifted to the receiver. As a result, the sender does not follow up, makes the assumption that all is well, and then blames the receiver if events do not go as the sender intended.

We see this regularly: a written memo or e-mail message goes out, but only half the people who were supposed to receive it ever do. For example, the education department notifies potential participants of an upcoming program for which they need to register, but the message doesn't make it to all intended recipients. Those who do not receive the message may appear resistant or negative because they do not take the required action or as complaining if they point out that they were left out of the loop. E-mail has contributed to this problem because it leaves no paper trail unless the communicator intentionally creates one. We quickly tap out messages and instantly distribute them with a single keystroke to multiple recipients. But the old adage, "Out of sight, out of mind," holds true. It is difficult to remember to follow up on something if there is no reminder.

If the relationship with receivers is fraught with distrust, the feedback the sender gets may not be entirely honest. The receiver may be embarrassed to admit that the e-mail, proposal, or vision statement was so filled with buzz-words, jargon, ten-letter words, or highly technical language or was just plain unintelligible that the receiver did not understand what it said. One speaker, scheduled to present at a statewide hospital association annual meeting, made this point in a clever way. Prior to his presentation, he asked to interview participants, who were mostly CEOs and other high-ranking hospital executives. He began the interview in a normal fashion and then began asking questions that were really just a string of words. There was no coherent thought or message in the words. They were truly gobbledygook. Watching these high-level executives try to answer these nonquestions was hysterically funny. It was amazing to see these executives responding in almost the same manner. In other words, they strung together a bunch of words and tried to formulate an intelligent response to an unintelligible question. Only two of the executives interviewed responded in a totally honest and forthright manner, turning to the interviewer and saying, "That didn't make any sense at all" or "I have no idea what you just asked." One point this illustrated is just how difficult it is to be honest when we don't understand but think we should.

The receiver may also find it difficult to admit that he or she did not get the message the first time because of distractions in the environment. As a receiver, I may feel at fault if I allowed myself to be distracted or didn't read the message carefully enough. One executive recently complained to her next-in-line that she hadn't been kept informed about a particular situation, to which that individual responded angrily, "I copied you on all of the e-mails." The information overload contributes to this difficulty in sorting through and differentiating between the mundane and the important.

Perhaps the sender responded in an angry and defensive fashion when the receiver gave negative feedback on a previous occasion, and the receiver is unwilling to endure such a response again. Trust in the sender is essential for accurate feedback to occur. When feedback is negative, a common assumption is that the receiver has an attitude problem. The conclusion may be that the person receiving the message purposely did not take the intended action and is being obstructive, resistive, or just plain stupid. Instead, to avoid this pitfall, the first question the sender might ask is whether there were technical or semantic problems with the communication. The sender must consider these first before assuming that the receiver has an attitude problem.

A parenting example makes the distinctions between different communication problems clearer. Similar examples exist in the work world.

CASE EXAMPLE 1
MISCOMMUNICATION

A family expects overnight company during the weekend, and on Wednesday the parents of sixteen-year-old Sarah ask her to clean her room so that the visitors can sleep in it. Friday arrives, and Sarah has not cleaned her room. A typical parental reaction is to assume that Sarah just didn't get around to it, didn't follow through, or was perhaps being rebellious in reaction to giving up her room or being told what to do (an attitude problem).

If Mom looks back, however, to see how she carried out her responsibility as sender, she might find other reasons for the miscommunication. For instance, she may remember that when she told Sarah to clean her room, Sarah was on her way out the door. Also, Sarah had stayed up late studying for a test she was very worried about, and she had overslept and was late leaving for school (internal anxiety—noise in the system). And as any parent knows, "Clean your room" may mean one thing to a sixteen year old and something entirely different to a parent (semantic differences). To Sarah, it meant getting everything out of sight: stuffed under the bed or in the drawers or the closet. To her mom, it meant emptying a drawer and making closet space available, as well as ensuring that clutter and odors emanating from under the bed wouldn't disturb the guests.

CASE EXAMPLE 2
MIXED MESSAGES

A three-hundred-bed hospital in the St. Louis area was in severe financial straits. Part of a larger system, the hospital was given six months to reverse these financial problems, or it would be sold. The director of education purchased modular education that the managers and supervisors (as internal facilitators) were to deliver to employees in the belief that this education would assist in an extensive downsizing and restructuring effort that was under way. An outside trainer arrived to present the modules for the internal facilitators beginning on a Monday afternoon.

On Monday morning, the internal facilitators were gathered together and received a message from the CEO regarding the corporate decision about a likely closure or sale, a planned layoff, and the reduction of management and supervisory positions by half. In the afternoon, these same people were expected to attend a learning and development session. Although they rallied and concentrated on how they could use the educational modules, the effectiveness of any communication that afternoon was greatly reduced by the presence of strong emotions (a technical problem) following the morning session. If administrators later labeled these managers and supervisors as resistant or nonsupportive because they had not used the modules, this example would closely parallel the parenting example in the previous case example.

Sometimes where the message is delivered is less than optimal and results in communication difficulties. How many important conversations take place in the hallway or in the minutes before or after meetings? There never seems to be enough time to communicate thoroughly, and yet the sender and receiver may end up spending hours to clear up miscommunication.

Communication and Leadership

Warren Bennis and Burt Nanus describe communication as the management of meaning (1985). When Max DePree (1989) talks about a leader's role as defining reality, it means that the leader and follower have reached a

CASE EXAMPLE 3
INAPPROPRIATE SETTINGS

A management development specialist told the story of feedback she received from her leader regarding an important project that the leader had asked her to undertake. Their offices were located in different cities, making face-to-face feedback difficult because of inaccessibility. It happened that both the specialist and the leader were attending a seminar together. The specialist decided to use this opportunity to obtain feedback on the project, but the only place and time available was in the women's restroom during a break. As one might imagine, the feedback left a lot to be desired.

shared understanding of that reality. Shared meaning is the very essence of communication. The leader communicates not only words and concepts throughout the organization but emotional tone as well. One of the most important things the leader communicates is his or her emotions. "Emotions are contagious, particularly when exhibited by those at the top, and extremely successful leaders display a high level of positive energy that spreads throughout the organization" (Cherniss and Goleman, 2001, p. 38). The emotional tone that the leader sets ripples out through the organization and affects the entire culture. And as presented in Chapter Two, the neuroscience research is now providing empirical evidence that validates this long-held recognition (Goleman and Boyatzis, 2008).

Although complete and totally accurate communication is probably impossible to attain, a more reasonable goal is to accomplish communication just clear enough to enable followers to act on ideas or information in a positive and forward-moving manner. The sender of the message retains responsibility until the receiver closes the feedback loop. Following up on feedback and assessing the message for technical, semantic, or attitude difficulties can prevent major miscues.

Information

Information is one of the most important things we transmit through communication. Information is like a lubricant in the system: without it, the different parts do not work well together. In an automobile, if there is not enough oil in the engine, gears grind, friction develops, and overheating can destroy the parts. The same thing happens in an organization. Margaret Wheatley, in *Leadership and the New Science* (1992), does a beautiful job of exploring the role of information in a system: "If information is not available, people make it up. Rumors proliferate, things get out of hand—all because people lack the real thing. Given the need for constant nourishing information, it is no wonder that 'poor communication' inevitably appears so high on the problems list. Employees know it is the critical vital sign of organizational health" (p. 107).

Part of the problem is that many people regard information as stable, factual, and something that will be the same tomorrow as it is today. Information instead is dynamic and ever changing. Even simply sharing it may essentially change it as it is passed along, much like the childhood game of telephone. "The function of information is revealed in the word itself: information. . . . For a system to remain alive, for the universe to move onward, information must be continually generated. If there is nothing new, or if the information that exists merely confirms what is, then the result will be death" (Wheatley, 1992, p. 104).

Leaders who treat information as fixed and static, failing to appreciate its dynamic quality, end up frustrated by the need to continually communicate with others. Followers who see information as stable have great difficulty understanding why the message today is different from the message yesterday. Some followers conclude that the leader was not being honest yesterday or did not have accurate information, because they find it hard to believe that the information could change that quickly. Mistrust grows quickly unless followers understand the true nature of information: that it is always in formation.

The leader's attitude toward sharing information is crucial to being an expert communicator (Wilson, George, and Wellins, 1994). At least five rationales, or internal messages the leader may be playing, affect the amount of information the leader shares with followers:

- Followers already know the information.

- Followers do not want to know.

- Followers do not need the information.

- Followers cannot understand the information.

- Everyone is on information overload.

Followers Already Know the Information

Sometimes we believe that the person already knows the information. This often happens in the area of behavioral expectations. We may not clearly articulate that we expect everyone to treat others with courtesy and respect because it is assumed that all employees understand this. We further assume that we all mean the same thing by the term *respect* instead of clarifying the behaviors that we mean when we talk about respect. One manager may not see it as disrespectful to not ask employees for their opinion about a decision or course of action, yet those same employees may feel quite disrespected when they aren't asked to participate. In another instance, a well-established and experienced CEO has the expectation when hiring new executives that the new individual will not speak up or participate for the first three months of tenure until he or she has settled in and knows the ropes in the new organization. New executives in this organization report feeling totally disrespected by this unusual expectation. What makes it worse is that this expectation is never verbally articulated; it is conveyed through negative, reactive body language.

Another common misconception that hampers many would-be excellent communicators is the assumption that because they shared the information once, the receiver understood the message. In fact, only a very unusual follower gets the message right the first time. With so much noise in our changing systems and with stress levels as high as they are, it is almost guaranteed that we need to repeat messages multiple times before they are received accurately. In fact, during times of great change in the organization, leaders should expect to repeat messages at least seven to ten times before receivers understand them.

Not only do the messages need to be repeated frequently, but using a variety of different channels will increase the likelihood that they will be received. This means using a combination of channels such as face-to-face dialogue, spoken presentations, written methods, and modeling the behavior we request. The greater the frequency and the wider the variety of methods used to communicate messages, the more likely they will get through. Another key principle is to encode the message with what it means for the receiver: why it is important and what the impact is on the receiver's life.

Followers Do Not Want to Know

In one organization, a benevolent, paternalistic leader's attitude was, "They don't really want the truth—they couldn't handle it." Even in a supportive, empowering leader, the thought that the truth would scare the followers can be a deterrent to open communication with them. Some leaders believe that part of their role is to shield followers from bad news. In fact, some employees do say: "You take care of that; we don't want to know the gory details." In these cases, followers are giving up their power and sense of control to the leader.

This leader attitude displays a lack of respect for followers. From the leader's perspective, it implies that the followers are not strong enough or able to handle difficult news or unpleasant information. "When we shield people we are acting as their parents and treating them like children" (Block, 1987, p. 91). It is better to err on the side of high expectations of others than to continue to weaken followers' self-esteem by keeping them from the truth.

Followers Do Not Need the Information

In some instances, the leader believes that followers do not need certain information, that it is privileged or confidential. The notion of sharing information openly is the opposite of the military model that "only those that 'need to know' should be informed" (Block, 1987, p. 90). Here's an extreme example from a southwestern community hospital. The executive team in this 320-bed facility spends several weeks each year involved in strategic planning. Team members analyze the organization's strengths, weaknesses, opportunities, and threats and plot out the steps for action over the next two to three years. The team is very clear about its direction and what the hospital needs to do to accomplish the plan's outcomes.

Interestingly, however, the executive team never shares the plan with employees or managers. The team is afraid someone will leak it to the hospital's competitor, a similar-sized facility in the same community. Employees and managers alike have directly and repeatedly asked over the years to see the plan, and they may have finally reached the conclusion that there is no plan. How this executive team expects to accomplish its strategic plan in isolation from employees and managers is a mystery. This situation has led to significant feelings of mistrust in the organization.

Instead, the goal should be to let followers know of plans, ideas, and changes as soon as possible. Plans cannot be implemented without the support and involvement of followers, who need to be included from the beginning. Robert Haas (quoted in Huey, 1994, p. 48), says: "In a command and control organization, people protect knowledge because it's their claim to distinction. But we share as much information as we possibly can throughout the company. Business literacy is a big issue in developing leadership. You cannot ask people to exercise broader judgment if their world is bounded by very narrow vision." These are examples where presumptive trust is very important. In other words, if we treat people as if they are trustworthy, they will be trustworthy.

Followers Cannot Understand the Information

Admittedly much of the information concerning the health care environment, the business climate, and community issues can be complex. However, the workforce today is better educated and informed than ever before. When Congress was debating U.S. trade agreements years ago, so were workers on factory room floors all over the country. Becoming well informed is as simple as turning on a television set or the computer and getting on the Internet. Increased availability of information through mass media, and especially the Internet, has resulted in well-informed citizens—when they choose to seek the information and take the time to differentiate between what is true and false. A growing cause for concern is the amount of misinformation on the

Web and in the news today. It makes it very difficult for people to distinguish accurate information from that which is blatantly wrong or purposely skewed. Moreover, once they have perceived something as true that is actually false, it is more difficult to accept or even recognize the truth when it is reported or shared.

Employees or followers are often capable of understanding a great deal more than they are given credit for. Increased appreciation for employees' capabilities has been a wonderfully liberating outcome for organizations that have successfully implemented models of shared decision making in their organizations, such as shared governance structures, unit councils, and process improvement and employee work teams and helped these employees develop a high level of self-direction and self-management (Manion, Lorimer, and Leander, 1996). Many think that traditional management responsibilities—such as departmental budgeting, interviewing and selecting new employees, planning, and managing supplies and inventory—are beyond the capabilities of the average employee. Yet these same employees leave at the end of their workday and assume these responsibilities in their homes. They manage financial resources, possibly serve on a church board undertaking a multimillion-dollar building project, help their children select vocational schools or colleges, and resolve conflict within the family. The next morning at work brings sudden dependence on a manager to accomplish very similar tasks.

In a Baltimore hospital, executives discovered the power of sharing increasingly complex information with employees. Over the years, the administration had made great strides in creating an empowering environment. Executives shared information openly and freely with employees. The hospital held town hall–style meetings, with executives and employees engaging in direct dialogue about issues of concern. In the early stages of this transformation, the questions employees asked executives at these meetings involved issues such as adequacy of parking space, health care benefits, and expected structural changes. As months passed and the executives shared increasingly more information, employee questions changed significantly. Executives began hearing questions such as: What's the impact of the economic downturn on our organization's investments? What's our current payer mix? What is the impact of recent legislative changes on our organization and community? How will our business structure change? The more information the leaders shared, the more sophisticated followers became, and the broader was their understanding was of the organization's reality.

Everyone Is on Information Overload

A common and often justified message playing in a leader's head is that followers are already on overload and too much information is potentially damaging. The leader's concern is that excess information may be overwhelming. There is no question that the overload of information exists and only worsens as each year passes. Hemp (2009, p. 83) reports, "Current research suggests that the surging volume of available information—and its interruption of people's work—can adversely affect not only personal well-being but also decision-making, innovation and productivity. In one study, for example, people took an average of nearly 25 minutes to return to a work task after an e-mail interruption."

No one is immune from the information explosion. The elderly remember days before television when radio was the primary media. Baby Boomers remember when only two or three channels were available on television. Now communication is possible virtually anywhere and at any time. Cell phones, texting and tweeting, beepers, fax machines, overnight express mail: all contribute to the immediacy of information. Computers and mass media, in addition to voice and electronic mail, have contributed to an information glut. It's no wonder everyone feels overloaded. The flow of information is an unrelenting bombardment that continues throughout nearly every waking hour.

This communication barrage causes repeated interruptions of work, leaving people feeling frustrated and overwhelmed. Appreciating this information overload is important, but it should not keep the leader from sharing as much as possible about a project or situation.

The Leader's Primary Responsibilities: Information and Communication

Because of the massive amount of information in the environment, an effective communicator knows that messages need to be simple and easy to understand. Using a variety of channels helps ensure reception. Analyzing how the information is important to the recipient gives the leader clues about preparing effective transmission.

Communication is a full-time responsibility for all leaders. A leader can never communicate too much. It is far better to err on the side of excess information even though it may create its own problems at times. "The fuel of life is new information. . . . We need to have information coursing through our systems, disturbing the peace, imbuing everything it touches with new life. We need, therefore, to develop new approaches to information—not management but encouragement, not control but genesis. How do we create more of this wonderful life source?" (Wheatley, 1992, p. 105). Many organizations today have chief information officers to help the system develop an approach to handling the massive amounts of information available. Learning organizations must be able to disseminate information widely in order to learn from all parts of the organization in a timely manner.

A leader must master three methods of communication—spoken, nonverbal, and written—in order to be an effective information disseminator. The more versatile the leader is in these three methods, the more congruent the message is and the more likely it will transmit clearly. This section explores principles of each method with ramifications for today's health care leaders. Not all followers are equally skilled as communicators, and the less skilled the follower is, the more highly skilled the leader needs to be.

Spoken Communication

Spoken communication is more than selecting the right words. For a leader to influence followers, there must be a way to exchange ideas and opinions, engage in dialogue about issues, and share concerns. This is usually done through oral communication. Successful communication includes the following aspects:

- Delivering the message clearly
- Creating a message with impact
- Getting the listener's attention

- Establishing commonalities with listeners
- Finding ways to be different
- Using gestures and movement
- Using symbols and graphics
- Using metaphors and analogies
- Storytelling
- Using the environment
- Listening
- Asking the right questions

Let's take at look at each of these aspects within a leadership context.

Delivering the Message Clearly

Leaders must be able to order their thoughts, choose words that impart the message clearly, and be comfortable and at ease with the spoken word. Inarticulate leaders often feel self-conscious and are less likely to express their opinions and ideas or engage in conversations with followers. This greatly reduces their effectiveness and results in the loss of synergy between leader and follower.

The ability to express difficult or technical concepts in simple ways is essential if the message is going to be received. Some people believe that the larger and more complex words a person uses, the more intellectual or important he or she sounds. Use of such language may be appropriate for presenting technical or highly complex information to a homogeneous, professional audience, but it does not apply when speaking to or with general audiences. Instead of the communication fostering a connection, the opposite happens: followers feel more distant from the leader. The gap widens, and followers focus on how they are different from and perhaps less informed, less educated, or less intelligent than the leader.

This ability to express complex concepts simply is not always a natural talent, but it can be learned. At a department head meeting with approximately seventy managers attending, an executive of a six-hundred-bed medical center gave a twenty-minute presentation on statistical tests of significance.

These managers represented all hospital departments, and less than a handful had any formal research background. The speaker explained difficult, complex research concepts during the presentation in a way that everyone in the room could clearly understand. When one person asked this executive where and how she developed this ability, her response was interesting. In her graduate work, she had a professor who would assign a paper but leave the choice of topic up to the student. Once she selected the topic—quality, patient safety, sustainability, just culture—she had to write the paper without ever using the word or term the paper was about. She explained how this taught her to find multiple ways of expressing the same concept.

An easy, conversational style of communicating establishes rapport with receivers, whether in a large group or a smaller, more intimate gathering. Ideas flow more freely, and speakers and listeners are less reserved about expressing opinions and disagreements. Bennis (1989) believes that a good leader encourages dissent, establishing a climate that encourages expression of contrary ideas.

Body language congruent with the verbal communication substantiates the message sent. If the speaker uses words that ring with sincerity but makes limited eye contact, has a stiff posture, and makes reserved gestures, these lessen the impact of the message. During a recent program, a speaker was talking about the importance of passion for our work. Yet because he was just developing his presentation skills, he delivered the message with no observable passion or enthusiasm in his voice. It wasn't that he felt no passion; rather, his overriding concern at the moment was delivering the content. But listeners were left with an odd sense of incongruency and less likely to get the important message he was trying to convey.

When verbal and nonverbal messages contradict each other, the listener will have trouble interpreting the speaker's meaning. The receiver may leave the situation feeling baffled but unable to put a finger on what is wrong. The words sounded good, but some sense or intuition tells the listener that the sender did not really mean what he or she said. At one meeting, the agenda was to review and discuss recommendations from a project team. The leader and several members of the team, all frontline employees with the exception of one manager, were to present their recommendations to the executive team. The CEO started out by saying how important it was to have employees involved in these project teams because of their perspective and proximity to the work and problems being discussed. He also reaffirmed the executive team's commitment to having employees become more involved in major decisions that affected their work.

The team presented its findings while the executives listened politely. They asked a few questions and then graciously thanked and gently dismissed the project team members. Behind closed doors, the real discussion began, and the executive team ended by discarding all the project team's recommendations. The executive team gave the following feedback to the project team: "Thanks for all your efforts," and "Your recommendations helped us clarify the issues and our thinking." Is it any wonder that members of the project team had mixed feelings? How were they to reconcile the courtesy and appreciation the executive team expressed with their feelings of exclusion and impotence?

Occasionally miscommunication is humorous, as the following story shows: "During his tenure as the director of the Federal Bureau of Investigation, J. Edgar Hoover once wrote in the margin of a draft letter: 'Watch the borders.' He intended only that his secretary widen the margins of the letter; what he got, due to a grand misinterpretation by some overzealous aides, was heightened readiness along the U.S.-Mexico border" (McDonald, 1997, p. 4). Of course, this story is funny only in retrospect. At the time, it was a fairly costly miscommunication. Mixed messages can be dangerous because we often do not consciously recognize them. They leave us with vague feelings of discomfort but nothing that we can pin down or examine. Often they create a sense of discord, and although mixed messages may not lead immediately to a breakdown of trust, loss of trust is an eventual outcome.

This next example helps illustrate the tremendous impact negative body language can have on followers. Tom, a well-experienced and well-intentioned CEO, had a habit of pointing his finger at people in the audience when he was trying to make a point or when he felt intensely about a topic. He was clueless about the negative effect this had on people. It was significant enough that he did get feedback from employees (through surveys and other methods) that his body language was a problem. However, he did not concretely understand the feedback. He became increasingly irritated with being told this, especially through anonymous surveys, and the body language just became more extreme. His voice would become clipped and abrupt, and the finger pointing took on the appearance of an angry parent.

In an executive team meeting, he expressed his frustration at being told about his body language because he felt he was an excellent communicator. As he was saying this to team members, he was becoming angrier and began pointing his finger at each of them as he emphasized his points. The room became deathly silent, and his tone increased almost to a rant. He was honestly frustrated and meeting a wall of silence. Finally, the chief nursing officer, John, who was sitting right next to him, reached out and gently put his hand over Tom's pointing finger and stopped it. Quietly he said, "Tom, *this* is what they mean." He got the message.

The only foolproof way to determine message clarity is for the leader to seek feedback from the receiver. If the response is negative or the receiver does not have clear enough understanding to act on the message, another attempt is in order. Ideally, through direct dialogue with the recipient, it may be possible to determine the source of confusion and clear it quickly. In any event, the communicator can resend the message, perhaps with additional information or a new explanation to increase clarity.

Creating a Message with Impact

Clear, concise information bolsters the impact of messages. And an effective communicator knows how to emphasize the key points of a message by getting listeners' attention; establishing something in common with them; finding ways to be different; employing gestures and movement for key points; using metaphors and analogies; telling stories; and employing symbols, graphics, audiovisuals, and the environment.

Gifted communicators use these methods effortlessly. Although some of these techniques are simpler and easier to use than others, all can become smooth with practice. Mastering these methods is worth the effort because they help receivers understand the message.

Getting the Listener's Attention

Gaining others' attention is an initial step in communicating. In formal presentations or discussions, a third party may introduce the communicator or the topic to the group. Most often listeners' eyes and minds focus on the leader because there is a natural beginning point. Just the presence of a known and admired leader may draw the attention of followers who are interested in communicating with him or her. In a few instances, however, the leader may need to specifically draw followers' attention in order to make a point. Effective ways of accomplishing this include using a hand gesture indicating the desire to speak or simply waiting for silence among the audience.

Establishing Commonalities with Listeners

Pointing out commonalities between the speaker and listeners is another way to gain attention and establish rapport or a sense of connection. This is difficult unless the leader knows something about the followers. The more familiarity the leader has with followers and their situation, the easier it is to identify common backgrounds, values, goals, and ideas. If the leader does not know a great deal about the followers, listening closely for free information is a useful strategy. This means being alert to information they share during conversations that may not pertain directly to the topic at hand but reveal something about the individuals in the group.

Dialogue between leader and follower often reveals many points of similarity. During the interchange of ideas, thoughts, and opinions or with the expression of concerns and fears, the leader who is in agreement with the follower, has had a comparable experience, or shares the follower's concerns or feelings can use these similarities. The leader may say something like, "Yes, I remember that when I worked in the lab on the night shift, I often felt left out of the loop." Done briefly, without drawing attention away from the speaker, this establishes a commonality and sense of connection. Selected self-disclosure is a gift of trust that the leader extends to followers. Telling the listener, "I know just how you feel," is detrimental because it sounds like a platitude or cliché. Some listeners may react with skepticism and anger if they do not believe that the person communicating understands. "When I was in a similar situation, I had some of the same feelings or reactions you are expressing" is a more realistic statement and communicates understanding without minimizing the uniqueness of the speaker's experience.

A dramatic example illustrates what happens when a leader emphasizes differences. Susan was the project director for a massive organizational initiative in a hospital in which she had been a well-known nurse manager for years. She enlisted the services of an external consultant to assist with employee education. At the first session, she introduced herself, saying, "I am the hospital administrator in charge of this initiative." To this audience of nursing employees, the message was clear: Susan no longer considered herself a nurse. Many among them were taken aback. Susan's attempt to distance herself from her background was successful: she was so distant from these followers that she became ineffective in her new role.

Finding Ways to Be Different

Although it sounds contradictory to the point just made, being different is another way to emphasize a message. O'Dooley (1992, p. 7) writes, "People remember the unusual better than the ordinary." This can be as simple as a leader's appearing informally instead of at preannounced, prearranged, and structured times; not using PowerPoint for a presentation; or acting out a skit to demonstrate a major point. O'Dooley gives an example from his years selling photocopying machines for IBM, when he wanted customers to remember him over his competitors from Xerox and Kodak. He introduced himself as "Patrick O'Dooley, reproduction specialist." It worked in spite of the odd looks he received. His goal was "to stand out in others' minds, do things a little differently than everyone else does them."

When one large medical center undertook a massive restructuring project, the senior executive staff performed a skit to help deliver a message about the importance of the project and the role of employees. The skit, which revolved around a pioneer theme, included these executives in western garb and on horses. The videotape of this skit was powerful—not just the overt message but the impact of seeing these leaders in blue jeans and cowboy hats on horses was dramatic.

Using Gestures and Movement

Accenting key points with gestures, movement, or tone of voice helps anchor the message for listeners. This is what Tom (in the previous example) thought he was doing when he pointed at people. Useful in casual conversations as well as more formal discussions and presentations, movement draws listeners' attention and increases the likelihood that they will remember the point. Controlled hand and arm gestures can be used to communicate emphasis. Effusive, broad gestures may raise suspicion about the speaker's level of sincerity and should be avoided. Changing the tone or volume of voice can be effective. Either softening or increasing the volume causes the receiver to listen more closely.

Using Symbols and Graphics

Using symbols, graphics, pictures, or videos can increase message clarity. A good graphic display often communicates a message in a way that makes words unnecessary. The graphic has to be one the audience can understand, of course. Audiovisuals are useful adjuncts to formal presentations, and many sources, especially training journals and materials, can provide ideas for making them more effective. PowerPoint presentations can be an effective tool but may be overused. One health care system banned executives and leaders from using them because of competition among presenters. PowerPoint presentations had become glitzier and more technologically advanced until they totally distracted members of the audience from the message meant to be communicated. And people started questioning the amount of time being allocated to just create the presentation.

Symbols are capable of motivating human behavior. They are very powerful and can be quite stirring. In an article about the use of symbols in health care, Clark (1996, p. 20) gives some evocative examples:

A firefighter carries a lifeless toddler from the bomb scene at Oklahoma City's federal building. In the South Bronx, the athletic shoes of youths killed by violent means are hung from fire escapes and clotheslines. In New Mexico, crosses adorned with flowers mark the roadside where a loved one has been killed in an alcohol-related automobile accident. Mementos left at the Vietnam Veteran's Memorial. The homespun patchwork of the national AIDS quilt. Blouses tied together to signify the women who have been battered and killed as a result of domestic violence. Yellow ribbons as a remembrance of someone missing from home, red ribbons for those who died of

AIDS, pink ribbons for the fight against breast cancer. . . . All these images represent the shared experience of Americans, with respect to our health and well-being.

With the passing years, the list of symbols can include even more contemporary images, such as the collapse of the World Trade Center towers or the images of a U.S. soldier holding an Iraqi prisoner by a leash.

The communication may use symbolic language or behavior without conscious intent or awareness. Termination of employees or announcements of major decisions on Fridays may symbolically distance the sender from receivers of the message by the physical separation of the weekend. Executive offices far from the workers may be practical for executives who want limited accessibility but create a daunting prospect for employees. The hierarchy often plays out consistently within the executive offices—the CEO is located farthest from the front door, buffered by layers of secretarial staff. In what ways does this symbolize the leader-follower relationship? The layers of automated directions within the telephone system can create a sense of distance and lack of focus on the customer. And some of these telephone systems make it impossibly frustrating for the person simply trying to find a real person to respond to a problem or need.

Using Metaphors and Analogies

Another way to increase impact is by using metaphors and analogies to help people relate their own experiences and understanding to the message. Metaphors are comparisons in which we describe something as if it were something else. Analogies involve a comparison between two cases or things and infer that what is true in one case is true in another. Songwriters and poets use metaphors and analogies extensively. So do effective leaders in health care organizations.

One hospital, which usually had eight labor and delivery rooms available, was undergoing major renovation in that department. The entire department seemed to be torn apart, and at one particularly difficult time, desk drawers from the central nurses' station were placed on the floor down both sides of the hallway. With ten patients in active labor in the department, there was absolute chaos. The leader remarked, "This is like having a dinner party for ten while your kitchen is being remodeled!" This humorous observation diffused some of the high emotion and created a picture in people's minds that helped them understand and appreciate their frustration.

Storytelling

Storytelling is one of the most effective tools a good communicator uses. There is magic in stories. Throughout history, people have relied on narration and storytelling to express ideas that are difficult to communicate any other way. Abraham Lincoln was a consummate storyteller and is a wonderful example of a leader who was able to use conversation, humor, and stories to make his point and convince listeners of his way of thinking. Phillips, in his fascinating book *Lincoln on Leadership* (1992, p. 157), writes: "Nearly everyone who came in contact with our sixteenth president heard him relate some kind of yarn. Lincoln, it turned out, had an overwhelming inventory of anecdotes, jokes, and stories; furthermore, he possessed the ability to instantly pull out just the right one for any situation that might arise. Lincoln was a master at the art of storytelling, and he used that ability purposefully and effectively when he was president of the United States."

Storytelling is "one of the world's most powerful tools for achieving astonishing results. For the leader, storytelling is action oriented—a force for turning dreams into goals, and then into results" (Guber, 2007, p. 55). Storytelling can be entertaining, but that isn't its primary purpose in a professional context. Leaders use stories to instruct and lead. Great storytelling is built on the integrity of the story. It emphasizes truth rather than make-believe. A great storyteller is authentic, and his or her actions are congruent with the story.

The best storytellers collect ideas and anecdotes continually. They are always looking for examples that make a point or that they can use to illustrate a complex or emotional concept. The excellent storyteller may use the same tale over and over again, but it is often slightly different in each telling, based on the audience and the situation. The astute leader knows that successful organizations and teams are "storied" organizations and teams. They listen to the stories circulating and think about what these stories say about the culture. Do the stories reflect positive values and aspirations of the organization? Do they create enthusiasm and loyalty among followers?

In one urban tertiary medical center, the organization mission statement and values were beautifully inscribed, framed, and strategically mounted in every office and conference room of the facility. They described a wonderful organization—words with heartfelt meaning that anyone would aspire to reaching. Amazingly, the predominant flavor of stories circulating in the organization was exactly the opposite. The favorite stories, repeated with great fervor, highlighted personal and professional corruption of the executive staff, unscrupulous maneuvering of managers against peers and employees, and malicious whisperings suggesting various unethical reasons for promotions. The stories revealed the organization's true culture. But stories do not have to be extreme to have negative impact.

People remember stories longer than they can recall data and facts. Students of leadership theory and effectiveness confirm storytelling as a strategy and emphasize the role of stories "as powerful motivational tools that spread loyalty, commitment, and enthusiasm" (Phillips, 1992, p. 158). Peters and Austin (1985, pp. 278, 281) note that "human beings reason largely by means of stories, not by mounds of data. Stories are memorable. . . . They teach." A leader who understands this pays more attention to the role that stories and myths play in communicating ideals, values, and direction.

In a southern 280-bed hospital, a massive renovation and building initiative was under way. There weren't enough staff, and patient care demands were high. During a particularly trying week, a serious flu epidemic hit the community, and the hospital census reached a peak. Employees had been stretched well beyond their capacity, tempers were short, and absenteeism due to the flu ensured that the upcoming weekend was going to be a calamity. On Saturday the vice president for patient care services was pitching in and helping out on the patient care units. One of the most pressing needs was cleaning the patients' bathrooms. People in the patient care departments were captivated and heartened to hear the story of how this vice president rolled up her sleeves and began cleaning toilets. The story of this doctorally prepared nurse doing what most needed to be done for patients' comfort and cleanliness still circulates in this organization. People here understand the organization's values of "patients come first" and teamwork.

Perhaps some of the most poignant stories come from times of disaster such as the San Francisco earthquake of 1989, Hurricane Andrew in southern Florida, the Oklahoma City bombing, 9/11, Hurricane Katrina, and the trapped miners in Chile. During these times of crisis, people rise to meet heartbreaking challenges, and leadership emerges. Rosemary Jacobson, then CEO of United Health Systems (now Altru Health System) in Grand Forks, North Dakota, describes the disaster of the record-breaking 1997 spring flooding:

> During the early morning hours of Friday, April 18, the dikes within the city began to fail, forcing mandatory evacuations of several large neighborhoods in Grand Forks and East Grand Forks. The state health officer called me Friday evening and informed me that the water system and infrastructure would fail. I still believed we would be able to keep United dry and open.
>
> It took only a few hours for realization to set in. I knew we would not be able to manage care of 197 in-patients without water or sewer for an extended period of time. Because of this, the decision was made to evacuate all 197 hospital patients and 371 nursing and retirement home residents from Medical Park and the Grand Forks community. This was accomplished within a 24-hour period.
>
> Our evacuation could only have been accomplished with teamwork. We spent many, many hours planning the Altru Health System, and it paid off. We functioned as a team anyone would be proud to know [personal communication to the author, May 20, 1997].

This emergency evacuation was the largest hospital evacuation since Saigon fell to the Vietcong during the Vietnam War. Stories about disasters endured and calamities shared can strongly bond people together. Even more riveting stories have come from recent disasters too numerous to mention. These stories survive and serve to inspire and hearten, as well as to illustrate the basic beliefs and values of the people in the organization.

Using the Environment

Creative use of the environment is another powerful method of making a point. A good example is one clever speaker's presentation to a group of human resource specialists, executives, and trustees about the cost of discrimination when an organization does not solicit members of minorities or other unrepresented groups for governing board positions. Knowing the audience would be approximately 98 percent male, the speaker had interspersed throughout the audience pairs of high heels in front of empty chairs—a visual reminder to this highly homogeneous audience of at least one underrepresented group.

John, CEO of a major health care system, was having trouble with followers who were regularly late to meetings. The group discussed punctuality as a team value repeatedly, but to no avail. Finally, John decided to communicate the message differently. On the day of his next meeting with the system vice presidents, John went to the boardroom and locked the door at the time the meeting was scheduled to begin. Ten minutes later, the first vice president arrived and was dismayed to find the door locked. Within twenty minutes, all attendees were gathered outside the boardroom, where they waited anxiously until the scheduled meeting was over. When John finally opened the door, he told them that if they weren't on time, he would make decisions without them. News of that locked door spread like wildfire throughout the organization. The message was clear and simply communicated through a locked door.

A different leader facing the same problem started her meetings on time regardless of whether anyone else had yet arrived. The impact of coming into a room to find the leader talking to herself, conducting the meeting with no participants, made a tremendous impression not just on the first follower to finally arrive but on everyone else who heard the story. People got the message.

Listening

A discussion of spoken communication would be incomplete without considering the skill of listening. As important as the ability to be articulate is the leader's ability to listen. "The common image of leaders is that they are great talkers, charismatic and articulate. Far more important is that they are great listeners" (Berry, 1992, p. 2). Giving attention to others' thoughts, ideas, and opinions allows a leader deeper understanding of the follower. Listening for emotions and feelings ensures that the leader understands a message fully, as these elements are difficult for many people to express verbally. Nothing is as powerful as a leader who has accurate facts and information and realizes that followers are an excellent source of both. Not only does it lead to better decision making, but it increases the shared meaning between leaders and followers. Other notable reasons for developing good listening skills are that the listener can learn new information, listening provides time to digest ideas and fully attend to the entire message, and listening communicates respect and caring to the speaker.

Listening Provides New Information

Exemplary listening skills enable the leader to learn and gather information not previously known. The comment, "When you speak you only repeat what you already know; it is when you listen that you might learn something," has been attributed to Abraham Lincoln. Not listening to others conveys an attitude of arrogance, intended or not. They will perceive the nonlistener as not needing input from anyone else because the leader feels all-knowing and correct. Listening to others generates ideas, especially for meeting any resistance to the leader's approach. New ideas blend with the leader's ideas and serve as a catalyst for a unique thought or strategy.

Listening Provides Time to Reflect

We think faster (about three to four times faster) than we can speak. As you listen, think about what the person communicating is trying to say. Does the individual's body language match his or her words? Does the message fit previous experiences you have had with this individual? How does the speaker's message fit with previous thinking on this topic? Do the ideas expressed stir any other thoughts or possibilities?

Listening Communicates Caring

Listening to an individual express ideas and thoughts has a powerful impact on the speaker. Perhaps nothing else the leader can do communicates respect and caring for the follower as much as showing interest in what the follower has to say. M. Scott Peck, in *The Road Less Traveled* (1978, pp. 81, 120–121), defines love as "the will to extend one's self for the purpose of nurturing one's own or another's spiritual growth." He continues: "When we love another we give him or her our attention; we attend to that person's growth. . . . When we attend to someone, we are caring for that person. The act of attending requires that we make the effort to set aside our preoccupations and actively shift our consciousness. Attention is an act of will, of work against the inertia of our own minds. . . . By far the most common and important way in which we can exercise our attention is by listening."

Increasing Listening Skills

Communication courses often teach the skill of listening, and leaders with a background in a discipline that emphasizes and requires listening ability, such as counseling or social work, are at an advantage with this skill. This is a personal skill and as such can be learned and improved with practice. It is common to overrate one's listening ability because it seems so simple. Peck (1978, p. 121) points out, "Listening well is an exercise of attention and by necessity hard work. It is because they do not realize this or because they are not willing to do the work that most people do not listen well."

The best leaders are great listeners. There are many helpful pointers for improving your listening skills:

- *Work at listening and continually attempt to increase your listening span.* Good listeners control any temptation to interrupt or draw attention away from the speaker. Some people grapple for the right words to express their ideas and may take longer to finish their thoughts. Interrupting them only extends this process and gives a speaker the clear message that the listener finds that what he or she is saying is not important enough to wait for its full expression. Our attention needs to be conscious and deliberate.

- *Take the time to listen.* Not everyone is able to speak extemporaneously in a clear and concise manner. Instead they may think out loud and gradually grope their way to their meaning. Their first statement may be only a vague approximation of what they mean. For the speaker to open up and crystallize the meaning of a message, the listener must convey a feeling that there is plenty of time to speak freely. Some leaders rationalize that they are too busy to listen. A good leader is too busy *not* to listen. The leader who does not take time to listen may miss crucial information and never achieve needed understanding. A good listener makes mental or actual notes of items to remember.

• *Listen for understanding rather than to reply.* Stephen Covey (1990, p. 237) believes that the most important principle he has learned in the field of interpersonal relations is to "seek first to understand, then to be understood." Instead of focusing on preparing a reply to the speaker or thinking about how to make himself or herself understood, the listener actively tries to understand what the speaker is saying. Sometimes by taking on the behaviors of being a good listener, we find that the act of listening may follow. A good listener stays alert, establishes eye contact with the speaker, leans forward if appropriate, shows interest by nodding the head or raising the eyebrows, and encourages the speaker to continue by asking thoughtful and appropriate questions. Effective listeners who don effective listening behavior may find it leads to that very behavior.

• *Listen in spite of the delivery method.* Some speakers are more difficult to listen to than others. The speaker may have been blessed with wonderful ideas and thoughts but have a boring, monotone voice or a face without much expression. Good listeners aren't as concerned about mannerisms or delivery but focus on the message itself. They ask: What can I learn from this speaker? They know that not everyone is a brilliant, witty conversationalist.

• *Listen in spite of the content.* If the content of the message evokes strong emotion in the listener, it can be very difficult to not respond emotionally and interrupt the speaker. The listener can become excited or upset, especially when what the speaker says ignites pet peeves or challenges personal convictions or prejudices. It is easy to judge the speaker's comments too hastily, and this can shut down further communication.

• *Remove external distractions and resist internal distractions.* Distractions create noise in the system and make communication even tougher for both speaker and listener. If this is an especially important conversation, move the dialogue someplace where distractions are at a minimum, even if it means delaying it. A good listener recognizes and admits internal distractions and suggests alternate times for the speaker to return. With the emphasis on an open door policy and total accessibility of the leader, it may seem contradictory to ask the person to come back at a better time. However, if distractions are just too great, it is better to be honest than to pretend and risk missing an important message. Of course, the listener must make certain that the follow-up conversation occurs.

• *Restate or paraphrase the message.* When the speaker is finished, the listener should restate what he or she heard and understood as the message. This is affirming to the speaker and also allows the speaker to clarify if the listener received an inaccurate message. This powerful technique is often referred to as reflective listening because it reflects back to the speaker on major points of the message as well as the emotion the speaker was communicating.

These suggestions can help increase listening effectiveness but probably even more important is that the leader continually evaluates his or her level of listening ability. Is it improving? Do followers believe they have been heard and understood? How often are miscommunications occurring as a result of poor listening? In addition to using these principles, effective listeners understand that there are levels of listening.

Levels of Listening

In *The Seven Habits of Highly Effective People* (1989), Stephen Covey identifies several different levels of listening:

1. *Ignoring.* The person is not listening at all. This occurs when we tune someone or something out totally.

2. *Pretend listening.* The "listener" may nod and behave in a manner that suggests listening without hearing a word. The standard example of this is when one's spouse is reading the paper or watching a favorite sports event on television and distractedly responds to questions that he or she does not even hear.

3. *Selective listening.* The listener is hearing only chosen parts of the conversation. The leader who is interested in agreement from followers may hear only positive elements of feedback and ignore or discount more unfavorable segments.

4. *Attentive listening.* The listener pays attention and focuses energy on the words being said.

5. *Empathic listening.* The listener understands not only the words of the message but its emotion and meaning as well.

Whether we call it active, reflective, or empathic listening, this highest level of listening is the only form that focuses completely on the listener and puts the listener in the speaker's frame of reference. Its purpose is to fully comprehend what the speaker is expressing, and it goes even further by adding the feedback loop to give the speaker a response that reflects this understanding. The power of this communication technique is that it gives the speaker the opportunity to correct misperceptions or misunderstandings immediately. When a listener uses reflective or empathic listening, the speaker feels understood and validated.

Use of this technique requires the listener's judgment and skill. Reflecting back the speaker's words and perceived emotion is a direct invitation to the speaker to continue. If the listener does not have time to follow through fully, use of this technique may send a mixed message. Practice and refinement of this skill are necessary so that the listener is not just parroting the speaker's words (an irritating and foolish thing to do). The listener may say something like: "Let me check this out. I thought I heard you say . . ." "Are you saying . . . ?" "It sounds like you're feeling . . . Am I right?" Until this is part of the listener's repertoire, it may feel uncomfortable, but the benefits are tremendous.

Using empathic listening helps a listener stay actively in the listening mode and focus solely on the speaker. If the listener has to repeat the essence of the message to the speaker, it focuses his or her attention tremendously. It puts the listener in the speaker's frame of reference and increases the listener's understanding of the speaker. Virtually no other technique is as helpful in building a solid relationship. The disadvantage is that the listener has no sense of control or efficiency. So although this method is effective, it may not feel efficient. It is efficient in the sense that it prevents miscommunications.

A signal that you are not using empathic listening occurs when someone conveys the same message repeatedly. The problem is that you may not have provided any feedback indicating that you received the message. An example of this occurred in a team of executives who attended a long-term learning program together. Members of the team were handpicked and were required to commit to attending a series of four three-day sessions over a year. As part of the selection criteria, all agreed that they would attend every session. After two sessions, Cal told his other team members that he would be missing the next session. His team members were justifiably angry and gave him that feedback. One member, Jill, told him directly that she felt he was letting the team down and she was very disappointed in him. He showed no response.

In another week, the team met again to discuss what they would do with Cal's decision to miss the next three-day session. Again Jill gave Cal the same feedback, and he showed no response. The team was having difficulty dealing with this dilemma and met one last time to decide whether Cal should remain on the team after the missed session. Again the teammates expressed their concern and anger, with Jill again directly telling Cal how she felt. Cal became very angry in return and said to Jill, "You've said that three times now. Will you stop beating a dead horse? I'm getting tired of hearing this." Jill was surprised and replied, "I didn't think you ever heard me because you showed no response."

Followers who believe they have not been heard do one of two things. They may stop trying, believing that the leader does not care or is not interested in their opinions or ideas. Or they become more persistent, continuing to repeat a message until the leader acknowledges it. To be effective listeners, good leaders pay attention, and if they are hearing the same message repeatedly, they ask themselves: "Why am I hearing this again? Have I acknowledged this message?"

Listening is a skill that takes time to develop and continual attention to keep improving. The payoff is tremendous. One of the most remarkable benefits of listening to others is that it becomes reciprocal. If leaders want to increase the probability that others will listen to what they have to say, they will start listening (Campbell and Inguagiato, 1994).

Asking the Right Questions

Few people consider asking questions an art form, and yet asking questions requires a much higher level of skill than most people think. The leader can use questions to gain information, obtain a different point of view, show respect for followers, and make them feel important and valued. And there is another benefit (Oakley and Krug, 1993, p. 150): "Smart communicators ask questions not only so they can hear the answers, but so the person asked can hear their own answers and thereby gain clarity for themselves or internalize something they have grasped only intellectually." Oakley and Krug describe questions as a gift to the person being asked, just as answers are a gift to the asker.

These tips for more powerful questioning techniques can increase the skill of the individual asking the questions:

- *State the reason for the question.* Letting the person know why you are asking the question can eliminate resistance or the feeling of unwarranted curiosity: "Help me understand this better," or "I would like to understand the factors you considered when you made this decision."

- *Make it enjoyable for the other person.* Be enthusiastic, and the person being questioned will feel positive.

- *Show interest in what the other person is saying.* Through body language, show an attentive attitude. This includes good eye contact, nodding or tilting the head, and appropriate facial expressions.

- *Use open-ended rather than closed questions.* Closed questions can be answered with a yes, no, or other one-word answer, which does not provide the breadth of communication the asker desires. It is the difference between saying: "Do I have your support on this project?" versus, "What parts of this project can you support? What elements will you have difficulty supporting?"

- *Avoid creating the feeling of the third degree.* Giving followers the third degree puts them on the defensive, even if they were feeling open in the beginning. One question after another delivered in a rapid-fire manner is certain to elicit a negative reaction in most people.

- *Ask for their opinion.* A very powerful question is one that simply solicits the person's thoughts about a particular issue or situation: "What do you think about . . . ?" Of course, the person asking the question has to be truly interested or risks sending a mixed message.

- *Repeat key words from answers and summarize thoughts.* This indicates to the person responding to the questions that you have listened to and heard him or her.

- *Share appreciation of responses.* Let speakers know that you appreciate their thoughts and the time they have given to answer your questions: "Thank you for going through this with me so that I can understand it better."

Sometimes leaders are afraid that if they seek opinions from others and listen carefully to their answers and ideas, they are communicating implicit agreement with these ideas. This is one reason that feedback to the speaker is important. It is possible to listen attentively and yet clearly tell the individual when there is disagreement on an idea. Good questioners continually monitor other people's reactions to their questioning techniques. Does their technique facilitate the flow of information? Do people open up more, or are they becoming quieter and more reserved? This feedback gives the questioner direct information on the effectiveness of his or her technique.

Nonverbal Communication

Intertwined closely with spoken communication is nonverbal communication. Sometimes referred to as body language, nonverbal communication is actually a broader term and can include the use of time, space, and the environment as well. Verbal and nonverbal messages must match, or they create confusion and frustration. Of these two channels of communication, nonverbal language can be more potent, as demonstrated by the childhood game of Simon Says. Simon gives rapid oral instructions while demonstrating the requested behavior. Participants follow the leader's movements, and the unlucky players who continue to follow the leader even in the absence of the phrase "Simon says" lose the game. The point is that people are more likely to emulate behavior than to follow words or directives.

The potential power of nonverbal language compels the effective leader to observe and understand the significance of certain body language and continually examine his or her nonverbal communication for the messages it sends. Leaders who are sensitive to these messages have greater control over their ability to communicate with clarity. In the same way, a leader becomes more skilled at interpreting others' messages by tuning in to nonverbal cues. It pays to be cautious, however, because body language can have multiple meanings. Important nonverbal messages can be conveyed in these ways:

- Use of time

- Touch

- Use of space

- Appearance

- Body motions and posture

- Choice of words and voice tone

- Eye behavior

Use of Time

The leader's use of time communicates a clear message about what the leader believes is important. This relates back to the concept of visibility and accessibility in the discussion of trust. Are followers able to reach the leader? Is there time to talk about important issues and concerns? With whom does the leader spend the most time? Who doesn't get any of the leader's time? Allowing enough time in a busy schedule to periodically have coffee or lunch with followers is a practical way of keeping in touch with what is happening. This can be difficult for more introverted leaders for whom casual, spontaneous conversation does not come easily. Sometimes scheduled, structured meeting times, even though the meeting itself is informal, can ease the way for this leader.

Touch

In the United States, the issue of touch is more complex because of the increased focus on sexual harassment. Anything that could be construed to be intimate or sexual is unacceptable. Even if it doesn't result in litigation, it leads to distrust between leader and follower. Casual contact, however, can actually improve the relationship because it connotes acceptance and caring. A famous classic research study involved a librarian who was asked to lightly and impersonally touch students on the arm when the librarian checked out books to them or answered their questions. The students in the experimental group whom the librarian touched rated the librarian as more helpful, intelligent, and personable than did the students in the control group. The librarian was the same individual and otherwise treated the students identically.

Cultural and familial differences influence the use of touch (Morris, 1979). North Americans and northern Europeans have noncontact cultures, which means that body contact and touch are not common except in prescribed arenas. Many Hispanic people are high contact and consider North Americans and northern Europeans reserved, cool, and downright uptight. Some people come from affectionate, demonstrative families where hugging is common. Other people are uncomfortable with hugging even in social situations because they reserve this behavior for their intimates. Paying close attention to a follower's reaction to touch alerts the leader to its appropriateness.

Use of Space

Both space and spacing are issues to consider when evaluating nonverbal messages. Space can connote status: the person with the best and most space usually has the highest status. A corner office with windows is often touted as the highest-status executive space. The size and location of the work space send a message indicating value and worth. Does the organization allot space for classrooms and adequate room for employee lounges? Do physicians have a separate dining room? Do executives and managers have reserved parking? In the same way, reserved parking for an employee of the month indicates value and esteem. What message is the organization's leadership sending?

Another issue related to space is that of territoriality (Morris, 1979). Humans are highly territorial, and this translates to an inherent compulsion to possess and defend space that they perceive as their property. Participants at a meeting or a conference choose a chair and put up boundaries to indicate to others where their space begins and ends. A strategically placed coat on the chair, a notebook, and a coffee cup all indicate possession of space. Employees carve out their space in the workplace and may then feel violated if they return to find someone else in "their" chair, at "their" desk, using "their" telephone or computer.

Respect for an individual's space is an important issue because organizations often show a complete lack of regard or concern for an employee's space, especially that of frontline employees. Departments are relocated, offices moved, and space invaded, often without any acknowledgment of the impact on the individual. To build trust between leaders and followers, each must show care and respect for the other's work and personal spaces.

Personal space is another concept the excellent communicator understands. North American adults who are interacting in a professional or business capacity generally have four basic and distinct distances of interaction (Morris, 1979):

- *Intimate zone,* ranging from actual physical contact to about two feet
- *Personal zone,* ranging from about two to four feet
- *Social zone,* extending from about four to twelve feet
- *Public zone,* stretching from twelve feet to the limits of hearing and sight

If someone violates an individual's space by coming too close, the result is increased tension and distrust. Common cues are that the individual reduces eye contact, moves away, or puts something (like a chair, table, or desk) between himself or herself and the speaker. Leader-follower relationships usually begin in the social zone and move into the personal zone after trust has been established.

Seating arrangements at a meeting send a message. A leader who joins others in the break room for a cup of coffee and always chooses to sit at the head of the table may be sending a message that he or she expects always to be in charge. In a formal meeting, with several people around the table, sitting straight across from someone who holds an adversarial position tends to increase conflict between the two parties. Sitting next to each other reduces the amount of conflict. A too-crowded conference or meeting room can increase hostility. Power is also ascribed to the person on whose turf the meeting is taking place. Does the leader go to where followers are, or do followers always come to the leader? Especially in resolving conflict, the leader can equalize power by using a neutral territory.

Appearance

An individual's dress and appearance send a message to others. Like it or not, physical appearance makes an impression on others within the first five to seven seconds of contact. Although this is not about dressing for success or impressing followers, it is a reminder to consider the importance of the leader-follower relationship and the need to establish rapport and trust with followers. Rapport is built when others perceive sameness rather than difference. If the leader is trying to impress those higher in the hierarchy, the dress-for-success model is appropriate. Peers or those who are lower in the hierarchy are more often impressed when they can see what they have in common with the leader. Some of these issues become clouded when formal hierarchy is part of the leader-follower relationship. A peer or employee leader is more likely to dress like the followers. If followers are in scrub clothes and uniforms, a leader in a navy blue business suit may inadvertently emphasize differences. On the other hand, if an employee leader normally wears scrub clothes to work and is now leading a more formal interdisciplinary task force, showing up in scrub clothes may reduce his or her effectiveness.

Body Motions and Posture

Body motions and posture send distinct messages. Posture and gestures clearly communicate passive, aggressive, and assertive behaviors. Slumped posture indicates passive behavior. Restrictive hand and arm movement, hiding the hands, gripping one arm with the opposite hand, and holding hands rigidly at the side reinforce an impression of a nonassertive individual. Clenched teeth suggest aggressive behavior, as does a jaw jutted forward, tight lips, flushed cheeks, flared nostrils, a thrusting arm with a pointed index finger (remember Tom), pounding of fists, hands on hips, or clenched fists. The assertive leader uses more moderate and less frequent facial movement that expresses emotion congruent with the communication. Hand and arm movements are fluid, with hands held open and in view.

Leaders who sit in relaxed positions are better able to influence followers, and followers will see them as more persuasive and active. They are generally better liked than those who sit tightly and in a closed manner with arms crossed and held across the chest. Standing over others is seen as dominance; although it is appropriate in some settings (giving a formal speech), it would be too intimidating in others (at an informal or spontaneous meeting).

Some gestures are considered universal signals: hands over the head for surrender, saluting, shrugging the shoulders, and blowing a kiss. However, leaders who understand cultural differences are aware of the importance of accurately assessing the followers' body language; otherwise signals from one culture may lead to misinterpretation by followers in another. Every culture has its own body language, and children learn these nuances as they grow up. A North American who had traveled in Japan related this story. He and his wife were very impressed with the politeness of the Japanese schoolchildren who would stand by the side of the road and wave at cars going past. On their third day, they commented to the hotel desk clerk about how polite the children were. Imagine their chagrin when he told them that Japanese children stand at the side of the road and wave to indicate that they want to cross the street! They had totally misinterpreted this simple behavior.

Leaders need to understand the significance of their followers' cultural behaviors, a tremendous challenge in today's multicultural and diverse ethnic environment. One south Florida manager had a difficult time talking with several workers from the islands about productivity and the need to move quickly as they always seemed to be "on island time" as she put it. Other managers report difficulty in coaching employees of Asian descent to take responsibility for direct communication with coworkers if they have been socialized to believe that directly addressing difficulties is rude behavior. The ramifications for the leader are significant. Anticipating and understanding cultural differences allow a leader to communicate more effectively. People do not hear the intended message if they are embarrassed, insulted, or intimidated.

Choice of Words and Voice Tone

This chapter has explored the effect of metaphors and use of language to evoke meaning. Health care is liberally sprinkled with military metaphors (Annas, 1996). People talk of doing battle with disease, patients are given shots or endure invasive procedures, and employees on duty are in uniform. In emergency departments, patients are triaged, and surgery takes place in the operating theater. "When we use language like this, the force of the metaphor powerfully conveys our values, past experiences, and what we consider legitimate. . . . The truth lurks in the metaphor" (Henry and LeClair, 1987, p. 23). For this reason, leaders need to be very careful about the words they use. Referring to comatose patients as "vegetables," to people who cannot pay their bill as "write-offs," to employees as "bodies, "full-time equivalents," and "drones" communicates the way the leader values people. One health care manager was well known in her organization for joking about wanting to "lobotomize" employees so that they would be more compliant. Although this conversation almost always occurred behind closed doors, it certainly affected her leadership ability and subtly reflected how she valued people.

Voice tone and volume also communicate congruence or discrepancy with the words being said. An assertive tone of voice usually has moderate volume and emphasis on words, a tone of voice appropriate for one adult speaking with a peer. Aggression is communicated with a loud voice, a heavy emphasis on certain words, and a parental tone. Nonassertive, or passive, voice is usually a soft, perhaps inaudible monotone or a childlike delivery.

Eye Behavior

Eye contact is culturally determined. North Americans are very careful about how and when they meet another person's eyes. An honest person looks another straight in the eye; shifty eyes connote dishonesty. North Americans avoid eye contact when walking down the street in a large city, when they are uncomfortable, or sometimes when they ask a question. In contrast, Israelis stare at each other on the street, not breaking eye contact until they have passed each other. In many Eastern cultures, direct eye contact is considered impolite. In England polite listeners fix the speaker with an attentive stare and blink their eyes periodically as a sign of interest.

Direct eye contact in North America is considered assertive, usually meaning the individual is comfortable with looking another straight in the eye. Too piercing a stare can be intimidating, however, and narrowing the eyes is often considered aggressive. Eyes flitting back and forth between objects can give an individual a scared-rabbit look. Not looking a person directly in the eye causes the listener to wonder what the speaker is hiding.

Understanding the nuances of nonverbal communication not only enables the effective communicator to transmit clearer, more congruent messages but also assists both speaker and listener in interpreting the signals they read. This process often occurs in retrospect, after miscommunication has occurred. Continually evaluating the effectiveness of your communication leads to better results later.

Written Communication

Classic management studies reveal that leaders who hold managerial or executive positions spend approximately three-quarters of their day in spoken communication with others (Mintzberg, 1980). Today, more may occur through electronic communications. Nevertheless, the point is that the majority of a leader's day is spent in communication. Ideas are not exchanged exclusively by word of mouth. Although oral communication skills are more often used, writing skills are just as pivotal in a leadership practice. The ability to choose words carefully, express thoughts in writing, and create a document that helps followers understand a message leads to better communication. Clear and confident expression of the written word is an asset for any leader.

Of the three methods of communication—spoken, nonverbal, and written—the written form is most troublesome, if only because of its formal nature. "It is received cold, without the communicator's tone of voice or gesture to help. It is rigid; it cannot be adjusted to the recipients' reactions as it is being delivered. It stays on the record and cannot be undone. Furthermore, the reason it is in fact committed to paper is usually that its subject is considered too crucial or significant to be entrusted to casual, short-lived verbal form" (Fielden, 1981, p. 42). For these reasons, a strong leader needs to be able to communicate effectively through writing.

The written word can be used to emphasize the importance of a message and serve as a record for future reference. Some people are visually oriented and prefer to see the message in writing to anchor it more solidly in their minds. Leaders today can write e-mails, blogs, memos, letters, announcements, bulletins, newsletters, and reports. The purpose and importance of the message determine which means to use. Because retrieving the written word once it is published is impossible, important written messages require a lot of thought and consideration. Abraham Lincoln, viewed as one of the best leader communicators of all time, not only wrote his own speeches but was an eloquent public speaker and wrote "thousands of letters and notes to anyone with whom he felt he needed to communicate" (Phillips, 1992, p. 145). He believed in thorough preparation, often writing his thoughts over a long time and refining them later. This is still good advice today.

Important messages deserve the necessary time to ensure that they are well written and communicate the desired meaning. Being overly cautious, however, can result in an unreasonably prolonged communication process. In one organization, the executive team decided that it needed to write a letter to communicate with employees about several significant upcoming changes. The members of the team were so worried about litigation that various attorneys and team members took months to review the document, which then appeared so late that it was virtually useless. In addition, most of the intended audience could not understand what it said. Remember to balance the need for accuracy, clarity, and caution.

Electronic Communication

Electronic means of written communication have revolutionized the way we communicate. E-mail and online social networking sites are proliferating. The new means of communication has many advantages, including speed and ease of sending information. These approaches enable closer and timelier contact between leaders and followers because it allows direct access to the leader. Sometimes the significance of this change goes unrecognized: "Power relationships are now dramatically reconfigured. Communication between executive, managers, and staff are now horizontal, vertical, diagonal, up-and-down historical lines of authority and chains of command" (Porter-O'Grady and Malloch, 2010, p. 35).

E-Mail

On the downside, e-mail has replaced face-to-face communication in some organizations precisely because it is so easy. As with any other written communication, a major disadvantage is that there is no tone of voice or body language to help the receiver interpret a message, and miscues can be serious. Tap out a message, hit the send key, and it is gone! This spontaneity has some disadvantages because it results in less thinking time. The final disadvantage of e-mail is also one of its benefits: it leaves no paper trail. Follow-up is more difficult to remember and yet more critical.

Too many people today depend solely on e-mail for communication and neglect to realize the importance of emotional intelligence and the effect of face-to-face interaction in communication between leaders and followers. The emotionally intelligent leader realizes that it is important to be present and observe the other person's response to the message and then make adjustments spontaneously, using the listener's feedback cues to increase the flow and accuracy of information. This is difficult to impossible to do with e-mail or texting.

Another disadvantage, which also applies to the use of cell phones and voice messaging, is that there is little universally accepted etiquette for these newer forms of communication. Until this etiquette becomes common practice, some people will unintentionally damage communication through newer technologies such as by misusing e-mail to communicate difficult messages better transmitted face-to-face; leaving lengthy voice mail messages with numbers and details that are difficult to capture completely; rambling on and on and producing quite lengthy e-mail or voice mail messages; blanketing the entire organization with e-mail messages that only a few individuals really need; and ignoring rules of grammar and courtesy because it is "only an e-mail." Wendy Leebov (2005b) offers some additional suggestions for e-mail etiquette:

- Limit the quantity and length of e-mails to the essentials. Keep your message to one screen or less.

- Consider the sensitivity of the issue. Controversial and sensitive issues must be resolved face-to-face.

- Check your e-mail regularly. If you aren't able to respond immediately, at least let the sender know you have received the e-mail and when you might get back to him or her.

- Consider the nuances. Reread everything, and consider possible negative connotations. Others cannot hear your joking tone, and sarcasm is easily misinterpreted.

- Consider sensitivity and confidentiality. In Leebov's words, e-mails are as confidential as a postcard.

- Remember that laws relating to written communication apply to e-mail messages as well.

- Sending an e-mail from your account is the same as sending out a letter on your organization's letterhead. Make certain the punctuation and grammar is appropriate.

Another major issue with e-mail is managing the amount of e-mail received. Hemp (2009) points out that the tremendous amount of information available today easily leads to information overload. Although there are possible technological solutions, such as software that automatically sorts and prioritizes incoming e-mails, there are other suggestions, for both sender and receiver, that Hemp offers to help manage volume:

- Turn off automatic notifications of incoming e-mail to minimize the distractions. Instead, establish specific times of the day when you check and take action on e-mails.

- Send out less e-mail. Hemp found that an outgoing message generates on average roughly two responses.

- Before you choose "reply all," stop and deliberately consider whether everyone on the list needs a copy.

- Minimize e-mail table tennis by making suggestions ("Can we meet at 9 am on Tuesday?") rather than open-ended questions ("When can you meet?").

- For very short e-mails, put the entire contents in the subject line (followed by "eom," for end of message). This eliminates the need for others to open the message.

- If possible, paste the contents of an attachment into the body of the message.

Norms for dealing with e-mail need to be developed at both the organizational and individual levels. Beyond agreement on appropriate etiquette, organizationally this would also involve agreeing on what are unnecessary e-mails and having an honest conversation about eliminating them. There aren't many material management departments that are open over Labor Day weekend, and yet the hospital sends an e-mail to everyone announcing that the department will be closed until Tuesday at 8:00 A.M. Copying everyone in the known universe on an e-mail at times becomes ridiculous. Who needs the information should be a deliberate consideration.

At the individual level, it's important for those who work together closely to come to agreement on protocol around e-mail. And if three or four e-mails have bounced around on the same topic, pick up the telephone and resolve the issue.

Perhaps more important, the unintended negative consequences of being too linked ought to be considered. Accessibility within a reporting relationship is a key component of forming a solid relationship. However, leaders who are too accessible may end up with followers who never learn to be comfortable making decisions on their own. An unintended negative consequence is that boundaries tend to be obscured. "Unbounded e-mail, CrackBerry, and cell-phone communications have turned civil society into an anarchic, free-fire zone of ceaseless incoming, stealing our time and invading nights and weekends. The volume of electronic messaging keeps mounting—without rules, limits, or traffic lights" (Robinson, 2006, p. 54). Robinson suggests what he calls an e-tool bill of rights. Included are items such as these:

- The right to be secure from unwarranted electronic work intrusions at home.

- Nights and weekends shall be considered unplugged zones.

- A person is not on vacation if he or she is checking e-mails and is in contact with the workplace.

Social Networking Sites

Online social networking sites such as Facebook, LinkedIn, Twitter, and MySpace provide the ability to connect easily with a larger community. These sites offer great promise for increased communication and collaboration through increased interaction and sharing of ideas. They create high value as they connect people in ways previously unimagined. Unfortunately, the increased use of these sites has often blurred the lines between what is professional business and what is personal. Hospitals and health care organizations are exploring new ways of using these sites for advertising and connecting with their specific audiences.

"Social networking sites offer the benefits of instant messaging, chat rooms, file sharing, photo storage, and blogging at one site. MySpace was created primarily for entertainment updates. LinkedIn was created specifically for business networking purposes and offers a variety of professional benefits such as online resume posting" (Klich-Heartt and Prion, 2010, p. 57). Facebook is a hybrid and allows users to limit accessibility to selected users.

Some organizations block employee access to these sites in the workplace. Others are looking for opportunities and ways to use this new form of communication. One hospital encouraged employees and supporters to connect with their site on Facebook. This allowed these users to stay informed about and engaged with the current building project and other organizational activities. Some managers use a blog as a way for their employees to stay up-to-date on departmental information and activities.

These sites have great potential for bringing people together. Many professional associations are using this means to bring members together to share ideas, reflect on their experiences, and learn from each other. Ethical issues are probably the greatest concern in using sites for these purposes. Any content available on a social networking site is considered to be in the public domain and is accessible to anyone. There have already been multiple instances where health care workers have posted private and confidential information about a patient. "Social networking sites may be the antithesis of federal regulations protecting privacy. Social networking encourages openness, dialogue, and connection of ideas and people, whereas HIPAA regulations protect an individual's privacy through strict expectations about how client information can be used and by whom" (Klich-Heartt and Prion, 2010, p. 57). An individual who is commenting on his or her own work may not be violating specific regulations; however, including any identifying patient information is a clear and flagrant abuse of client trust and confidentiality.

There may also be unexpected consequences when a person shares personal information on one of these sites. Although it may increase a sense of connection between people, suddenly personal information shared on a Web site may be readily available to others. In some instances, a potential employer has checked out an individual's Facebook page and rejected the job applicant because of objectionable content posted on his or her personal site.

Twitter is newer and finding popularity in some health care settings. A rapidly growing Web site, Twitter allows users to post "tweets": succinct messages of 140 or fewer characters. The posts are received by followers, other Twitter users who are signed up to receive and respond to other members' updates. Although Twitter has been around since 2007, it has gained significant notoriety because many celebrities are using it. In health care, an increasing number of hospitals are using it to communicate with patients. The most common update on hospitals' Twitter pages in spring 2009 was about the swine flu outbreak (Bush, 2009). Other Twitters have ranged from updates during live surgical procedures to at least one hospital CEO who tweets about activities in his executive practice. Other reported uses include the search feature, which serves as a resource and communication tool (Ambler, 2009). Ambler also suggests potential use in the future for sending tweets about recalls or safety alerts regarding medications or equipment.

Improving Writing Skills

Several classic and timeless principles are useful to consider when evaluating business writing. They apply to all forms of written communication. Fielden (1981, p. 42) identifies four categories:

- Readability
- Correctness
- Appropriateness
- Thought

The relative importance of each of these categories differs with the writer and situation, but considering each will increase a writer's effectiveness.

Readability

Readability depends on a clear style of writing. The leader needs to know the audience for whom he or she is writing in order to write clearly. The more general the audience, the simpler the sentences, and the less use of jargon, or shop talk, the more readable the document is. Liberal use of paragraphs, each beginning with a topic sentence, helps readers grasp content quickly, and simple language increases their comprehension of the material.

Another aspect of readability is the ability to lead the reader in an intended direction. The effective writer develops a skeleton structure first and later fleshes it out with descriptive words. Clearly identifying the purpose and using transition sentences between paragraphs increase readability. Staying focused on the communication's main points takes less effort if the writer has clearly thought through what needs to be said.

Correctness

Correctness refers to much more than grammar and punctuation. Coherence and the ability to correctly position sentences and paragraphs increase the smoothness of the communication. Sentences that logically flow from one to another result in clearer understanding. An easy way to evaluate coherence is to ask someone with no knowledge of the topic or situation to review the document and give feedback. E-mail seems so innocuous that people often delude themselves by thinking correctness is not as important in this form of communication. But in a professional setting, e-mail is a business communication.

Appropriateness

Appropriateness is related to how the writer presents the content. A leader writing an e-mail or memo announcing a major initiative must first clarify in his or her own mind the communication's intent. Diplomacy is important: the reader who finds the tone of the document insulting or condescending will less easily accept the message. Giving enough information and using straight talk is better than employing flowery, convoluted language that passes for communication but is really just semantics.

Thought

The thought content of the communication is the last category to consider when writing. Content must be accurate and well organized. "Much disorganized writing results from insufficient preparation, from a failure to think through and isolate the purpose and the aim of the writing job. Most writers tend to think as they write; in fact, most of us do not even know what it is we think until we have actually written it down" (Fielden, 1981, p. 46). A carefully considered outline is of tremendous value to producing logical, well-presented information.

Careful analysis, bias-free evidence, and identification of working assumptions are all components of the written communication's content. If facts are part of the document, the document must carefully analyze them, and these facts must support the conclusions it draws. The writer may experience a tendency to state a conclusion without sharing any of the relevant facts with the reader, perhaps fearing that the reader would not draw the same conclusion. Supporting evidence that is logical and clearly presented serves to guide readers in the direction that the writer seeks. The writer can share opinions if he or she identifies them as such and does not consider them hard evidence for a particular argument.

It is also the writer's responsibility to succinctly state any assumptions that are operating in the situation. This gives the reader the opportunity to agree or disagree with the assumptions and prevents potential disagreements with the actual content. A steering committee overseeing a major organizational cultural initiative conducted a review of employee opinions about the process. In crafting a response to employees that was intended to share the results of the survey as well as further actions, one of the first sections included the committee's assumptions:

> The underlying principles are accepted by everyone in the organization as the right things to do.
>
> Respondents to the survey were positively intentioned, even when delivering negative or critical feedback.
>
> Becoming something different is as important a goal as dealing with day-to-day issues.
>
> Leaders must model the desired behaviors.

Simply identifying these assumptions generated tremendous dialogue within the steering team. As they talked through each assumption and examined the current reality of their system, they achieved increased clarity of issues and needs, and the communication plan for employees helped them understand the committee's thinking more fully.

Leaders communicating through written words need to avoid an effusive "con man" presentation meant to manipulate others. Simple words that ring with conviction and enthusiasm for an idea and for understanding the reader's point of view go further to convince readers of important points than flowery language. Keeping readability, correctness, appropriateness, and thought content foremost results in clearer written communication.

Too often a written communication strategy is hastily conceived and just another task to check off the list. Instead it should be carefully strategized and, in the case of crucial communication documents, written with the expertise of those highly skilled in this area. Furthermore, the effectiveness of our communication strategies needs to be continually evaluated. If there is a major communication campaign to inform frontline employees of an initiative or project, or key results of organizational efforts, follow-up efforts can be employed to determine the campaign's success. For example, several weeks after the campaign, employees can be questioned during walking rounds and asked key questions about the major points of the communication. Determine what level of knowledge is acceptable ahead of time. For instance, can 70 percent of all those questioned relate the key principles of the cultural change initiative?

Summary

Effective communicators are skilled and versatile in all three modes of communication: spoken, nonverbal, and written. The leader must judge each situation to determine the appropriate means of sending a message and continually scan the outcomes of every communication to evaluate the effectiveness of the message transfer. Exemplary leaders know that the highest impact of message delivery occurs when the message is congruent for all three modes.

Special Communication Issues

Today's leader faces many challenges in attempting to communicate with clarity to all followers who need information:

- Communicating during change
- Communicating across geographical separations
- Communicating with teams

Communicating During Change

Health care is undergoing tremendous changes, in some instances almost cataclysmic in nature. The basic principles and techniques of good communication become even more important during times of rapid change because people seem to have an almost insatiable need for information at these times. Principles especially applicable during change include the following:

- Be available, visible, and accessible.

- Find multiple ways of describing a concept.

- Articulate complex concepts as simply as possible.

- Communicate relentlessly. Repeat key messages at least seven to nine times.

- Share stories that communicate desired key values. Make an appeal. Draw on people's loyalty and the values you know they hold dear.

- Make certain that the metaphors you use fit what you need to communicate.

- Scrupulously avoid mixed messages; they are deadly in times of change.

- Ask for feedback to ensure the message was received.

- Remember that people are in a state of high emotion, which creates noise in their systems.

- Separate resistance from learning and seeking information. Make room for doubts.

- Respect the old; never dismiss it out-of-hand.

In addition to these principles, a key strategy during change is to develop specific communication approaches for key stakeholders. In *The Empowered Manager* (1987), Peter Block does a beautiful job of describing this strategy. He points out that a stakeholder is anyone who is needed for the success of the project or who can influence the project significantly. The first step is to identify the issue or change project and any key stakeholders whom this initiative will affect. The next step is to assess the stakeholders by the degree to which they agree with the project and the level to which they are trusted. The leader should not assume that a stakeholder agrees with the project. If the leader does not know the stakeholder's level of agreement, evaluation occurs after the leader sits down with the stakeholder and talks about the vision, purpose, or goals of the project or endeavor. This dialogue helps confirm or deny the stakeholder's agreement.

The leader then determines where the stakeholder fits into a specific matrix (Figure 4.2), depending on the level of trust present and the agreement the individual has with the change. Both of these factors influence the communication strategy and effectiveness of message transfer. Opponents differ from adversaries only in the area of trust, but this difference dramatically affects the selection of communication strategies for each. A strategy for working with opponents is to keep communication lines open and to engage in frank and honest dialogue with them. Opponents are important because they value and trust the leader; they just do not agree with this particular initiative.

With adversaries, however, there is not only a lack of agreement but a lack of trust. Dialogue is not particularly helpful because the leader does not believe the adversary will be honest. Leaders using this model should be aware of a common error in judgment: assuming that anyone who disagrees is an adversary. If the leader treats opponents like adversaries, they may in fact convert to this less desirable category. This can occur when a supposed leader sees opposition as negative and all resisters as untrustworthy. A summary of appropriate strategies for each category is provided in Table 4.1.

Some difficulties are inherent in using this dynamic—not static—model. Through ongoing interchanges with stakeholders and continual reassessment of both their status on the matrix and the effectiveness of a

Figure 4.2 The Stakeholder Matrix

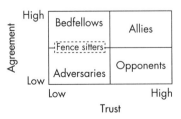

Source: The Empowered Manager by Peter Block, © 1987. Reprinted with permission of John Wiley & Sons, Inc., Hoboken, N.J.

Table 4.1 Strategies for Categories of Key Stakeholders

Allies	Treat them as "one of us."
	Ask them honestly what they believe and see happening; listen to what they tell you.
	Continually discuss the project, vision, plan, and so on.
	Reaffirm the quality and importance of the relationship, especially that you appreciate their honesty.
	Acknowledge the doubts and vulnerability you feel.
	Ask for advice and support.
	Have regular meetings and ask them how they perceive things are going and what they need.
Opponents	Reaffirm the quality of the relationship and the fact that it is based on trust.
	State your position; keep communication lines open.
	State in a neutral way what you think their position is.
	Engage in some kind of mutual problem solving.
Bedfellows	Reaffirm any agreements.
	Acknowledge the caution that exists.
	Be clear about what you want from them in terms of working together, and ask them to do the same.
	Try to reach some agreement on how you will work together.
Fence Sitters	State your position.
	Ask where they stand, and encourage them to express their opinion without judging them.
	Apply gentle pressure.
	Encourage them to think about the issue, and let you know what it would take to give you their support.
Adversaries	State your vision for the project.
	State in a neutral way your best understanding of your adversary's position.
	Identify your contribution to the problem.
	End the meeting with your plans and no demands.

Source: The Empowered Manager by Peter Block, © 1987. Reprinted with permission of John Wiley & Sons, Inc., Hoboken, N.J.

particular communication strategy selected is critical. Something in the environment or within the individual may have changed that alters his or her placement on the matrix. One business office manager, Jim, whose organization was widely implementing employee teams, was resistant to the idea of teams in his department. The leader identified Jim as an opponent according to Block's matrix (1987). Jim's daughter visited over the holidays and told him about her experiences with employee work teams at her bank. She was enthusiastic, and after that weekend he became an ally. All it really took were concrete examples from a similar business, and he could see the possibilities. It also helped that he trusted his daughter explicitly and that she had no ulterior motives for trying to influence his opinion in this case.

A second drawback relates to accurately identifying where the stakeholder fits on the matrix. Some groups of stakeholders are so large that it is difficult to determine where each individual falls. To use this model, the leader must be able to talk directly with each stakeholder to determine agreement and choose a communication strategy based on this knowledge.

A cardiopulmonary leadership team in one organization used this model successfully for communicating with key physician stakeholders during a massive change initiative in their service center. The team consisted of the executive leader and the managers reporting directly to her. First, the team identified all key physician stakeholders and placed each on the matrix. In one or two instances, no one had enough information to make an accurate determination, so the team assigned each of those physicians to a team member. The team member's responsibility was to engage in a dialogue with the physician to determine that physician's understanding of the change being planned and level of support.

Once the team located all the physician stakeholders on the matrix, they determined an appropriate communication strategy based on levels of trust and agreement for each. The team assigned all key stakeholders to a member of the leadership team to provide primary communication regarding this change initiative. This spread the responsibility of physician communication among all team members and allowed a more individualized strategy for each stakeholder. The team implemented this project with greater support from more physicians than this team had previously experienced.

Communicating Across Geographical Separation

Today's leader has a new challenge: leading people from afar. Recent mergers, acquisitions, and consolidations of health care facilities have resulted in fewer stand-alone organizations (Blouin and Brent, 1997). With each passing year, the likelihood that leaders will be geographically distant increases. Leaders are managing and directing projects with representatives from multiple sites, which may or may not be within the community; more executives and managers today have responsibility for multiple facilities and departments; and the ascent of the virtual office coupled with the outsourcing aspects of health care all combine to create the need for leaders who are effective in spite of geographical distance from their followers.

Geographical distance from followers creates significant barriers to applying any of the interpersonal competencies. Forming and nurturing a quality relationship can be difficult if two people are not physically proximate at least periodically. Talking over a computer or telephone line is not the same as face-to-face interaction. Distance makes communication more difficult and complicated. Pinchot and Pinchot (1996a, p. 18) articulate this issue well:

> As organizations become more complex, more geographically distributed, it becomes harder to create enough common vision and community spirit to guide the actions without increasing reliance on the chains of command. When people are separated by distance, vast differences in power and wealth, and conflict over resources and promotions, political struggle often replaces community. As the power of community is stretched thin, the chain of command becomes more prominent, and sense of community declines further.

The savvy leader applies the basic principles of communication and pays special attention to them when distance complicates the situation. In *Knights of the TeleRound Table* (1994), Kostner shares insights for executives who must manage from afar. Many of the principles she identifies are equally applicable to long-distance leaders. She points out that "the key way to build high performance across distance . . . is to build trust. Be obvious that every word, every action, every initiative on the virtual team builds trust" (p. 169).

The paradox is that in these long-distance relationships, trust is more difficult to build but is even more important.

Here are some helpful tips for establishing effective long-distance leader-follower relationships:

- Use strong symbols as a way of uniting people who are not in the same workplace.

- Establish ways to help people learn more about each other so that they collaborate even when distant, such as on-site visits, kickoff meetings for key projects, and teleconferencing.

- Use a computer network, e-mail, teleconferencing, or other technology to link people across distances.

- "Be scrupulously fair in treating all team members, near and far, equally. Even appearances or suggestions of favoritism break trust" (Kostner, 1994, p. 171).

- Rely equally on followers whether on- or off-site (there is often temptation to rely more fully on those sharing the same geographical location).

- Expect high performance equally from followers, not allowing distance to impede dealing with performance issues.

Leading from a distance is a growing challenge in today's workforce. We cannot overstate the importance of good communication. "Miscommunication, inequities of information, and unequal access to information are significant trust-breakers. . . . The impact of these remote problems may not show up for months, but will always negatively impact productivity and profits across distance" (Kostner, 1994, p. 172). Continually flowing communication and diligent sharing of information can counteract the out-of-sight, out-of-mind syndrome.

Communicating with Teams

In organizations that have converted to a team structure in their departments, leaders face the challenge of communicating with teams in addition to communicating with individuals or work groups. In each situation, the leader must be sensitive to the question: Is this an individual issue or a team issue? If it is a team issue, the leader must decide carefully how to communicate and with whom. Executives especially need to be careful about not usurping the team's responsibility and authority. There is often a strong tendency to access previous lines of communication and simply pick up the telephone and contact the manager to whom the team is responsible. Most managers willingly follow up and attain information or take the action the leader requested. Results are speedier and seem to simplify communication. However, the team may end up resenting the fact that the manager intervened in what the team members consider their work. An astute manager may put the leader directly in touch with the team so that the communication is as direct as possible.

When working with a group of individuals who have been selected as team representatives, a good leader makes certain they are clear about their role. Too often team members participate on ad hoc problem-solving teams or committees within the organization and forget that their role is to represent all of their teammates' interests and ideas. A simple reminder at each meeting helps these people focus on their need to return to their team and communicate with their colleagues. When the group discusses issues, asking attendees about their teammates' thoughts and ideas also reinforces their roles as team representatives.

Communicating with teams can complicate matters in an organization. The increased feeling of ownership and responsibility, as well as the improved outcomes that teams attain, usually outweighs the difficulties. However, there is a strong tendency for leaders to want to simplify reporting and communication relationships and to stay with the methods they have used in the past. A vivid example of this took place in a large medical center that was four years into the process of converting to a team-based structure. Employees in the risk management department had begun working together as a team. They were cross-trained, self-directed, and self-managing. The director, Sammie, had been asked to investigate a particular problem, and she had turned the project over to the team.

These highly seasoned team members investigated the issue thoroughly and produced an outstanding report. Each proudly signed the work and asked to present it to the executive team. The executive team declined the team's request to present the report and instead asked Sammie to do the honors. Then, unbelievably, the executive team refused to accept the report with the team's signatures and insisted on the department director's signature only. Their reasoning was that the department director was solely accountable in case of any future problems. This demoralizing blow to an excited, enthusiastic, fully engaged team was devastating. It created a tremendous ripple of distrust and cynicism throughout the organization that these executive leaders never recognized. Employees in this organization no longer believed that executive leaders understood what it meant to be on a team. And in fact, today their team initiative is essentially defunct.

Conclusion

This chapter has addressed one of the most crucial issues for any leader: how to communicate effectively. Without this skill, the other leadership competencies are virtually inoperative, relationships are not healthy, it is impossible to gain commitment to a cause, processes cannot flow smoothly, and the leader is unable to develop and nurture others. An effective leader understands the facets of spoken, nonverbal, and written communication and the barriers that must be overcome. Every day brings a leader numerous opportunities to improve his or her communication skills, as well as new challenges in creating shared meaning with followers. Beyond mere skill development is the need for the leader to have insight into his or her own philosophy of communication and its impact on leadership effectiveness.

DISCUSSION QUESTIONS

1. What is the philosophy of communication in your organization? In your department? Is the communication transparent and honest? Is communication timely, open, and free flowing? Is information closely guarded?

2. What is *your* philosophy of communication? Do you believe that employees have the right to and need for virtually all the information the manager has? What information, if any, do you think they should not have?

3. What types of communication challenges or difficulties do you see in your organization? What kinds of problems have they created?

4. If you are a manager, what are the predominant methods you use for communicating with your staff? What communication strategies are you most comfortable with? Why? How could you increase your communication with employees?

5. What are the common thoughts or reasons you have for not communicating more fully with employees?

6. How effective are your listening skills? How often do you have other people repeat the same message you have already heard? Are you ever accused of not listening? What behaviors do you think led to this accusation?

7. What bad habits related to listening do you have? What could you do to increase your listening effectiveness? How often do you use reflective listening?

8. How comfortable are you using questions in conversations with others? How do others react to your questioning technique? Do your questions facilitate the flow of information? Do people open up more, or do they become more reserved and quiet?

9. In what ways do you use nonverbal language to enhance, rather than detract from, your messages?

10. With your group of coworkers or employees, develop a list of etiquette tips for the use of e-mail and cell phones (the easy way to start is to list your pet peeves). Do you violate any of these when using these forms of communication technology?

11. What is your level of skill with written communication? What are the kinds of problems you experience? How could you improve your written communication?

12. Do you use any of the online social networking sites in your professional life? How could you use any of these sites to increase your communication effectiveness?

13. Practice multiple ways of explaining the same concept without using jargon or buzzwords. How could you use storytelling more effectively as a way of communicating?

5

The Art of Effectively Facilitating Processes

CHAPTER OBJECTIVES

- Discuss the four sequential elements of empowerment.

- Compare the four levels of authority.

- Identify common effective and ineffective methods of conflict resolution and discuss why they are ineffective.

- Relate the steps of an effective negotiation process.

- Discuss the six steps of creating an effective team.

- Identify the five phases of the energy model as it relates to change management.

- Compare and contrast the concepts of change and transition.

Solutions . . . reside not in the executive suite but in the
collective intelligence of employees at all levels, who need to
use one another as resources, often across boundaries,
and learn their way to those solutions.

R. A. HEIFETZ AND D. L. LAURIE, "THE WORK OF LEADERSHIP"

Transformational leaders are skilled at guiding key processes in order
to obtain synergistic, extraordinary outcomes. Process facilitation is a
critical competency for a leader because of the increasing complexity of work
and the accelerating competency of workers. The old command-and-control
approach to leadership and management was effective in the past when
workers did not have the scope, skills, or ability to make decisions other
than basic ones directly influencing their work. Today's workforce is better
educated, more sophisticated, and increasingly interested in being involved
in planning and making decisions that directly or indirectly affect their
work. Ramifications of these changes for leaders are significant. Good leaders
develop relationships, gather information, involve others, engage in dialogue,
guide discussions, build commitment, empower others, and recognize when
a decision needs to be a group effort and then gain consensus. In short, they
are capable and skilled at facilitating a variety of processes.

Facilitating processes as a leader is not as easy as it might at first appear.
In the past, managers were often rewarded for a get-it-done mentality and
approaches that were decisive and outcome oriented. How they achieved a
result mattered less than the fact that they did so. In fact, individuals who
focused on the process in achieving outcomes often reached those results more
slowly and were thus judged not very effective. Today's business climate adds
pressure to managing processes in that it reinforces the need for quick action,
decisive leaders, and an outcome-oriented approach. Courage is a necessary
asset for leaders who are pressured for a decision but believe better results are
possible when they and followers make a collective and collaborative decision.

In the first edition of this book, this chapter was titled "The Art of
Effectively Managing Processes." The term *managing* implies that one can
control the process, which discounts what we know of systems theory. An
organization, a department, a team, and an individual are all open systems.

An open system is one that continually takes in information, transforms it, and changes as a result. It is in a constant state of emergence. As such, emergent systems are anything but controllable, and our future is not just unknown but incapable of being known (Stacey, 1992). To the degree that the environment is stable and there is certainty about a particular outcome, there is a sense of control. Leaders understand that although our systems are continually in an emergent state, and thus unpredictable, wisely facilitating the inherent process as it unfolds can increase the certainty of outcomes. Porter-O'Grady and Malloch (2010) do a thorough job of describing the nature of our complex adaptive health care systems in their book *Innovation Leadership: Creating the Landscape of Health Care* and note that organizations have moved well beyond complicated to complex in ways almost too difficult to fully grasp.

The leader's judgment throughout the unfolding of a process is crucial. Tichy and Bennis (2007) believe that "the leader's most important role in any organization is making good judgments—well-informed, wise decisions that produce the desired outcomes. When a leader shows consistently good judgment, little else matters" (p. 94). Multiple decisions must be made throughout any process. The consequences of the leader's judgment calls are magnified exponentially because they influence the lives of so many others and determine an organization's success or failure.

This chapter explores several key tenets underlying the leadership skill of facilitating processes. The first is to understand and respect the process. The second refers to the role of leaders in persistently seeking to improve current situations by continually challenging the process. The final tenet establishes the leader's role in facilitation. To illustrate, the chapter examines several fundamental processes as they relate to health care leadership practice: empowering others, resolving conflict, creating teams, and facilitating the processes of change and transition. Chapter Six addresses the key process of problem solving and discusses it with other approaches for getting needed results.

The Key Tenets

Three tenets underlie the leader's ability to effectively facilitate a successful process.

Tenet One: Understand and Respect Process

This tenet is twofold: not only must leaders understand basic processes that are operative in particular situations, but they must also respect the processes, allowing them to unfold in their own natural time frames. Both elements of this tenet are important. First, it is necessary to recognize the process and demonstrate knowledge of it through the application of logical, methodical, or other appropriate steps. A major cause of an ineffective process is skipping or eliminating an important step, as this chapter will illustrate.

Leaders need not always apply the steps to these processes in exactly the manner they are outlined here. Any effective process is more likely to unfold in a nonlinear fashion than in the linear way it is explained here for clarity. Through practice, trial and error, and continual evaluation of outcomes, a leader gains experience as well as judgment and may develop his or her own processes. However, most processes have certain key elements— in some instances, a structure that will improve outcomes when it is consistently applied.

Process requires patience. The leader and followers may spend more time in preparatory groundwork, but when they make decisions or formulate solutions, those involved are thoroughly committed to carrying them out. With the directive or command-and-control approach, after the leader makes a decision or determines a solution, he or she must spend time convincing others to comply—a never-ending cycle of explanations, persuasion, and monitoring of behavior.

Respecting the process means that the leader understands approximately how long a normal process should take and allows the necessary time for the process to unfold naturally. This requires a significant amount of judgment because a little nudge or push may sometimes be required to get things back on track. People who express an aversion to processes likely have been involved too frequently in a previous process that seemed never ending. People inexperienced or unskilled in facilitating processes sometimes let them drag on, never bringing closure or producing needed results. Following a process simply for its own sake is numbing and demoralizing. The purpose of facilitating process is to make it meaningful. And to be considered meaningful, a process must result in effective and beneficial outcomes.

Respecting process is similar to understanding and respecting the principles involved in a situation. In *Principle-Centered Leadership* (1990), best-selling author Stephen Covey describes principles as abiding laws of nature that never change. To explain the concept, Covey uses farming as an example. A farmer cannot take it easy in the spring and summer—procrastinating and not planting—and expect a bountiful harvest in the fall. The farmer must plant the seeds in the spring and cultivate and fertilize the fields during the summer to be rewarded with a crop in the fall. Unable to hasten the growth of the crop or to control all the external elements that affect the crop's bounty, the farmer respects and awaits the unfolding of the process. In the same way, a leader who understands and respects the natural flow of a particular process does only what he or she can to influence results but knows that he or she cannot accelerate the process unnaturally or control it completely. There needs to be trust that the process will unfold.

A senior leader, Della, who is responsible for leading a massive organizational cultural change effort in her system, recently shared an example. She worked with an outside facilitator who led the initial process of a group of over two hundred organizational leaders (management and staff) whose purpose was to determine the guiding principles of the new culture. Della's personal leadership style is a combination of a no-nonsense, "just get it done" approach, coupled with a genuine regard for and enjoyment of people and relationships. She said she was extremely anxious the evening before the work session because the process felt too loose and not directive enough. During the morning session, participants participated enthusiastically and generated over sixty concepts they felt were important. Della said that at that point, "I stood there and thought . . . oh my gosh! How are we going to get this down to six or seven key principles?" Inside she felt total dismay. However, the process continued with active group participation, and they pruned the list down to a manageable six concepts, which still has Della shaking her head in amazement. She cannot look at these principles without feeling a tremendous sense of pride in the work her colleagues did during this process. In some cases, one of the most important things a leader can do is to relax and trust the process to unfold as it needs to. People really do have most of the answers they need, and facilitating the process helps them discover their own answers.

Examples demonstrating a lack of respect for process are common in today's health care organizations. Unfortunately, the external climate creates a sense of urgency and need that can easily affect the leader's ability or desire to patiently let a process unfold. Take, for example, the formation of a healthy relationship between followers and leaders. Establishing and developing this relationship is a developmental process that cannot be rushed or developed suddenly when a crisis generates a need for it. Yet observe what happens in an organization in which employees threaten collective action through a union-organizing attempt. The organization hires consultants to coach managers about what they can and cannot say. Overnight, managers are available and visible to employees, listening to what employees are saying and asking for input. But it's often a matter of too little, too late. Employees often receive managers' sudden flurry of relationship building with cynicism. Worse, the managers' behavior may reinforce the thought that threatening union organization causes management and administration to finally listen to employees. The parties are more likely to resolve issues to their mutual satisfaction if they have established healthy relationships built on mutual trust and respect over the years. This means that leaders have always been listening to employees and employees and managers work together as full partners. When a volatile or critical situation develops, followers will extend trust to a leader who has built a trusting relationship over time.

Empowering employees is a process, and there are many examples of failure to recognize this. One midsized hospital brought in consultants and paid hundreds of thousands of dollars for a reengineering and restructuring project in the 1990s that was believed to be essential for the organization's survival. Employees were cross-trained and placed in teams and expected to assume responsibilities not only for their own work but for that of management and supervisory positions that the organization had eliminated. All this might have been reasonable except that the organization had never invested in employee or management education and development. Neither employees nor managers were prepared in any way for the tremendous change this project represented. The organization needed these people to be empowered yet had never taken time or allotted resources to develop them. Instead of empowering and strengthening the organization, the initiative failed miserably;

the hospital went on the market and later closed. Earlier investment in its people's development could have been the turning point for this organization's survival.

Tenet Two: Continually Challenge the Process

Leaders do more than simply understand the operative process and allow it to unfold within its natural time frame. Leaders continually question the process, looking for opportunities to improve it and methods that increase its effectiveness. "Challenge is the opportunity for greatness. People do their best when there's the chance to change the ways things are. Maintaining the status quo breeds mediocrity. . . . [Leaders] motivate others to exceed their limits. They look for innovative ways to improve the organization" (Kouzes and Posner, 1987, p. 29).

Challenging the process requires continually evaluating the effectiveness of outcomes and identifying lessons learned from the manner in which the outcomes were obtained. What went well, and what actions created problems? Did the process flow smoothly or drag on? Did the leader intervene at appropriate times? Was enough time allotted? Did members of the group or team participate fully?

Questioning the status quo often identifies opportunities for improvement. Too many times we do things in particular ways in an organization simply because we have always done them that way. A leader challenges this thinking by questioning the traditions: Does it make sense to continue doing things the old way? Is there a better way? Leaders are always on the lookout for something that is not working well or can be improved. Kouzes and Posner (1987, p. 32) clearly describe this role:

> The root origin of the word lead is a word meaning "to go." This root origin denotes travel from one place to another. Leaders can be said to be those who "go first." They are those who step out to show others the direction in which to head. They begin the quest for a new order. In this sense, leaders are pioneers. They are people who venture into unexplored territory. They guide us to new and often unfamiliar destinations. People who take the lead are the foot soldiers in the campaigns for change.

Another way leaders challenge a process is to encourage risk taking. They take risks themselves and grow from the lessons they learn and the accomplishments they achieve. Leaders also encourage risk taking when they talk about their own failures and mistakes and treat these as opportunities for learning. They support followers when they make errors and expect them to learn from their mistakes. The overall attitude in the organization is similar to the sentiment that silent-film actress Mary Pickford expressed: "If you have made mistakes . . . there is always another chance for you. . . . You may have a fresh start any moment you choose, for this thing we call 'failure' is not the falling down, but the staying down" (*Quotable Women*, 1989, p. 22).

A risk is simply the act of seeking to achieve a goal that exceeds the usual limits. Risk is inherent in any change initiative or innovation. Exemplary leaders and followers are familiar with risk taking because it is part of their very nature. Uncertainty and danger are a normal part of this process. Taking a risk is central to everything worthwhile in life. No one can grow without taking a chance. In every risk there is an unavoidable loss—something that one has to give up in order to move ahead. Not risking is the surest way of losing. If an individual or organization continually shuns new experiences or experiments because they are risky, the result is a person or organization that is comfortable with fewer and fewer stretch experiences. Not taking risks is a sure way to become stagnant and ill prepared for the future.

Part of a leader's role is to understand and become comfortable with risk taking. Although careful planning reduces risk considerably, no one is ever completely prepared to take a big risk. But we gain nothing if we venture nothing. One of the changes today's managers most need is "to cultivate the imagination and courage to innovate—that is, to question received wisdom and constantly look for a better way. Too many managers are still afraid of innovation" (Kanter, 1997, p. 7).

Unfortunately, this is true not only of managers and employee leaders but also of many systems. Difficulty letting go of the hospital mentality and traditional modes of service can lead to an aversion to risk sharing among physicians, community agencies, and hospitals. Board members may also be averse to taking risks. Many board members have traditionally focused on narrow financial concerns and must now refocus and reorient themselves toward expressing the voice of the community (Chawla and Renesch, 1995). Their role is changing, and speaking for the community may mean accepting higher levels of risk for the system.

Tenet Three: Facilitating Process

In addition to understanding and challenging the process, the leader has a role in intervening to facilitate the process flow. Facilitation skills such as managing and leading group process, addressing difficult or negative group behavior, getting participation from everyone involved, asking the right questions, and guiding a group to consensus are necessary. However, a leader might use additional techniques to facilitate process. Teaching others the elements and logical steps of a process may be necessary. Rather than assuming that followers or participants understand the process, the leader encourages followers to learn the elements and sequential steps and know what the leader expects. This smoothes the process because followers become knowledgeable enough to support the process and can work in partnership with the leader.

Another subtle but critical manner in which a leader facilitates process is by providing the time needed to engage the process fully. A patient leader encourages patience in others. He or she does not look for results too early yet urges progress based on realistic time frames and gives reassuring and reinforcing feedback . If the leader is a manager, this support can be concrete, such as allotting time for employees to work through a process while being clear about expected outcomes. In a laboratory department, for instance, an employee action committee was working with another department on solving a particular problem. The manager not only approved employee time away from the department but assisted in finding replacement help for committee participants. She was also available to coach the employees, who had limited committee experience.

Removing barriers in the department or organization is another way a leader facilitates effective processes. This may be as simple as providing any training that followers need. Being clear about parameters, expectations, and levels of authority also reduces barriers. The leader may need to communicate and pave the way with other leaders or managers in the organization.

Again using the example of the laboratory department, when the employee action committee was initiated, the leader made certain that several members were skilled in using an established process improvement model. At the first meeting, the leader taught other members of the committee the same model. The group established expectations and levels of authority for carrying out their responsibilities at the second meeting. The lab manager also contacted several peripherally involved department managers and introduced committee members to them, asking the managers for their support and assistance should committee members call on them.

This chapter has already briefly discussed the final way to remove barriers, which is to reduce risks in the process by using trial periods and properly measuring results. Expecting and planning for mistakes and stops and starts provides an opportunity for damage control. Modeling accepting behavior when mistakes occur and helping sort out the reasons for the mistakes and ways to correct it removes yet another barrier: the fear of failure and punitive consequences.

These three tenets, or principles, can be applied to all types of processes. In addition to developing healthy relationships with others, some additional processes necessary for leaders to master are empowering or transferring responsibility to others, resolving conflict, solving problems, making decisions, creating teams, and managing change and transition. All are key elements to increasing a leader's ability to influence others in a manner beneficial to the organization and people involved. This chapter and the next examine each process in some detail and illustrate it with recent real-life examples to show its importance, as well as common pitfalls.

Empowering Others

One of the most important processes that any leader can undertake today is transferring responsibility to others, often known as empowering them. Unfortunately, empowerment is also one of the least understood of the key processes. Although *empowerment* became a buzzword in the 1990s, many never went beyond giving lip-service to the concept. Use of the term today often brings cynicism and horror stories that seem to substantiate the ineffectiveness of empowerment. However, leaders who found ways to operationalize the implied promise of empowerment can point to dramatic results.

The definition of *empowerment* is "to be given the legal authority to." The word *power* means "the ability to act or to produce a result." These two definitions combined are "to be given the legal authority to act or produce a result." Gibson (1991, p. 351) defines *empowerment* as "a social process of recognizing, promoting, and enhancing people's abilities to meet their own needs, solve their own problems, and mobilize the necessary resources in order for them to feel in control of their lives." This is similar to the definition of *leader* provided in Chapter One.

Empowerment is both a process and an outcome. As a process, the sequential ordering of steps in empowerment promotes a greater likelihood of success. Empowerment is dynamic because it is transactional, meaning that it occurs as a result of interaction between two or more people and therefore cannot be completely predictable. Empowerment is a developmental process because it is directly influenced by the increasing ability of an individual to accept higher and higher levels of responsibility.

The importance of empowering people in organizations cannot be overstated. Empowered employees are fully engaged in their work, contributing at a much higher level than their counterparts who see their work as simply a job. With the constantly shifting business climate and increasingly challenging external conditions facing health care, every organization needs the ability to respond rapidly. Quick response is virtually impossible from a workforce that has to constantly be told what to do, is basically uninformed and unused to making decisions, and has never before participated in collaborative planning. Organizations that have dedicated resources to continually developing their people and treat their employees as intelligent partners in the delivery of services are much more likely to have individuals who are able to respond quickly when external and internal conditions change. These employees are not dependent on the manager or leader for direction or decisions; they can function independently and interdependently when they need to.

Many organizations develop and empower not just frontline employees but also first-line managers. This creates a tremendous ripple effect in the organization. Rosabeth Moss Kanter, a professor at Harvard Business School who has been on the frontier of management and leadership for over thirty years, points out the dangers of not empowering managers in the organization: "Managers with power accomplish more because they have greater access to information, resources, and support in the company. Being busy, they pass the information and resources to subordinates. Thus, powerful leaders are more likely to delegate responsibility and reward talent. Powerless managers who can't easily get access to resources and information are frustrated and weak. The result is often petty, dictatorial managers who wield the only power they can: oppression of subordinates. It is powerlessness, not power, that corrupts" (1997, p. 6).

Empowerment does not occur simply because a leader says, "You are now empowered; go perform!" There is no Harry Potter magic wand to wave or incantation to chant so that people suddenly begin behaving differently. "Empowerment takes planning, patience, trust, and time. It's not something you can do overnight. If you want it to work, you have to commit to it. You must be willing to invest in it, support it with systems, and approach it in a logical, determined way" (McCarthy, 1997, p. 7).

The Process

As a process, empowerment begins with an understanding of four interrelated concepts:

- Capability

- Responsibility

- Authority

- Accountability

The sequential application of these four concepts leads to empowerment. First, let's clarify the meaning of each of these terms.

Capability

Capability refers to the ability, knowledge, and willingness of an individual to carry out the task, assignment, or responsibility. Ability is not only personal competence comprising skill and experience but the availability of needed resources. An individual may be willing to accept a particular responsibility but simply not have the time, equipment, or resources necessary to do an adequate job. Or the opposite may be true: the person may have ability—both personal competence and resources—but lack willingness. All must be present, or empowerment fails.

Responsibility

Responsibility is the clear allocation or assignment of a task or piece of work to be accomplished. It also implies that the individual accepts this allocation. The person to whom the leader has given the task or assignment must accept ownership before this responsibility truly occurs. For instance, a team accepts responsibility for carrying out its work, monitoring and controlling work flow, and making necessary decisions within its members' scope of responsibility and authority. The members are responsible for maintaining an acceptable standard and continually searching for ways to improve their processes and outcomes.

Authority

Authority is the right to act in an area for which one has accepted responsibility. In order to carry out a responsibility, an individual must have a commensurate level of authority. According to Miller and Manthey (1994), there are four commonly accepted levels of authority:

Level one. This is the authority to collect data or gather information. The individual takes no action on the data or information, and the person assigning the responsibility and granting the authority remains the decision maker.

Level two. Once the individual collects the data or information, he or she also reviews it and makes a recommendation based on his or her assessment and previous experience. The person assigning the responsibility and granting the authority continues to make the decisions but considers the gatherer's recommendation in making the final decision.

Level three. The individual collects and reviews the information, makes a recommendation, and discusses it with the person assigning the responsibility. After their discussion and agreement, the individual proceeds to carry out the action.

Level four. The individual can initiate independent action. He or she has the right to gather information, determine what needs to be done, and take necessary action. The person accepting the assignment has the authority to act in place of the delegating individual.

In addition to these levels of authority, the individual's responsibility or authority may be limited by constraints or parameters of a particular situation. For instance, the individual may have responsibility for making a purchasing decision with a level four authority but must stay within the constraints of an established dollar amount. Or a person may have the responsibility to make a decision and determine necessary action but only after getting agreement from certain key stakeholders.

Accountability

Accountability is the retrospective review of decisions made or actions taken to determine if they were appropriate. Did the decisions or actions achieve the desired outcomes? If results were not satisfactory, what corrective action would remedy the situation? This attitude of continual review is characteristic of a lifelong learner, a learning team, or a learning organization.

Applying the Process

When a leader applies this empowerment process sequentially, it goes something like this. Before expecting a follower to take on a responsibility, the leader assesses the individual's ability and willingness. Does the person have the knowledge to carry out this responsibility? Are necessary resources such as information and time available? Has training or education been provided? Once the leader determines that capability is present, he or she clearly defines and communicates the responsibility. Assumptions are not enough; the assignment must be clear to both the party accepting the responsibility and the other people whom this assignment may affect. The parties discuss the applicable parameters and reach agreement on the appropriate level of authority. Finally, they determine outcome measures to monitor success. If the outcomes are not satisfactory, the individual who has accepted the responsibility takes action to remediate the situation.

The significance of empowerment as a developmental process is now clear. As an individual becomes more capable and highly skilled, he or she can accept increasingly more responsibility. The leader gradually increases the level of authority following successful performance of a responsibility. The leader may expand parameters and constraints as his or her comfort with an individual's performance increases. It would be highly foolish, and even dangerous, to give a novice performer a level four authority and no constraints the first time that he or she takes on a responsibility.

This process appears simple, yet it contains pitfalls and there are many missteps in organizations today. When people feel disempowered, leaders can use this process to assess the source of the problem and sort through solutions for correcting it. Here are some of the more common examples of pitfalls with each of these elements of empowerment.

Pitfalls: Capability

The first pitfall has to do with the sometimes heard complaint from employees who are resisting a new job expectation: "But you didn't tell me that was going to be part of my job when I was hired." Job requirements change as a result of new needs in the organization, yet people stay in their positions even though they are no longer able to do the work required. This leads to an environment of entitlement rather than earned responsibility and authority. Organizations can communicate new expectations in the workplace, provide education and training, and give employees time to adjust and meet new standards. However, at some point it is necessary for the leader to expect these individuals to develop the abilities required or face a change in roles.

Another problematic situation occurs when individuals accept responsibility for something they are not capable of doing. Perhaps they believe they have the ability, but in reality they do not. The result is frustration for both the individual and the leader, along with lengthy and potentially costly delays in completing the task. This can be difficult to address if the employee is genuinely interested and wants to volunteer for a responsibility.

Some individuals are simply unwilling to accept more responsibility, an admittedly difficult situation for a leader or manager. With reductions in staffing levels and downsizing of organizations, everybody has to pull his or her own weight. The organization needs the highest levels of performance from every individual, and others cannot continue to absorb shortfalls from those not contributing fully. Although you cannot force someone to accept responsibility, you can make acceptance of responsibility a job requirement; an individual who does not accept responsibility may need to be separated from the job.

Also, there may be insufficient resources for people to capably accept certain responsibilities. Time, equipment, money, education, training, or coaching may not be available, although individuals may be willing to accept additional responsibility. Organizations that attempted to convert to team-based structures in the 1990s are a good example. They accomplished redesign of work and determined team structures. They assigned employees to teams and expected them to carry out their work in a new way without preparation in the form of education or training; furthermore, the employees reported to managers who were inexperienced at and, in some instances, at least, incapable of coaching a team. This created a no-win situation for all involved.

Pitfalls: Responsibility

The most common pitfall with responsibility is that leaders do not clearly define it but instead assume that followers understand their responsibility. For instance, a manager-leader makes the mistake of assuming that the job description clearly and completely defines what the organization expects the employee to do. Leaders do not always realize that the position holder will be held accountable for numerous other responsibilities and that the leader must clearly articulate them. For instance, newly hired employees should be told: "You are responsible for two things as an employee in this organization. The first is to do the work for which you were hired at an acceptable level of quality. The second is to form and maintain healthy working relationships with everyone else here." This means employees and managers are responsible for relationship issues in the workplace. This ranges from resolving conflicts in a positive manner to having open, honest, and direct communication with coworkers. Yet how many organizations have clearly and directly given employees this expectation? Most employees believe that relationship management is the job of the manager.

Another problem with the element of responsibility occurs when responsibilities overlap significantly. It can also happen as a result of carelessness. In one organization, the chief operating officer (COO) was a cautious individual with a bad habit of asking multiple managers to do the same tasks. A manager whom the COO asked to investigate and follow up on a problem would discover that the COO had asked others to assume the same responsibility. The managers found this duplication of efforts irritating and demoralizing. In some rare instances, having several people share a responsibility makes sense. But in order to avoid a disempowering and discouraging situation, the involved parties need to clearly discuss who is doing what. Few people appreciate wasting time. Excessive managerial layers also lead to confusion about roles.

In some instances, individuals have an exaggerated sense of responsibility and take ownership beyond what the leader intended. This can lead to frustration and discouragement for all involved. One organization created a team of internal trainers to provide the education and training for a major organizational initiative in process improvement. In the beginning, the team mistakenly believed that its role was to lead this initiative. Team members felt responsible for the effort's success or failure; managers in the organization did not help matters when they abdicated their responsibility for leading the process. Conflict and difficulties were significant until each set of parties clearly defined its responsibility.

Pitfalls: Authority

Problems and confusion occur most frequently with the concept of authority. Many people believe that empowerment occurs only when they have level four authority and that anything less than independent action is disempowering. Nothing could be further from the truth. The level of authority has to be high enough for the individual to carry out the responsibility, and when these two are commensurate, empowerment results. Even a CEO or system president does not have level four authority for every aspect of his or her work. In any role, some responsibilities rightfully entail a lower level of authority.

A second source of confusion around authority comes from the mistaken but commonly held belief that lower levels of authority are not as important as those at higher levels. People in organizations today make many mistakes and poor decisions because of this misconception. Leaders ask employees to give their opinion or gather information, but because the employees are not making the final decision, they do a half-hearted job of collecting or giving the requested information. The poor quality of the input creates a disadvantage for the leader who is making a final decision. Each level of authority is critical, and individuals must take seriously the responsibilities that come with each level.

Both performers and leaders may inaccurately assume levels of authority unless they specifically discuss and agree to them. Conflict occurs when disagreement becomes apparent. Quality or process improvement teams often run into this situation. In one organization, this occurred in the nursing department with a very visible employee team that had been asked to develop a clinical career ladder for the department. The team worked diligently for months and created an entire program based on extensive research from other hospitals.

When the team was on the verge of implementing the program, the corporate human resource department stopped the process because of compensation issues and a need for equity across the entire system. The proposed program had neglected to include other key services, such as the clinics, home health, hospice, and long-term care, and no other professional departments from the system had been considered. This team had unwittingly exceeded its level of authority; as a result, a significant amount of resentment and frustration developed among the hospital nursing department, corporate human resources, and the rest of the system.

Changing levels of authority in the middle of a project is sometimes necessary but should be avoided if at all possible. A leader may give an individual or a group a responsibility, and the parties may have agreed on its level of authority, only to have the leader recall or decrease the level of authority when the individual or group does not carry out the work in the way the leader expected. There are, however, multiple ways of achieving necessary outcomes, and a confident leader recognizes the need to relinquish control and let followers find their own way. Snatching a project or assignment away midstream may dismay the followers and leave them unwilling to accept further responsibility.

New authority-related problems are appearing today with the major structural changes in the workplace. In the past, managers clearly had a certain level of authority, and their reporting relationships were delineated and unambiguous. For many people in today's health care system, this has changed completely, as it has for a nurse executive who is responsible for the nursing function throughout the system. The responsibility has become increasingly difficult to carry out now that it is dispersed among a variety of operational leaders, some of whom have no professional nursing background and may report directly to a different executive. Communicating the essence of nursing issues and ensuring quality standards in the absence of line authority requires strong leadership skills.

A final problem related to authority is the reversal of authority. This occurs when the work of an individual or group is undermined or disrespected by others—either peers or leaders. The recommended decision or solution is disregarded. This happens most frequently when the leader has neglected to identify key parameters at the start, so the individual or group made the decision with incomplete information. Less frequently, the leader may have had no intention of relinquishing control but wanted others to feel as if they had participated.

In the early days of the quality movement, employees frequently learned this lesson the hard way. One quality team worked for six months on a specific problem. Its recommendation cost $200,000 to implement and included the addition of four full-time-equivalent positions to the annual personnel budget. No one had thought to tell the team that any recommendation could not exceed the current budget. Unfortunately, the experience led team members to conclude that administration was not serious about involving employees in decision making and that quality was not a primary concern. Although leaders had selected the team members because of their interest and commitment, these employees became unwilling to participate in any further projects after this negative and demoralizing experience. These budget constraints might have been more acceptable to the team if leaders had identified them in the beginning stages of work.

Sometimes group members attempt to undermine decisions. A medical clinical affairs committee discovered this in one organization. The director of medical affairs was given the authority to solve a problem within a certain dollar amount. Two weeks later, he reported on his actions. Two physicians who had not been present at the previous meeting began questioning and second-guessing his decision. The chair of the committee firmly reminded them that the committee had given the individual the authority to solve the problem and that it would respect and support his decision.

Pitfalls: Accountability

Although problems with authority are the most common, issues of accountability are often the most serious. This element may well be the weakest link in the chain. If organizations do not hold people accountable for their behaviors and actions, whatever they may do through the first three steps can be quickly negated. One reason so many things go right in organizations today is that many employees and leaders feel a high level of personal accountability, continually reviewing their outcomes and learning from them. People who are continual learners demonstrate a high level of internal accountability. Nevertheless, there are many problems with external accountability, that is, the formal, traceable lines of accountability in the organization.

Most organizations have only limited systems of accountability. Ascertaining what went wrong and why is often very difficult because of the extreme complexity of our systems. Large numbers of part-time staff and per diem or temporary employees have made determining who is responsible when a problem occurs rather complicated. Assignments of employees are often not consistent, and many handoffs from caregiver to caregiver and department to department increase the difficulty of tracking.

Another issue hampering accountability is the tendency of managers and leaders to protect employees. When an individual or team makes a mistake or poor decision, the real role of the leader is to coach and support them in their efforts to correct the situation. Too often the manager steps in and takes responsibility for correcting the problem. Consider what happens in a situation in which a physician goes to the manager with a complaint about an employee or a team. If the manager takes care of the problem, the employee or team has learned little except that it does not have to deal with its customer service problems or is not capable of resolving them. If instead the manager coaches the individual or team to work directly with the physician to resolve the issue, both the team and the physician benefit. The manager's behavior is sometimes motivated by his or her satisfaction in solving problems or in some cases by expectations within the hierarchy. Many established bureaucracies have only limited tolerance for these situations and simply want them resolved in the quickest fashion possible.

The final major pitfall for accountability is that the consequences of mistakes or poor judgment are too often punitive rather than corrective. Many organizations blame and accuse people when things go wrong. These negative, punitive responses are probably the fastest way to squelch any desire to accept responsibility. People are quick learners, and they also watch what happens to their colleagues and coworkers. Swift retribution designed at extinguishing poor performance actually extinguishes all performance. Few people are willing to take risks in a harsh and unforgiving environment. This is precisely why so much work has been done in the area of creating just cultures.

Summary

This process for empowering others is key to transformational leadership. It offers an effective mechanism for delegating responsibility and developing people. Without leadership's astute application of these skills, people in the organization are less likely to contribute at their highest potential.

Resolving Conflict

Conflict in the workplace is on the rise as major change disrupts comfortable and known routines, accelerated expectations require greater job performance, and the workforce shrinks as a result of changing demographics and economic woes. People going through change and transition experience a wide range of intense emotional reactions, heightening the potential for conflict. Skill in conflict resolution is crucial for today's leaders.

Common Reactions to Conflict

Most people react to conflict negatively for a variety of reasons. These include early socialization patterns, when parents admonished children for being angry or fighting with siblings, or past negative experiences with conflict. Perhaps the individual remembers how it felt as a child to hear his or her parents argue and fight with each other. If the arguments and conflict ended in physical abuse or divorce, the message the child retained may be that conflict is bad and has horrible consequences. Or if a child never saw or heard his or her parents disagree or argue with each other, the child might believe that conflict is to be avoided at all costs. The child may never have seen parents take steps for healthy conflict resolution and conclude that conflict does not exist in healthy relationships. Another factor influencing an adult's reaction to conflict is the normal need to feel in control of situations. Intense conflict is frightening for many because it is unpredictable and hard to control.

To effectively assist in resolving conflict, leaders with insight into their own reaction to conflict are an asset. Each leader has unique conflict resolution skills. For instance, one leader may be especially skilled at mediating, whereas another may be a skilled negotiations coach. One may stay calm under attack, whereas another needs time away to separate emotions before intervening. Knowing and tapping into our strengths increases our ability to assist others.

Understanding and accepting one's limitations are also vital. Very few people enjoy being involved in open conflict, but a strong leader recognizes that conflict is part of everyday life in any organization or workplace; every relationship has within it the elements of potential conflict. People often avoid conflicts because emotions run high, egos respond defensively to attack, people feel hurt, and solutions seem elusive and difficult to reach.

The Positive Side of Conflict

When we consider conflict a normal part of the environment, it takes on a more positive aspect. Gutbezahl (2010) identifies two types of conflict. Relationship conflict, which is often based in dislike and distrust, is negative. However, task or cognitive conflict "originates from differences in perspective about how to perform a task. Studies show that groups that generate task conflict and manage it well perform better than do groups that have little task conflict" (para. 4). Organization development literature reports widely the stages of team development, noting that teams go through a normal stage of development called storming in which the predominant characteristic is conflict. Members argue about everything, disagree with the team leader and each other, and resist even good ideas. Healthy teams learn how to resolve conflict from these experiences as they work out these issues together. The team becomes stronger by addressing differences and conflicts rather than avoiding or ignoring them. What is true for teams is also true for individuals. Too many people believe that avoidance is the best approach for dealing with conflict, but all it does is delay the inevitable: the need to deal with the conflict. The best relationships and the best teams are those who have found effective ways to respond when conflict arises. In fact, task conflict unresolved often deteriorates into the more detrimental relationship conflict with its strong emotional component.

Conflict can serve as a positive, driving force for change and improvement. It often exposes true feelings, which leads to a better frame of mind and increases the likelihood that resolution will occur. When one party shares honest feelings, the others understand how strongly that individual feels. Open conflict can save time in an organization because excessive politeness and courtesy may mean that the parties accomplish nothing. Conflict over procedures, policies, or systems in place forces examination of the status quo. Conflict helps us identify our boundaries more clearly. We usually experience conflict when someone has impinged on something important to us. Maybe something needs to change in order to prevent a serious problem later. An honest dispute often engenders a greater mutual respect among individuals and a clearer understanding of the positions of both sides. Seeing others disagree and work out conflicts encourages the more timid to express their opinions, which they might otherwise have never shared.

The benefits of open conflict were demonstrated clearly by a clinical information systems team in a midsize hospital in the South. For the first six months, the team members worked beautifully together, becoming a strong team and establishing their purpose and working approaches. At this point, however, a major conflict about working approaches erupted during a team meeting in which the external leader was not present. The team had agreed on a specific procedure for documenting help calls it received from customers that would allow the team to measure outcomes and evaluate their service. One team member, the clinical laboratory's computer systems person, continued to document her help calls in the manner she had been accustomed to prior to the team's formation, thus creating problems for the team in tracking their outcomes.

When the rest of the team discovered this, open conflict exploded between this individual and other members; the team spent the entire meeting trying to work through this issue. Weeks later they still expressed negative feelings about the conflict and believed that they should have handled the situation better. In exploring these feelings, the leader asked the team to identify what they had learned from the situation. They came up with thirteen specific positive learnings about either how they had handled the conflict or what they had learned from the experience. This discussion immediately shifted their perception from "conflict is bad" to "conflict can help us grow." The leader's perception of conflict influences how others see it. Recognizing a positive side to conflict conveys an important message.

The Leadership Role

Joni and Beyer (2009) write about how to pick a good fight. They believe that strong leaders may actually create conflict because it can lead to increased creativity and innovation. This is more likely task or cognitive conflict. They identify three characteristics that a leader can evaluate to determine whether a conflict is healthy. The first is that the stakes have to be high enough to motivate those involved. This is based on the belief that no matter how conflict averse some people are, most are willing to really fight for something they believe in. Joni and Beyer say "a fight is material if it creates lasting value, leads to a noticeable and sustainable improvement, and addresses a complex challenge that has no easy answers" (p. 50). The second characteristic is that the fight is future facing rather than focusing on the past, affixing blame, and dissecting causes leading to the conflict. "A good future-facing fight has three qualities. It speaks to what is possible, shifting the debate away from what happened to what could happen. It is compelling, focusing people on real, achievable benefits . . . and it involves uncertainty, because if things are certain, there's no need to fight" (Joni and Beyer, 2009, p. 52). And the final characteristic is that the conflict needs to be about something that makes a true difference: a noble purpose. These are the conflicts that produce most of the positive benefits of conflict already presented.

Relationship conflict can result in negative outcomes. However, when it is handled appropriately, positive benefits can result. In organizations that empower employees, those employees assume responsibility for having healthy relationships with others in the workplace, which means being responsible for effective resolution of conflicts. In organizations with teams, team members are responsible for resolving conflicts that occur. In both instances, however, employees need a leader to coach them as they learn these skills and, at times, to serve as mediator. The leader's role is to develop others in their conflict resolution skills and intervene only as necessary. The leader carefully assesses the situation and does not hesitate to intervene when the situation requires the use of the manager's legitimate authority, such as in cases of bullying. Employees can be taught skills to deal with bullying behavior; however, extreme examples may require intervention from management and even human resource staff.

Ineffective Methods of Conflict Resolution

Some methods of conflict resolution are ineffective. These strategies may seem effective over the short term, but because the solution is not mutually beneficial to the involved parties, not all are committed to supporting the solution. The following strategies may appear to solve the conflict but instead produce frustration, distrust, and a feeling of being treated unfairly:

- Competition
- Coercion
- Intimidation and dominance
- Persuasion
- Procrastination and avoidance
- Coalition building
- Accommodation

Competition

Competing is an ineffective strategy for resolving conflict because it encourages a scarcity mind-set in which there is never enough (time, resources, money) to go around. It creates a win-lose rather than a win-win situation. The parties do not even consider sharing for mutual benefit when they are pitted against each other because for one to win, the other must lose.

Coercion

Either overt or covert coercion may seem to settle the matter quickly but actually results in resentment. Leaders must be careful when they are serving as mediators not to use coercion. Because the manager has legitimate authority, his or her expression of an opinion can feel like coercion to others. This legitimate authority can give unfair weight to the manager's opinion. Coercion can also occur among peers. One individual may feel coerced into accepting a disagreeable point of view in the interest of preserving harmony within the group. More tenured staff may intimidate and coerce those with less tenure. A physician's voice may carry more weight than the staff member's.

Intimidation and Dominance

Similar to coercion, intimidation and dominance are pressure tactics based on power relationships. In the short term, they may seem to be effective, but many people find them distasteful. Intimidation and dominance can destroy trust in a relationship because of the use of unfair advantage.

Persuasion

Persuasion is a strategy that articulate, charismatic people commonly use. The problem with persuasion is that the persuader ends up psychologically superior to the persuaded individual. When an individual uses persuasion, keeping people focused on the solution becomes more and more difficult over time. Greater doses of persuasion are needed as people begin thinking for themselves and questioning the solution they were persuaded to accept.

Procrastination and Avoidance

Putting off any real resolution of the disagreement or conflict is the basis of this strategy. It usually causes the conflict to feed on itself and become worse with time. People often use a short delay in dealing with the conflict to see whether it will work itself out. Although this is appropriate and effective in some instances, leaders should use delays in addressing conflict judiciously and not allow them to interfere with effective resolution of the conflict.

Coalition Building

Alliances, in the positive sense, are often needed to get something accomplished. As a means of resolving conflict, however, building coalitions can be negative because people are forced into choosing sides, which increases the likelihood of head-to-head battles. Unfortunately, this is one of the more common approaches to resolving conflict in health care today. Employees who feel unable to obtain what they need through their own efforts talk to physicians in an attempt to engage them in the cause. Department managers in conflict with one another often talk to other managers in an attempt to build support for their positions. Some view this as an effective executive strategy: getting all their ducks in a row before a key meeting. Purposely talking with others to bring them to a certain point of view is building a coalition, which may work well when the group is planning or making a decision. But it is ineffective over the long haul in resolving active conflict.

Accommodation

Accommodation as a strategy is helpful at times but easy to overuse. It means that one party is giving up its rights or desires and allowing the other's rights or desires to take precedence. In some instances, this may be appropriate in order to benefit the whole. One problem with accommodation is that the same individual or group tends to allow this and eventually grows to resent the situation. Accommodation can result in perceptions of uneven status and foster long-term resentments. Individuals who usually seek harmony may begin to feel that others are taking advantage of them.

Effective Methods of Conflict Resolution

Although in the real world a perfect solution to conflict simply does not exist, parties in conflict can turn to several potentially effective strategies. These enable them to deal with the conflict in an open, positive manner while limiting the negative impact of the conflict. These are effective methods of resolution:

- Appeal
- Mediation
- Superordinate goals
- Peaceful coexistence
- Negotiation

Appeal

This strategy allows any party to take a decision to a higher level or to someone who is not emotionally or directly involved with the situation. Appeal is powerful because when both parties in a conflict realize that they can appeal a decision, it inspires them to seek resolution more honestly. The grievance procedure that exists in most organizations is a good example of an appeal process. However, a team or individuals can use it more informally by simply agreeing to take the decision to an uninvolved third party for a decision. When using the appeal, both parties must agree to support the third party's decision.

Mediation

Mediation, in contrast, requires the involvement of a knowledgeable and trusted third party to act as an intermediary for all involved in the conflict. The mediator's objective viewpoint can often diffuse emotions and serve as a catalyst to reach a mutually agreeable solution. When the leader serves as a coach or facilitator for conflicting parties in a conflict, this is an example of mediation. In some instances, each party has its own coach.

Superordinate Goals

Finding a goal that transcends the special interests of both parties is an excellent strategy for resolving conflict. This is a superordinate goal, which leaders use frequently, perhaps without even realizing it. Asking people to forgo minor differences and stay focused on the overriding purpose and goal is an example of this approach. The urgent deadlines and immense challenges facing a work group often pull them together and facilitate the speedy resolution of conflicts that arise.

Peaceful Coexistence

This strategy is useful in situations when the parties in conflict can stay on their side of the fence without negative impact. If two employees, for instance, find each other abrasive, they can still agree to work together peacefully if there is some separation, such as working on different shifts or in different departments or not having a significant amount of interdependent work to do. The leader gets the involved parties to agree to the old adage, "I don't have to like you to work well with you." This approach works only if the parties establish clear expectations and agree to work within them. This approach puts more onus on the manager, who must be vigilant that these attitudes have not affected the work group's effectiveness and productivity.

Negotiation

Negotiation is a process of mutual agreement based on a win-win problem-solving approach, in which no one involved has to give up anything that is essential to him or her. It thus takes place with a spirit of cooperation rather than conflict. It is the most powerful strategy for conflict resolution because in any work situation, the parties involved are likely to interact with each other over the long term. If they find win-win solutions, each will be committed to supporting these decisions. If they instead try one of the ineffective strategies, such as coercion, a subsequent conflict among the same people will be much more difficult to resolve. The party who lost in the first round is likely to be waiting for the next opportunity to get even.

Nierenberg and Ross (1985) outline a specific process for negotiating that they refer to as a negotiation map (see Figure 5.1):

1. Define the issue.

2. Clarify objectives.

3. Gather all relevant information.

4. Identify alternatives.

5. Select strategies.

Step One: Define the Issue   The need to define the real issues in a negotiation may seem self-evident, but a good negotiator makes no assumptions. For example, when a team and manager are experiencing conflict about a decision that the manager has made, the real issue may not be the outcome or decision but the fact that the manager made the decision rather than allowing the team to do so within clearly identified parameters. These are two very different issues; the real issue that is being negotiated is the team's decision-making authority.

The first step is to determine that both sides of the dispute share an understanding of the issue. This requires honesty and the ability and willingness to disclose hidden agendas. Both parties must trust each other enough to share information openly, without fearing that the other party will use the

Figure 5.1 The Negotiation

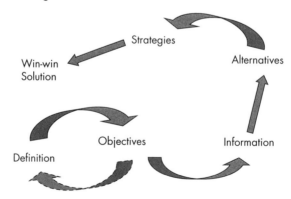

information in an adversarial manner. Hidden agendas and personal issues can destroy individuals' ability to negotiate effectively.

One newly formed senior leadership team was in the process of negotiating its members' assignments when a hidden agenda blocked their progress. Following a major restructuring of executive ranks, five new executives had been appointed but were not yet assigned to specific services. In a meeting to determine division of responsibility, one of the new team members, Lynette, was operating with a hidden agenda: she did not want to be assigned to the ambulatory services. Throughout the discussion, every comment and suggestion she made was based on her desire to avoiding taking an assignment to ambulatory services rather than focusing on what was best for the organization. The meeting ended in a stalemate with Lynette in tears. Her teammates were flabbergasted because the decision was not emotional in nature for them and they were not sure what was happening. The team decided to think about the possibilities over the weekend and return on Monday to discuss the issue further prior to making a decision.

When the facilitator talked with Lynette and discovered the important personal agenda she was keeping hidden, she advised Lynette to be open with her teammates and share her strong feelings. When she did so, the team was able to rapidly reach a decision that was good for both the organization and each team member. A major decision-making criterion for the group became that no one had to take his or her least-liked area.

Step Two: Clarify Objectives   In this second step on the map, each party determines what it desires. This sounds somewhat simplistic, but people often limit themselves by limiting their objectives. Thinking broadly about objectives may extend the possibilities available to consider in negotiation. Each side in fact may have a range of objectives that would be satisfactory.

An example of this step arose during the annual performance appraisal of an excellent department secretary in a home health agency. Renee was a superbly skilled secretary but functioned more as a direct assistant to the administrator of a special program. During her annual review, she requested a promotion to an executive assistant position. The manager knew this was impossible in the current setting because the agency's structure allowed only one executive assistant position. In talking with Renee, the manager asked why she was interested in the promotion. What was important to her? The title? The increase in pay? The type of work included in the job? Renee's response was interesting: she had noticed that the executive assistant was the only secretarial or clerical person who attended an annual workshop at the company's expense. Renee valued continuing education and wanted the same opportunity. Fortunately, this was something that the manager could provide, so once they had identified this objective, they easily achieved a win-win solution.

Once the objectives are identified, there may be a need to go back to step one and make certain that the subject to be negotiated is correctly identified. In some instances, this second step forces clarity that may not be there initially.

Step Three: Gather All Relevant Information   This step encompasses gathering relevant facts, identifying operative assumptions, and determining the needs of the involved parties. Facts are important because they determine how negotiable certain positions are. The more facts the parties share, often the more successful the negotiation is. Checking out the assumptions of all parties is absolutely critical because people often make decisions based more on assumptions than on facts. When both parties share openly before and during an active negotiation what they need, the likelihood of a successful win-win negotiation increases. Parties should not confuse priority needs with peripheral needs. For negotiation to have lasting results, both parties must have their priority needs satisfied so that each has a stake in the continued success of the solution.

When a physician asked a laboratory manager to have lab results available for early morning rounds, she discovered that to draw the lab specimens early enough, patients would have to be awakened before 4:00 A.M. Most patients would be highly dissatisfied by this early awakening. Furthermore, although the physician had made it sound as if was important to many of the physicians, investigation revealed that only one or two other physicians had been involved in the request. Another false assumption was the physicians' belief that this request would have no effect on the budget. Also, in terms of needs, it initially appeared to require a major shift in the laboratory employees' schedule. But the manager checked the facts and discovered that the physicians really were requesting this because of a problem on Sundays, when the physicians involved wanted to attend early church services and therefore to make rounds earlier than usual.

Step Four: Identify Alternatives   In this step, the parties consider all possible alternatives. As when identifying objectives, widening the range of possibilities makes finding a mutually acceptable solution more likely. After brainstorming to uncover all options from both parties, it is appropriate to begin to whittle them down to acceptable alternatives.

In the previous example of the lab manager and the physicians who requested earlier lab reports, the parties considered numerous ideas. Was there a technological fix? Was the lab already considering newer, faster equipment? Could floor or lab employees change schedules easily enough? Was no change actually best for all involved? Could lab services be decentralized or redeployed to smaller, more local labs nearer the patient units or to phlebotomists assigned to the patient care unit?

From the list of possible alternatives, the parties should generate at least two, and preferably three, reasonable alternatives. Locking on to only one acceptable alternative can be a trap in negotiation because it results in an ultimatum. Multiple alternatives allow for true choice.

Step Five: Select Strategies   Once you have identified acceptable alternatives, determine the action to take. Strategies are the actions to be taken both during and after the negotiation and include the type of climate to set for an effective negotiation. Climate should be fluid and dynamic in every negotiation. Nierenberg and Ross (1985) believe that the party controlling the climate has more influence over the negotiation and that the other party generally accepts positive climates and resists negative climates.

The lab manager in the previous example thought through the information she had and how to present it to the physicians. Part of her strategy might have been to discuss their needs more fully and share the assumptions she discovered. Sharing the facts she had collected might have helped appeal to the physicians' logic and critical thinking abilities. She also considered strategies for establishing a positive climate. Would the discussion take place in her office, the physician's office, or a hospital conference room?

This negotiation map works best when it is treated as a dynamic process. To prepare for a negotiation, each individual works through the map first from his or her own perspective and then from the other party's perspective. The most effective negotiators are those who are clear about their own positions, not overly accommodating, yet flexible when the other party has a valid point. Parties most easily assume this role when they have fully considered each step of the negotiation process. Clear expectations between the parties for obtaining a win-win situation can result in effective negotiation. In a clear example of this, organizations were attempting to negotiate a multisystem integration. The law firms for the parties involved were told they must find a win-win solution. This powerful message clearly avoided the development of adversarial posturing and positioning. This process helps prepare for actually negotiating the win-win solution.

Pitfalls of Conflict Resolution

The most common pitfall related to conflict resolution is a tendency to avoid dealing with the conflict. Although few people approach a conflict situation with enthusiasm, some individuals abhor conflict of any kind and thus greatly reduce their effectiveness because they won't deal with it or become immobilized in the face of it. Modeling this behavior as a leader sends the wrong message to followers, who will think, *If the leader cannot effectively deal with conflict, why should we bother?*

The experience of one health care entrepreneur is a good example of this pitfall. A visionary head of his company, Bob had attained great success in spite of an inability to deal with conflict. In his organization, he had retained several costly employees who consistently underperformed, yet he dreaded addressing their performance issues. Not only did they contribute significantly to a high overhead, but the company had lost several excellent performers who were not willing to continue to work hard to create revenue to cover the nonperformers' salaries.

Bob worked diligently to expand the company's services, and one strategy was to partner with other companies. These relationships began with great enthusiasm and high hopes, but at the first sign of any conflict (and what relationship is without it?), Bob would withdraw his support and sever the relationship. Needless to say, the company's reputation began to deteriorate. The source of all of these problems was Bob's intense discomfort with conflict and his inability to deal with it effectively.

A second common pitfall exists when a leader is so emotionally attached to an outcome that objectively identifying possible alternatives becomes difficult or impossible. Too often these situations reach an impasse, at which point one party delivers an ultimatum—rarely, if ever, a healthy way to resolve conflict. A midsize hospital in the Southwest averted such an impasse. Liz, the vice president of patient services, had the explicit trust of John, the CEO to whom she had reported for years. John supported her decisions and valued her judgment. On this occasion, a recruiting process for a new director of perioperative services was under way. Liz saw no viable internal candidates, and recruiting efforts had brought forth only two external possibilities. Suddenly a couple of the anesthesiologists decided they would recommend one of the operating room staff nurses for promotion. The suggestion fell on deaf ears: Liz felt the individual was not qualified for this promotion for a number of valid reasons. When the physicians were unable to achieve their goal through Liz, they descended on John's office. Although John sent the physicians back to Liz, he also talked to Liz directly about the recommendation and came very close to telling her to hire the internal candidate. Although Liz did not tell him directly at this point, her immediate response was concern that if John told her she must hire this internal candidate, Liz felt she would have to resign. She did not believe she could continue in her position if John interfered in such a way with her authority.

After discussing the situation with an objective and trusted colleague, Liz identified several alternatives that helped prevent the situation from escalating into an out-and-out conflict based on ultimatums delivered. Liz set up an interview process that included employees, other managers, surgeons, and anesthesiologists. They identified selection criteria ahead of time, and interviewers evaluated each candidate for the position against these measures.

As a result, the anesthesiologists realized for themselves the limitations of the internal candidate they were promoting.

The final major pitfall with significant consequences is seeing conflict only in a negative light. This creates an organizational culture in which people do not express disagreements openly because of fear that they may damage a relationship; employees repress conflicts; and people do not express their honest reactions to ideas or events because of possible repercussions. When this is the organizational culture, managers and leaders have little experience using the effective methods of conflict resolution because they view conflict as something to avoid at all costs.

This described the organizational culture in one eastern seaboard medical center that was part of a large system. One of the system's four hospitals underwent a major work redesign initiative. Planning took two years, with employees and key stakeholders heavily involved. Implementation of the new design began on the first two patient care units and, as is normal during major change, multiple conflicts arose. Implementation did not proceed as smoothly as anticipated, and physician and patient complaints increased. Some saw the conflicts as a sign that the change was not working, and the chief operating officer pulled the plug on the entire project. Years of work and hundreds of thousands of dollars were lost because the conflict was interpreted as failure rather than a normal step along the process. The impact on leadership credibility in the organization was profound.

Facilitating conflict resolution is probably one of the biggest challenges that leaders today face. It occurs at every level in the organization and with increasing frequency. Developing effective skills in this area has a direct impact on the leader's effectiveness.

Creating Teams

Creating and developing high-performance teams is another key process that today's leaders must master in order to be effective. "Teams make sense in today's world for many reasons: the increasing complexity of our work; the changing values of the workforce; the increasing need for immediate organizational response to difficult external marketplace changes and internal challenges;

and our desire to create a healthy, satisfying workplace for employees" (Manion, 1997, p. 31). Exemplary leaders understand the concept of the team and determine when a team can do a better job than an individual. Even more important, effective leaders have the skills to facilitate a team's development. "Health care is a team sport, but all too often practitioners act as individual players" (Weinstock, 2010, para. 1). Studies from the Joint Commission, Veterans Health Administration, and others all cite poor communication and lack of teamwork among caregivers as one of the top causes of medical errors and near misses.

Defining Team

Team and *teamwork* are terms that people often confuse and use as synonyms, but they are two different concepts. The word *team* is overused today, loosely applied to exhort others to perform in a particular manner, usually through teamwork. Teamwork is a way of working together, and it may mean different things to different people. For most, it implies cooperation, open communication, and pitching in to help each other out. A team, in contrast, is a structural unit—a group of people designed and drawn together to complete certain prescribed work. How team members carry out the work can be described as teamwork. As adapted from Katzenbach and Smith's definition in *The Wisdom of Teams* (1993), a team is "a small number of consistent people with a relevant, shared purpose, common performance goals, complementary and overlapping skills, and a common approach to its collective work. Team members hold themselves mutually accountable for the team's results and outcomes" (Manion, 1997, p. 31).

Types of Teams

Organizations today have several types of teams:

- Primary work teams
- Ad hoc teams
- Leadership teams

Primary work teams are permanent structures organized around a department's primary work. In a business office, the teams may be organized around business functions, such as credit verification, billings, and collections. Teams in a patient care department are organized around patient care. And teams in a clinical laboratory are often designed around specialized functions, such as microbiology, hematology, and chemistry. The emergency department may have a trauma team or urgent care team. In the perioperative services, there are many specialized teams such as the cardiovascular, orthopedics, or eye teams. These work teams are sometimes described more loosely as those doing the day-to-day work of the department (Kalisch and Begeny, 2005).

Ad hoc teams are temporary teams created to perform a particular piece of work; after the work is completed, the team is dissolved. Quality or continuous process improvement and project teams are good examples of ad hoc teams, which can last for years and yet not be considered part of an organization's permanent structure.

Leadership teams are formed to provide collective leadership for a project or initiative, department, service, or organization.

Distinguishing Between Teams and Work Groups

Grasping the distinction between a good work group and a true team eludes many people. The transformational leader is clear about the differences and as a result is able to capitalize on the tremendous energy and passion that exist within a true team. Katzenbach and Smith (1993) take great care in distinguishing between the two. A work group is often a cluster of people who come together to coordinate, communicate, and cooperate but less often do any shared work that is capable of impelling the organization to excellence. A good work group has a strong and clearly focused leader, and each member of the group is responsible for his or her individual work products and usually accountable to the leader. The primary contract exists between the group member and the leader who is often a manager or person with a higher position in the hierarchy. There is often good discussion, but the actual work of the team is done elsewhere. The group measures its effectiveness based on the ability of members to do their individual work more effectively.

A true team goes well beyond coordinating and communicating. Some piece of work (a plan, development of strategies, decision making) is accomplished together by the members. Leadership is shared. The same person may not always lead the meetings and leadership for key projects and initiatives is rotated. Furthermore, who takes the lead for a particular strategy is decided by the team rather than based simply on positional status or specialized expertise.

Probably the biggest difference between a work group and a true team lies in the area of accountability. In a true team, members are accountable to each other rather than primarily to the leader. Added to the already present individual accountability of each member, there is also a high level of shared accountability for team outcomes. If one team member is having difficulty, it affects everyone because the team shares ownership of issues and problems.

Much of the biomedical engineering department's work, for example, is individual work. If the clinical laboratory calls because of a problem with a piece of equipment, one of the biomed engineers takes the call, does an assessment, takes needed action, and is responsible for the outcomes. At a department meeting, there may be discussion of common issues, information shared, evaluation of work assignments, and other steps taken to deal with the day-to-day functioning of the department. This has the earmark of a good work group.

If the biomed employees are functioning as a team, the day-to-day work may be similarly accomplished by individuals. However, these staff members may function as a team within the department if they share accountability for meeting expected outcomes of their function. Their shared work may include developing a strategic plan for meeting the biomedical needs of the system, including all locations, reviewing and disseminating critical information about new regulatory demands or requirements, planning a strategy for accomplishing necessary preventative maintenance work, and determining their goals in alignment with the organizational cultural initiative of service excellence.

Essential Elements of a Team

Leaders today may need to create a team for a specific purpose (such as sharing the leadership function for the department) or may redesign the work flow in their department into one based on teams. Teams outperform individuals when systems issues require multiple approaches, a variety of experiences, and diverse thinking patterns. Regardless of the type of team, there are concrete steps to use in creating an effective team.

Step One: Define the Work

Prior to selecting team members, the leader must define the work he or she expects of the team and then delineate what the team is expected to do by considering certain questions:

- What is the primary work this team is to accomplish?
- Is this a process improvement team focusing on a specific issue or a project team formed to design and implement a new service or system?
- Is this an employee council for making decisions that affect professional practice?
- Is the team's work to provide collective leadership for the department or for the organization?
- What will be required of this team? Will systems thinking be required to challenge mental models and initiate breakthrough thinking?
- What are the general goals and objectives of this group?

This step forces the leader to be clear about the reasons for initiating a team.

Step Two: Select Members

Based on the work the team is to do, potential members are identified and then selected based on their potential contribution to the team's work. The team member may represent a particular segment of the system (such as a department or function) or have certain skills that the team needs. In some cases, it is impossible to obtain all the skills the team needs, and members may be selected for their skills potential. If so, then development of those skills is paramount. Perhaps no one in the organization has exactly the skills needed, but the team can develop those skills through its work. "Having the right team members may also determine the team's ability to overcome barriers encountered when developing or executing the project" (Weaver, 2008, p. 109).

Go widely to find the right people for the team and be ruthlessly honest about what team members are good at and what they aren't. "When putting together a team, I make sure it's spiky. And when people complain that their differences will cause problems I'll bluntly disagree" (Bürkner, 2007, p. 21). When Bürkner gets push-back about who he's selected for his teams because of the diversity, he tells the team leader, "Find out what he's best at, and show his strength to the team" (p. 21).

Edmondson, Bohmer, and Pisano (2001) found that the way teams were put together and how they drew on their experiences greatly influenced the team's success at learning. In their article on speeding up the team's learning, they found that improvements in the team's performance were directly related to their ability to adapt to a new way of working. Most teams become proficient over time and execute existing processes efficiently. However, when it comes to implementing new processes, they have far more difficulty. Cardiovascular surgical teams were studied, and several factors were directly related to their ability to learn quickly. The first factor was selecting the team members. The choices made were deliberate and intentional; members were selected because they had certain characteristics, not simply because they were available. During the learning process, the team membership was kept consistent; no substitutions were allowed. This reemphasizes the need to select the right members.

The most effective teams are those with a small number of consistent team members. Teams of more than twelve members run into more logistical problems than do smaller teams. In larger groups, members too easily disengage and remain anonymous, and finding a common time to meet is more problematic. Consistency of membership is critical. Frequent changes in team membership have a negative effect on the group's synergy and the quality of work that team members complete. When team members leave and are replaced, the team usually regresses in its effectiveness until the new member is brought up to speed and fully assimilated into the group. Consistency of membership also refers to consistent attendance at team meetings. Frequent absenteeism also stalls the team's ability to produce high-quality outcomes.

Step Three: Define the Team Purpose

When the team comes together for the first time, its initial work is to define its purpose. Although the leader may have given the group some preliminary direction (based on his or her thoughts from step one), it is critical that the team develops its own mission or purpose statement. This describes what the team does and for whom and clarifies the reason for the team's existence. Teams that are handed a completed purpose statement or are simply told by the leader why they exist never develop the same level of ownership as teams that take the time to reflect and do this work. If the team is given a mission statement describing its work, one way to ensure relevancy and identification with this purpose is to have the team modify it to fit its beliefs. Even small modifications increase team members' feeling of ownership. Team members simply do not engage with the work if they do not find the team's purpose relevant. "*Meaning* and *motivation* are derived from an understanding on the part of the team of its mission, and the vision" (Porter-O'Grady, Alexander, Blaylock, Minkara, and Surel, 2006, p. 215).

It is important for the leader to stay actively involved with the team during development of this mission statement in order to prevent the team from heading in the wrong direction. The team's purpose must also be congruent with the organization or department purpose. If the two are incongruent, the team is headed for trouble. An actively participating leader does not mandate the team's purpose but is involved in guiding and setting the general direction.

Step Four: Establish Common Working Approaches

Once the team is clear about its mission and reason for existence, the next step is to determine and agree on the approaches it plans to use in doing its work. "A common approach means that team members discuss, delineate, and agree on ways they are going to work together to accomplish their purpose. Common refers to the collective effort that is required, not an approach that is ordinary or average. There is nothing common nor ordinary about a highly effective team" (Manion, Lorimer, and Leander, 1996, p. 64).

Some examples of early decisions to make about working approaches include the following:

- *Logistics of team meetings.* How often will the team meet? When will it meet? Where? Will an agenda be circulated? How is the agenda developed? Who facilitates the meeting? Will minutes be needed? If so, who will take them?

- *Methods for communicating.* This includes both formal and informal methods of communicating. Is there a need for frequent team huddles? Are team members readily accessible to each other? Do they need to be? How will they communicate between meetings?

- *Problem-solving approaches.* How will the team tackle problems? Is there a specific process improvement methodology to follow?

- *Decision making.* What types of decisions will the team make? What are the boundaries in regard to the team's work? Which will be individual decisions, and which should the entire team make? Will the team make decisions by majority vote or by consensus? When will a subset of the team be authorized to make decisions instead?

- *Doing the work.* Are there certain processes and approaches the team agrees to do a certain way? Does there need to be consistency in practices? (In the conflict resolution section earlier in this chapter, the clinical information team that agreed on how to record the help calls that members received is an example.)

The team also needs to discuss members' roles and responsibilities. Do team members need to fill specific roles to ensure that work is completed—for example, a meeting coordinator or a facilitator and process person? Some teams identify a celebrations role to ensure that the team recognizes and cheers key events and accomplishments. If there are any needed roles, the team must define specific responsibilities of each role clearly. Some teams identify the role of challenger: "the team member who openly questions the goals, methods, and the ethics of the team, who is willing to disagree with the team leader, and who encourages the team to take well-considered risks" (Parker, 1997, p. 8). This role is critical for most teams because the challenger is honest in reporting team progress and identifying problems.

This individual, however, backs off and actively supports consensus within the team if the team does not accept his or her views. In other words, this person is not always in an adversarial role. Another common role is the team recorder, who generates the minutes of meetings and circulates them; this is often a rotating responsibility.

The final components of establishing common working approaches are the discussion of and agreement on what team members expect of one another. Identifying and articulating behavioral expectations are key steps early in team formation for several reasons. These expectations lay the foundation for the development of trust within the team. In addition, being clear about the expectations one holds of others is instrumental in preventing unnecessary conflicts. Too often people do not meet others' expectations because they did not know the expectations even existed. The group discusses what members expect or need from one another in order to do a good job. This often includes expectations for appropriate meeting participation, communication techniques, and acceptable team behavior. The following example from a real team demonstrates expectations related to these areas:

> We expect team members to:
>
> - Be on time and prepared for meetings and to fully participate as evidenced by an attentive attitude, asking clarifying questions, and remaining open-minded about the contributions of other team members
> - Communicate openly, honestly, and directly with each other, especially if we fail to meet each other's expectations
> - Work toward the goals of the team and support the success of the team first and individual work second
> - Stay focused on our goals and complete tasks and projects within agreed-on time frames (communicating any unavoidable delays to other team members as soon as possible)

Clear expectations help formalize the team's norms, one of the first steps in building and creating the team's emotional intelligence (Cherniss and Goleman, 2001). Being willing to address another team member's failure to live up to established norms and expectations is a crucial sign of the team's emotional intelligence. Fear of conflict and confrontation is a common dysfunction of ineffective teams. Seen as accountability, team members' willingness to call their peers on performance or behaviors that might hurt the team and its performance is essential for effective functioning (Lencioni, 2002).

Step Five: Specify Performance Goals

Closely related to the team mission are the team's performance goals. Larson and LaFasto (1989) examined high-performing teams and found, without exception, that these teams had clearly identified performance objectives and goals. These can also serve as a measurement of the team's outcomes, giving a team the ability to hold itself accountable.

Team goals are distinguished from system, organizational, or department goals. "Teams take broad objectives or directives from the organization's management and shape them into specific, measurable goals for the team. Specific goals are stated in concrete terms so that it is unequivocally possible to tell whether or not they have been met" (Manion, Lorimer, and Leander, 1996, p. 63). The most powerful goals provide for small wins along the way, and these intermediate victories serve to motivate and reinforce the team's direction along its chosen path.

Motivating goals are often those with stretch, forcing the team to extend itself and reach beyond what it had previously dreamed of. These ambitious goals produce momentum, growth, and commitment within the team. "Teams that face a significant challenge, or that develop their own ambitious goals, have a greater sense of urgency that forces them to focus their efforts in a unified direction. . . . The true strength of a team is realized when it faces and overcomes seemingly unbreachable obstacles to attain a worthy goal" (Manion, Lorimer, and Leander, 1996, p. 63).

Step Six: Hold the Team Accountable

A final and essential step is to hold the team accountable for its outcomes. This is a constant process of reviewing outcomes and determining whether the team has met established standards and obtained expected outcomes. If the team has not obtained desired outcomes, it evaluates its process and its work to determine what went wrong and then takes corrective action.

"Mutual accountability differentiates a real team from a working group. In both teams and working groups, individuals hold themselves accountable for the outcomes of their assignments. A team, however, takes the next step—members hold themselves mutually accountable for the team's outcomes or results. They continuously measure themselves against their established goals and objectives" (Manion, Lorimer, and Leander, 1996, p. 77). The team reviews its decisions for effectiveness and its processes for beneficial outcomes. All team members are equally accountable for the team's outcomes.

These six steps provide guidance for the leader who is establishing a team. However, presenting this process as linear makes it seem overly simplistic. These six steps serve to describe the underlying structure of an effective team. However, the truth is that the process unfolds in a much more nonlinear fashion with all of these essential elements important and crucial, yet continually interacting in a completely dynamic fashion. Step six, holding the team accountable, is an essential element of a high-performing team. However, accountability is an element that must exist throughout the development process, not just at the end when everything else seems to be in place. The team holds itself accountable for clarity of purpose and serving its true mission. Team members hold each other accountable for the expectations and common approaches on which they have agreed. And so it is true for each of these steps. Although it makes sense to consider these sequential steps, it oversimplifies the process.

The leader's involvement with different types of teams in the organization depends a great deal on the leader's placement in the organizational hierarchy, the culture of the system, and the leader's span of control. At the very least, every leader would do well to exercise the option of developing a leadership team that serves to provide collective leadership within their span of control. These teams can be the most difficult to guide to their fullest potential for a variety of reasons. The primary reasons are a lack of understanding of what collective leadership really means and an unwillingness, either conscious or subconscious, to disseminate power and control.

Leadership Teams

Leaders who are serious about developing colleagues and creating a strong foundation for shared leadership within their span of control will consider formalizing a leadership team structure. Composition of a leadership team varies widely. If the leader is a department manager, the team may be a small group of assistant managers or selected employees who work with the manager to provide the department's leadership function. For example, in the laboratory, the leadership team could include the manager, the supervisors of the different functions (chemistry, blood bank, hematology, and so on), and perhaps the employee responsible for quality improvement processes or the person who leads the employee governance council. In a patient care department for inpatients, the leadership team could consist of assistant nurse managers or charge nurses, the department educator, and the manager. If there is a unit-based shared governance structure, the chairperson of the unit council may serve on the department's leadership team. The team's purpose, rather than a particular formal title, determines the membership. In some instances, a member of an off-site facility or another shift may be an appropriate team member.

Creating a leadership team within his or her scope of responsibility is a way for the leader to broaden and deepen the area's leadership capacity as the members of the team are introduced to broader ways of thinking and considering issues and involved in more complex and far-reaching issues. A highly functioning leadership team can also serve as a foundation of the department or organization's succession plan. "As emerging leaders work together in a leadership team, they are learning skills and developing capabilities that will serve them well as they progress in their careers" (Manion, 2009b, p. 208). The team environment and the member's involvement offer an opportunity for assessment of the individual members and their leadership potential.

A leadership team offers many other benefits. It can serve as a tremendous source of support for the manager, who may otherwise feel alone in shouldering the tremendous burden of responsibility for everything related to his or her area of responsibility. A team that becomes an effective decision-making unit improves leadership thinking and effectiveness. Commitment to decisions made is stronger because of group ownership and accountability. It can also free up the manager to learn other skills and take a more strategic approach to focusing on the issues and challenges of the department or service.

The toughest hurdle for any leadership team is to truly understand the concept of shared or collective leadership. Jim Collins, in his seminal work *Good to Great* (2001), studied the differences between organizations that were good and those that became great. In 2005, he released *Good to Great and the Social Sectors* that added his most current thinking on their earlier findings. He notes that leadership in business and industry is quite different from that seen in the social sector, specifically in health care. Social sector leaders face a diffuse and complex power map without concentrated decision-making authority. He refers to this type of leadership as "legislative leadership." It's the type of leadership in play when no one has the necessary authority or enough structural power to make the decisions alone. The conclusion is that it is virtually impossible to be an effective health care leader without the ability to actualize collective or shared leadership.

Shared or collective leadership is a major shift for most formal leaders in organizations. Their promotions in the past have been based on personal characteristics, individual competencies, and leadership capacity. To become part of a collective entity and "give themselves up to the team" can be incredibly difficult. They are used to being in charge, making the decisions, and being responsible. However, the primary purpose of a leadership team is to collectively lead an area of responsibility. And there will be times when an individual member will need to support the collective decision of the team. On the plus side is the tremendous support that team members provide for each other as they carry out their responsibilities.

Pitfalls of Creating Teams

Using a team should be considered only when the potential benefits are clear. The process is not as easy as it appears.

A common problem with creating an effective team is the inconsistency of membership. Especially in hospitals, scheduling employees for a 24/7 operation means there is little consistency in which team members are present at any given time. This is less of a problem in departments that do not provide employee coverage 24/7. In most departments that provide 24-hour coverage, a variety of shifts are used, resulting in even less consistency of team membership. Research has found that effective teamwork and continuity of patient service is difficult, if not impossible, to achieve under these conditions (Kalisch, Begeny, and Anderson, 2008).

CASE EXAMPLE
A PATIENT SERVICES LEADERSHIP TEAM

A patient services leadership team was created in one midsize community hospital. The members were the directors of the clinical laboratory, medical imaging, respiratory therapy, pharmacy, perioperative services, and the various nursing divisions. They established their structure and began the work of shared leadership for patient care services. Although these people had long worked together, this was a new approach for them.

Ellen, director of the laboratory, agreed to be team leader. One of the biggest challenges facing the team was the need for improving patient satisfaction scores throughout the organization. In the past, this would have been identified as a responsibility of individual directors and managers and mostly in nursing. But because of serious concern about the low satisfaction scores, this team was assigned the leadership responsibility for this initiative. Although their work is only briefly summarized here, their approach illuminates this concept of collective leadership.

One of the strategies they developed was that each team member would accept responsibility to serve as a mentor for the staff in specific in-patient care units. Ellen, as the director of the laboratory, for example, began to serve as a mentor for one particularly challenging patient care unit that was currently without a manager. Patient satisfaction scores had plummeted right along with employee morale. She began rounding in the department, helping staff troubleshoot issues, and coaching them in service recovery when there were problems. The results were quite impressive. Not only did the patient satisfaction scores rise, but employee morale improved dramatically. Ellen's leadership capacity deepened significantly, and she became recognized for attributes that had not been apparent in her work as laboratory director. It was quite remarkable to see the results of this shared accountability.

Often when a team is in trouble, the leader gives a pep talk or brings in a dynamic, charismatic speaker who generates enthusiasm and excitement within the team. But this is a quick fix, and the results never seem to last long enough to get the team through the next crisis. More effective in turning the team around is facing a challenge that creates a sense of urgency. Giving the team a stiff work assignment that its members see as important does more to mobilize stagnated energy and turn it into a productive force than any motivational speech could possibly do.

Not recognizing the special needs and unique challenges based on the type of team is a second common error. Each of the three major types of teams (primary work, ad hoc, and leadership) has unique challenges, and to assume they are all similar is to underestimate the difficulty a particular team may have. For instance, most leadership teams find defining their work and purpose to be problematic. This may seem contradictory because this type of team is composed of leaders who as individuals are usually self-directed and focused clearly on their work. However, most leadership teams confuse their work as a team with the work of the organization as a whole (for example, ensuring the delivery of safe, quality patient care to members of the community versus leading others and creating a positive environment in which employees deliver safe, high-quality patient care to members of the community).

An ad hoc team formed to lead a change initiative often has difficulty in handing off the project to those who will actually implement it (usually managers) because team members feel a large degree of ownership. This is a basic principle of innovation: the people who implement a change are not as attached to the change as are those who create it. We have seen this repeatedly in health care organizations. Quality improvement initiatives and cultural change projects in organizations are often designed by people on project teams who then hand off the implementation to managers who did not have the same investment or interest in the project. In many cases, full conversion and implementation fails because no one anticipated this pitfall. Actions can be taken to overcome this difficulty by involving implementers more fully in the process and providing ongoing support during the implementation.

Understanding the unique challenges of each type of team alerts the leader to potential problems. A more complete discussion of these types of teams is available in *Team-Based Health Care Organizations: Blueprint for Success* (Manion, Lorimer, and Leander, 1996).

Ignoring or not establishing any one of the key elements in creating teams is another major pitfall, but this one is relatively easy to correct. For example, a team that had frequent and recurring problems finally called in an external consultant to help. During this work, the consultant discovered that the team had never established members' expectations of one another or agreed on common working approaches. Simply doing these two things cleared up about 90 percent of the conflicts.

Minimizing the time to develop a team is another common barrier to success. Too many managers and leaders believe that if they simply call a group a team, it somehow becomes one. Not taking the time to apply the proper steps of team development often creates a situation in which the group struggles needlessly, trying its best but unable to determine why it's not being effective. Unless team members come together to accomplish their work collectively, they do not become a team. The most effective teams are those that are emotionally intelligent, able to recognize and process emotion within the group, and regulate themselves in response to daily organizational events. For a team to become emotionally intelligent, it is helpful and perhaps necessary that at least some individual members have a high level of emotional intelligence (Cherniss and Goleman, 2001). However, the mere presence of emotionally intelligent team members does not ensure that the team as an entity will collectively be emotionally intelligent or effective in its performance.

Being able to create high-performing teams is one of the most critical challenges facing leaders today. Virtually every future organizational structure (matrix, network, or clustered organization) is based on the premise that teams are to be a prevalent structure. Leaders must have the ability to tap into and release a team's potential. Being able to create successful learning teams is also a strategy identified as effective in dealing with the complexity of open systems. It increases the likelihood that the organization can respond nimbly to the unfolding challenges it faces.

Facilitating the Processes of Change and Transition

We now turn to the interrelated processes of change and transition, which create significant challenges for leaders. Change today is faster than ever before and promises to continue accelerating well into future decades.

The continual onslaught of technological improvements has altered the very nature of work. Service delivery is rapidly shifting from acute hospital care to ambulatory, home care, and even Internet-based services. Health care services are moving from a residency-based to a mobility-based model (Porter-O'Grady and Malloch, 2003). The rapid rate of mergers and acquisitions in the 1990s resulted in fewer and fewer stand-alone, independent health care organizations and continues today. Solutions are shorter lived. The very changes organizations institute to solve problems today may become tomorrow's problems. Health care reform and new government regulations create great uncertainty for the future. We must realistically view any major change in an organization today as only a stepping-stone to the next change, and these stepping-stones are getting closer and closer together.

Change Versus Transition

Leaders face the challenge of these tumultuous times, and without an understanding of the underlying processes of change and transition, the situation they face could appear hopeless to them. The first step for any leader is to clearly differentiate between change and transition. Change is an external event that causes an alteration or modification in what has previously existed; transition is the internal process that an individual experiences during a psychological adaptation to the change (Bridges, 1991). Transitions take longer than change and may not be evident to others because they are internal. Change is complex, being both a process and an outcome. Leaders effectively lead both.

The Change Process

Research shows that 75 percent of all change initiatives fail. It has been found that managing change often sets up a struggle within leaders between managing business operations and managing the needs of their people (Bunker, 2006). Understanding change as a developmental process aids the leader in recognizing important sequential steps (Cox, Manion, and Miller, 2005; Manion, 1993; Manion, Lorimer, and Leander, 1996). We can differentiate five phases (illustrated in Figure 5.2) based on an energy model adapted for organizations by organization development consultant Nancy Post (1989):

1. Preparation

2. Movement

3. Team creativity

4. New reality

5. Integration

Each of these five phases involves several key issues or concerns. Imbalance is created when a key issue is ignored or passed over or if overemphasis of one issue overshadows the others. Not following the process sequentially results in a prolonged and less effective change process. When a leader understands these five phases and adequately addresses the key issues within each phase, implementing change takes less energy. (This model is explained more fully in Cox, Manion, and Miller, 2005.)

Phase One: Preparation

The two major issues in this phase are setting the direction and allocating resources. Addressing both of these issues during initiation of a change lays the foundation for a successful effort. In their enthusiasm to begin immediately, however, many initiators of change pay only scant attention to this

---

Figure 5.2 The Five Phases of the Change Process

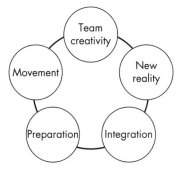

Source: From "Chaos or Transformation" by Jo Manion, © 1993, *Journal of Nursing Administration*. Used by permission of the publisher: Lippincott Williams & Wilkins, Baltimore, MD.

stage. Once the leader shares the direction, it is easy to forget to review available resources and obtain those necessary for implementation. Yet both issues—setting the direction and having the necessary resources—are equally important.

The leader must examine the purpose of the change. Why is this change needed or appropriate? How will it affect patients, key customers, employees, or the long-term viability of the organization? Will this change help the organization meet its basic mission? By clearly defining and articulating the purpose of this change, the leader sets the direction for those who will implement it.

Having identified the purpose, the leader considers resources required to implement this change. Although money and financial support are key resources, the lack of other critical resources can be devastating to a change initiative. These other important resources include adequate time; availability of coaches, mentors, and other support people; employees' and managers' skills; and interest from those who must implement the change. One aspect of this phase is to determine whether there are key individuals within the organization who could undermine its success if they are not in alignment with the initiative (Miles, 2010). Strategies for working with these individuals will need to be considered and established quickly.

Phase Two: Movement

During this phase, the two primary issues are developing a vision and providing a decision-making structure that enables implementation of the plan. Vision, as described in Chapter Three, is a compelling picture of what the situation will be in the future. A leader's ability to envision a different future, one that is energizing and desirable, makes creating a new reality possible. The most powerful visions are those of a preferred, rather than predicted, future. The envisioned future is a stretch and a challenge. Equally important is a plan that will create this new reality: a specific, concrete, step-by-step plan with time frames and a structure that move the vision from dream to reality. The plan may not unfold in exactly the manner conceived, but the thinking and strategic work accomplished serves the initiative well as it unfolds.

The leader also determines a decision-making structure at this phase. What is needed to move from idea to concrete change? Is a project team or committee necessary? What is the decision-making authority of the people involved? How does the change affect the current organization or department structure? What measurements or outcomes will determine success?

Phase Three: Team Creativity

This is the most dynamic of the five phases and marks the beginning of actually making the change. Prior to this point, most of the work is preparatory and sometimes considered tedious by enthusiastic and eager leaders. Without the work in the first two phases, however, this phase would not result in lasting change. The four major issues for this phase are coordination and cooperation, setting priorities, communication, and climate formation.

Change initiatives fail under the burden of poor coordination and lack of participant cooperation. If coordination is weak, participants may come to believe that the left hand doesn't know what the right hand is doing, eroding trust and confidence in leadership. During extensive change, those affected are likely to become more egocentric and focused on themselves. Unless leaders are prepared for this phenomenon, they can easily feel anger toward normally cooperative employees and departments that suddenly seem obstructive and resistant.

Clearly identifying priorities encourages both leaders and participants to stay focused on the change effort. It is a leadership function to continually evaluate pressing priorities and restate them as often as necessary to help others remain focused on the change. Congruency between leader behavior and stated beliefs is of utmost importance at this time. Because change is difficult and demanding, people implementing a change continually read the signals to ensure that their effort is worthwhile. Leaders must avoid becoming distracted by a new project or the next change, which could cause participants to conclude that the change they are working on is no longer a priority.

Communication is important during all phases of a change initiative, and at this point it becomes critical. A defined communication plan must be conscientiously implemented, including strategies for keeping key stakeholders abreast of changes. (Chapter Four includes a more extensive discussion about communication strategies during major change.)

Creating a corporate culture or climate supportive of the change is essential. If the change requires people to behave in a manner incongruent with the culture, the change is unlikely to succeed. Efforts to create employee motivation and full engagement are crucial for success (Miles, 2010).

Phase Four: New Reality

Once the change has been made and the situation altered, the true impact begins to sink in. Stabilizing the change at this point so that it is anchored for the future and achieving the desired results from the change are the major issues of this phase.

Stabilizing and sustaining the change are of paramount importance. Loss of focus during execution is a common issue. The leader must execute specific measures to anchor the change into the current reality because without constant pressure, people will revert to their previous behaviors. Methods for this "include formalizing structures or processes that were used during a trial period, establishing new routines, or formally communicating the new processes to key stakeholders" (Manion, Lorimer, and Leander, 1996, p. 202). An even more powerful method of anchoring the change is to modify the reward system to ensure that the organization reinforces new behaviors. Reward systems include recognition and compensation mechanisms.

The second key issue in this phase is achieving desired results so that the organization regains acceptable productivity levels. Few plans unfold as they were designed. Moreover, some work, and some don't. Sorting through to find the successful strategies and eliminate those that are unsuccessful is part of the work of this phase. Leaders must be patient with declining productivity during this trial period.

Phase Five: Integration

Integration, the final phase of the change process, means reviewing quality measures, evaluating results, and managing closure. Unfortunately, it is easy for leaders to undervalue or simply overlook this phase.

The leader now reviews the quality and outcome measures established during phase two (movement). He or she then evaluates results and outcomes obtained using these measures to determine the initiative's success. Were desired results achieved? Did any intolerable, undesirable consequences occur? What was the impact on the system, organization, or department? Has quality of service improved? In addition to reviewing quality indicators, the leader should evaluate the actual change process. What organizational learning occurred as a result of this process? How resilient were employees? What leadership skills emerged? How were emotional reactions handled?

The skill with which the leader deals with closure is instrumental in positioning people and the organization well for the next change. "Closure is often the least understood and most often overlooked issue of the entire developmental cycle" (Manion, Lorimer, and Leander, 1996, p. 205). Celebrations are appropriate and help mark the transition. However, closure often also includes grief, during which leading others can be difficult. Allowing and supporting any feelings of grief promotes respect for the natural progression of any change and models healthy adaptive behavior.

The Change Process: Five Steps for Success

This five-phase process for implementing change is applicable to change projects of any size. It has guided mergers of hospitals, as well as closures, and been used to implement change in a single department. Understanding the key issues of each phase helps leaders determine progress and prevents common missteps.

Following the phases sequentially reduces the amount of effort and energy that making a change requires. (For a more thorough explanation of each phase, see Cox, Manion, and Miller, 2005; Manion, 1994; and Manion, Lorimer, and Leander, 1996.) Because leaders too often do not consider key issues, major problems may arise later in the process. How many times do organizations embark on changes without enough resources to follow through or without even considering key but less obvious resources such as leadership skill and coaching abilities? How often does a dynamic, charismatic leader grow excited and enthusiastic about a change, exhorting followers to embark on the change—but without doing necessary preparatory work? How often has everyone been excited about a change—but later it did not unfold as planned, with nothing put into place to anchor the change, resulting in one more thing the organization did not follow through on?

The Transition Process

Change alters the way something is done, whereas transition is the psychological adaptation to change. The transition process exists within the change process, but for clarity, we address transition here as a separate entity. Bridges (1992) identifies three stages of transition (Figure 5.3):

- The ending
- The neutral zone
- The beginning

Stage One: The Ending

Bridges (1988, 1992) has studied people's reactions to transition for years. He points out that once a leader understands the dynamics of transition, he or she begins to see the need for endings almost everywhere: "Every change in leadership terminates relationships and plans that had been central to people's lives. Every merger takes away power and status that people had built their worlds upon. Every change in product lines or services brings to an end the functions and competencies that made people feel valuable and the groupings that made them feel at home. Even promotions cause people to

---

Figure 5.3 Stages of Transition

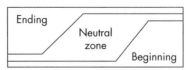

Source: From *Participant's Guide to Managing Organizational Transitions,* © 1992. Used by permission of the publisher: William Bridges & Associates, Mill Valley, Calif.

leave behind their familiar worlds. In short, every change causes loss, whether the change is large or small" (1988, p. 37).

This first stage of transition is painful because it entails saying good-bye to the world we once knew. Valued relationships may end with this change, and individuals lose the comfort of the way things used to be. This stage begins with the awareness that change has forced a closure, even a destruction, of the known world. This is unsettling—and often frightening—to most people.

People in this stage of transition are difficult to work with because they are experiencing the emotions of grief. Anger, irritability, depression, negativity, resistance, and resentment are common during the lowest emotional periods (Manion, 1995). Employees and leaders alike feel vulnerable and out of control. Indeed, in many workplaces, expressing anger is not safe because people fear retaliation. Employees' fear increases if they are angry with the person to whom they report.

Stage Two: The Neutral Zone

At first glance, this stage seems anything but neutral because it is characterized by disruption, confusion, and fear. "The neutral zone is the psychological in-between time, when it isn't the old way anymore, but it isn't the new way yet either. The old identity is gone but the new identity isn't clear. The old procedures and systems, the old values and norms, the old expectations and priorities are no longer operative or valid, but the new ones haven't taken shape yet" (Bridges, 1992, p. 45).

For most adults, the neutral zone is the most uncomfortable of the transition stages. It can cause tremendous frustration and anxiety because it exists between two worlds: the comfortable known and the frightening unknown. Even if the past was undesirable and fraught with unhappiness, individuals may now romanticize it and remember only its good elements. Compared with the unknown quantity of the future, the past can look pretty rosy. Because the change is in place and the situation has altered, many people assume that internal adaptation will follow at the same pace. Nothing could be further from the truth. Internal adjustment always takes longer.

There is a tremendous urgency in organizations going through change to push people through these first two stages because the characteristic emotions and behaviors are so discouraging. However, transition is not complete unless people experience these two stages; they only suppress the negative feelings. The more this occurs, the less likely it is that the organization will achieve the positive, creative side of transition.

Oddly, the second predominant characteristic of the neutral zone is creativity. Because everything is up in the air and uncertain, tremendous potential exists for transformation. Chaos and confusion abound, from which creative and innovative ideas arise. "During any period of significant change, one of the leader's most important tasks is to use the change as a challenge to all the assumptions and practices that got the organization to where it is" (Bridges, 1992, p. 51). In times of profound crisis, this challenge reaches to the very core of the organization. What is its mission? How does the organization identify itself? In the face of less significant change, it may simply be an opportunity to ask: Is there a better way to do the things we do?

Stage Three: The Beginning

Bridges (1992) differentiates between the start of something (the change itself) and the new beginning. The beginning implies that people are comfortable with the change and their new identities, and they have rebuilt their world. With a new beginning, comfort and ease have returned; people feel at home again. This is the easiest stage of transition to manage, although it must not be overlooked. At this time, anchoring and stabilizing the change are important.

Pitfalls: Leading Through Change and Transition

There are many pitfalls to navigate when dealing with these processes. Not recognizing the difference between change and transition often leads to ignoring one or the other. Although these two processes are highly interdependent, the value of separating them is to ensure that the leader uses specific interventions to manage each. Change can take place, but when people do not successfully make their transitions and adapt to the change, the change is compromised. People who never adapt to the change have the potential of undermining and destabilizing the change, whether intentionally or inadvertently. In the same way, mismanaged change affects people's ability to adapt successfully to an altered situation.

Examples of this pitfall abound in health care today. Hospitals down-size, merge, or unmerge; organizations implement a patient safety, service excellence, or continuous process improvement initiative, or they develop an integrated system—all requiring the shifting or changing of internal orga-nizational culture. But when leaders poorly handle or ignore shaping a new culture and managing people's transition to this new reality, the organiza-tion does not gain the full benefit of the initiative. Is it any surprise that the full promise of integration within health care systems has yet to be realized or that most work redesign and reengineering projects in the 1990s failed? In the past decade, how many organizations embarked on a massive organi-zational cultural change such as service excellence, only to be frustrated in their attempts to truly change their internal culture?

The most common mistakes in leading change and transition are ignor-ing the process and rushing people through the stages. Because certain stages result in unpleasant emotions and potentially strained interpersonal relation-ships, there is a natural desire to pass quickly through these stages or bypass them completely. Although this seems effective in the short term, it only slows the process later.

Less effective managers and leaders mistakenly believe that managing transition, the people side of change, is an expensive and time-consuming luxury. In one organization, managers were upset and concerned about the multitude of changes occurring. They believed that their executives were discounting the managers' observations and feelings. When the managers attempted to talk with executive leaders about their concerns, they were told in no uncertain terms that the change was a speed bump and they should just get over it. The managers felt chastised, belittled, and devalued. One would have to question the effectiveness of these executive leaders, because it is the management staff who usually leads the rest of the organization through change. How was this group of executives planning to gain support for the widespread changes after alienating this group of people?

Accepting the emotional issues of transition is simply not in the con-sciousness of the just-get-it-done leaders who are not process oriented. They often ignore the presence of messy emotions and decide they won't let them affect the implementation of change. In the words of one CEO, "I don't want my people being told about these emotions—it's just too negative." Unfortunately, not informing people about what to expect does not prevent the feelings or make the emotions go away. An emotionally intelligent leader recognizes and realizes that emotions, sometimes strong emotions, are part of our workplace environment. To try to separate these emotions from the people who experience them is futile.

During times of change and transition, leaders often exhort people to be more creative and come up with ideas for dealing with a difficult reality. This can create a no-win situation if the leader is not aware of where employees are in the stage of transition. If employees are trying to cope with closure and are experiencing the emotions of grief, asking them to be creative often results in a demoralizing, self-defeating situation and stronger feelings of disconnect.

Some leaders mistakenly expect these processes to be predictable. Although there is a predictable sequence, no one can accurately forecast the full effects of a change on another person. The change that triggers the emotions of transition may be different for different people. Although one individual may experience a title change as a significant loss, another barely notices. Moving a work space may upset one individual tremendously, but for another, changes in relationships are far more significant.

"It must be considered that there is nothing more difficult to carry out, nor more doubtful of success, nor more dangerous to handle, than to initiate a new order of things" (Kotter and Schlesinger, 2008, p. 130). Yet truly transformational leaders learn to lead during times of transition and periods of unprecedented change.

Conclusion

Transformational leaders are highly skilled at leading process. They recognize and understand the operative process and are able to guide it in a way that ensures relevant, synergistic outcomes. When process bogs down, they are able to assess the problem, intervene, and redirect the process. Good leaders respect the sequential nature of process and allow it to unfold within its natural time frame. They have the judgment to determine when a process needs a little extra nudge or redirection. Tomorrow's transformational leader is a master at empowering others, resolving conflict, creating effective teams, and managing change and transition.

DISCUSSION QUESTIONS

1. Where in your professional life do you see examples of disrespect for process (not recognizing the underlying developmental process that must occur)? What is the process involved? What have you seen are the consequences of misunderstanding the basic nature of the process?

2. How comfortable are you with facilitating key processes? What are your strengths and weaknesses when it comes to being involved in a process? Are you impatient with process, or do you enjoy the challenge? Do you find yourself bogged down, or do you force its closure prematurely?

3. What are examples of times you have challenged the status quo? Were you successful? What were the consequences? Would you do it differently today?

4. Think of a time when you delegated or transferred responsibility to someone else and the outcome was not what you wanted or expected. What went wrong? Consider the four elements of empowerment (capability, responsibility, authority, and accountability) and determine where the problem was. What would you do differently today?

5. How can you use your new understanding of the concepts of capability, responsibility, authority, and accountability to assess situations in the workplace that are not going in an acceptable manner? Where do you need to relinquish control and transfer responsibility to others? How can using these four concepts help you do so?

6. How do the four concepts of empowerment (capability, responsibility, authority, and accountability) relate to establishing a new committee, project task force, or team?

7. How do you feel inside when you know a conflict is building and you are going to be involved? What are your physiological reactions? Your emotional reactions? What do you do especially well in dealing with conflict? Where could you improve your skills?

8. What is the most common approach for dealing with conflict in your organization, your department, your life? Is it effective? What are the consequences of these approaches?

9. Think of a time when you used a negotiation process for resolving a conflict. What worked? What were the difficulties? Did you reach a mutually agreeable win-win solution? If not, what happened? Use the negotiation map to approach a conflict situation.

10. Where do teams exist in your organization or department today? Are these teams effective? What was their process for development? Do you have a leadership team in place? How would you go about developing a leadership team for your area of responsibility?

11. Think of changes you have gone through in your organization or department. Did you use a sequential process? What changes were successful, and which changes failed? Why did they fail?

12. Think about the last major change you went through. Can you see the three stages of transition? How can you use the transition model to facilitate people's transition during changes?

6

Getting Results

- Describe proactive behavior.
- Distinguish between first- and second-order problem solving.
- Compare the five types of group decision-making styles.
- Relate the four steps of an appreciative inquiry process.
- Define the concept of polarity management.
- Explain the polarity grid and the process for using it to reach action steps.

Leaders are proactive—and able to make something
happen under conditions of extreme uncertainty and urgency.
J. W. KOUZES AND B. Z. POSNER, *ENCOURAGING THE HEART*

S avvy leaders understand that process simply for the sake of process is not
acceptable. How we achieve results is important, but achieving results,
solving problems, and making improvements are ways that effective leaders do their job and create commitment and credibility with their followers
(Boyatzis and McKee, 2005; Manion, 2004b). A proprietary study found
that leaders who help employees find solutions to their problems at work
have a significant impact on both employee initiative and commitment.
A recent study focused on a manager's effect on employees' perceptions, emotions, and motivations. One of two effective behaviors that the researchers
discovered was that the manager engaged in activities that enabled the person
to move forward in his or her work. Results revealed that on the study participant's best days, the most important differentiator was a sense of being
able to make progress in his or her work. "Achieving a goal, accomplishing
a task, or solving a problem often evoked great pleasure and sometimes ela-
tion" (Amabile and Kramer, 2007, p. 81). Completion of projects and tasks
was important, but making good progress toward achieving a goal could
elicit the same emotions.

Furthermore, getting results is tightly connected to the other interpersonal skills this book addresses. For example, in *Execution: The Discipline of
Getting Things Done*, Bossidy and Charan (2002) report that the first essential
skill for getting things done is to know your people and continually expand
their capabilities through coaching. Creating alignment between employees
and the organization's values, mission, and vision generates passion and the
energy for accomplishing needed results. Effective communication skills
are required in order to achieve desired outcomes, and so on.

Getting results is much easier to talk about than to achieve. Today's
health care organizations are complex almost beyond our ability to comprehend.
The scope of many issues is often beyond what an individual manager can
influence alone. Common examples include problems with patient throughput

that results in congested emergency departments and backups in related areas; complex layers of management and bureaucracy that overlook vital information about emerging problems and are anything but nimble in dealing with issues; and workarounds that employees develop to compensate for operational failures such as ineffective processes and inadequate supplies or working equipment. Although these problems can be solved, it takes proactive leaders with high-level decision-making and problem-solving skills who are committed to working with employees, peers, and senior leadership to make forward progress.

Unfortunately we become habituated to that which occurs commonly. Just because something is common, such as inadequate or missing supplies, nonworking equipment, incomplete requisitions, or illegible handwriting, doesn't mean it is acceptable. These problems result in disruption of work flow for first-line employees and represent not only a tremendous amount of organizational resources in terms of lost employee time, but also incredibly high levels of frustration on the part of employees. These situations often result in what is referred to as first-order problem solving. This means that the person who encounters the situation (supplies aren't there when needed) usually does whatever it takes to obtain the supply in order to provide the service required. So the problem is solved for the now, but there is no second-order problem solving, which occurs when the person not only solves the existing problem but also takes steps to address the underlying issues or institutes a problem-solving or process improvement team to deal with the issue so it doesn't keep reoccurring. Few first-line employees have the time to initiate this second-order problem solving, so the presence or easy accessibility of the leader has a significant impact on whether this occurs. Managers who are present in the workplace are more likely to be aware of the problems through their own direct observations and more likely to make a connection between the problem and the organizational steps that can be taken to help solve it. This chapter's primary focus is on approaches for addressing second-order problem solving.

The leadership quality of proactivity is discussed briefly to set the context for this chapter. The rest of the chapter explores several approaches that leaders can use in getting results. It offers a generic problem-solving process that is congruent with the quality improvement methodologies in many health care organizations today. The chapter also discusses group decision making and identifies some common pitfalls. Finally, this chapter offers two alternative approaches for tackling tough organizational issues: appreciative inquiry, which focuses on what is going right, and polarity management, which recognizes that not all issues are problems to be solved but some are polarities to be managed.

Proactivity

Proactive behavior is a key leadership characteristic. When we are active in our behavior, we are better able to change the world around us. Individuals who are reactive simply wait for events to occur and then respond to them. In today's world, reactive behavior is often accompanied by emotions of frustration, fear, anger, and feeling overwhelmed. Moving from reactive behavioral patterns to a proactive approach leads to a sense of self-efficacy and empowerment. Proactive behavior requires contemplation of the situation and possible alternatives and a certain level of preparation in dealing with the event. It implies that action will be taken and steps assumed to ensure the maintenance of the new behavior.

Proactive people demonstrate personal initiative. They don't wait for direction from others; they take action on their own. Vestal (2009b) describes personal initiative as the ability to choose a course of action and take the necessary steps to implement it. It is a can-do spirit that motivates a person to get something done. Proactive leaders are future oriented and always scanning their environment for opportunities and problems. They spend the majority of their time preparing for their future. They are also persistent and overcome barriers that stand in the way of their goals. In some instances, they may adapt to overcome problems, but they always actively deal with problems rather than giving up.

Frese (2009), who has studied the relationship between proactivity and engagement in organizations, has found that personal initiative correlates strongly with work engagement. When the level of employee engagement is high, people are more proactive. Individuals actively attack problems;

when things go wrong, they immediately search for solutions; and they more readily embrace change. In other words, a proactive individual who is not happy with a situation will do something about it rather than simply react. Frese also found that a low-initiative climate negatively affected the financial health of organizations.

The relationship of proactivity to getting results is self-evident. The leader who assumes a high level of personal initiative for his or her work and workplace always seems to be trying new things to resolve issues and handle problems. Some of the characteristics this leader demonstrates are curiosity, an open and challenging attitude, and a strong interest in learning. They are also self-directed and comfortable in challenging the status quo in a constructive manner (Vestal, 2009b). Proactive leaders can also seek these characteristics and qualities in their employees by watching for these during the hiring process. These are qualities to recognize and acknowledge in the staff. Employees who take the initiative to participate and solve problems with new ideas and different approaches should be recognized and rewarded.

The benefits of proactivity are significant. Frese (2009) reports that leaders with high personal initiative enjoy higher employability and have more effective career plans that they are more likely to execute. They find jobs faster when they are looking and enjoy increased levels of innovativeness. Unfortunately for organizations, leaders with high levels of personal initiative also have a higher propensity to become self-employed. Frese also found that individuals grow in initiative when their work is fun and enjoyable. Higher personal initiative leads to higher performance, a stronger sense of self-efficacy, and higher life satisfaction levels. Proactive people engage in problem solving.

Problem Solving

Problem solving occurs at the individual level as well as in groups. The process followed is similar, although group problem solving has an added layer of complexity. In hierarchical, top-down organizations, problem solving is limited in terms of both the people involved and the kinds of problems around which groups meet. Group problem solving is a bottom-up process that requires a visionary leader—one who can relinquish control sufficiently to create an environment for employee empowerment. When problem-solving groups are prevalent in an organization, it is a good sign of employee involvement. And knowledgeable leaders understand that individuals have difficulty feeling empowered if they have no tools for solving pressing problems that directly affect their ability to do their work. Seeing improvement in their daily work life creates a sense of momentum and hopefulness for the future in the work group and ensures future participation in these activities. Many quality or process improvement groups are essentially problem-solving groups.

Most effective problem-solving processes include some variation of the following five steps (see Figure 6.1):

1. Problem identification and analysis

2. Statement of a desired future

3. Solution generation and analysis of alternatives

4. Action planning and implementation

5. Evaluation

Figure 6.1 A Problem-Solving Process

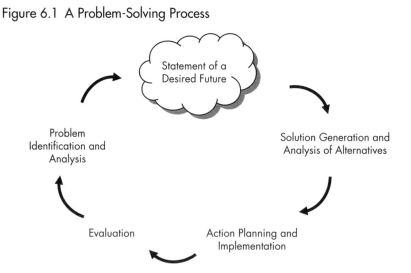

Regardless of how these steps are named, a skilled leader understands that this process must be both sequential and methodical. All steps must be included in the appropriate sequence in order to obtain a quality outcome. Often what passes for problem solving is some spontaneous, inconsistently applied brainstorming technique that follows no proven methodology and misses one or more important steps. This problem-solving process can be effective for individuals and groups, although this discussion focuses on group problem solving.

Step One: Problem Identification and Analysis

The discussion for describing, analyzing, and ultimately defining the problem typically begins with descriptions of symptoms or other evidence of a problem as it affects various members of the group. In many instances, initial statements of the problem are vague and confused. Sometimes the group needs additional information before it can write a problem statement.

It is important to bring to the surface as many characteristics of the problem as possible at this point and to avoid jumping to hasty conclusions. Psychologists who have experimented with thinking for over seventy years have discovered that once a person offers an explanation, he or she has difficulty revising or dropping it, even in the face of contradictory information. In early social psychology experiments, subjects were shown an out-of-focus thirty-five-millimeter slide of a fire hydrant. The psychologists found that if a person wrongly identified the object when it was out of focus, he or she often could not identify it when it was brought sufficiently into focus so that another person (who had not seen the blurry slide) could easily recognize it. Their conclusion was significant: more evidence is required to overcome an incorrect hypothesis than to establish a correct one. Individuals who jumped to a hasty conclusion were less sensitive to new ideas and information (Adams, 1986).

Questions often help to define the problem more fully. What are signs and symptoms of this problem? Whom does it affect? Does it affect them directly or indirectly? How often does it occur? What are all the possible causes or factors involved? The group may determine that it needs more information or data. Many of the techniques taught through quality improvement programs, such as using histograms, fishbone diagrams, Pareto charts, and process and scatter diagrams, can be helpful at this point (Byers and White, 2004).

During this first step, another important issue to consider is ownership. How have the group or individuals within the group contributed to or created the current problem? This is a critical consideration because focusing on the alternatives over which the group has control brings a higher rate of success. This is difficult for many groups, which often begin by believing that the fault for the problem lies elsewhere. By pushing themselves, however, they usually begin to see how they have helped create the current situation.

Caregivers in one organization were angry because they often did not have enough clean linen in the morning to complete changing patients' bed linens. They clearly attributed the problem to the linen services department. Even when they were pushed to look at their own role in creating the problem, they continued to insist that the other department was at fault. Nevertheless, with persistent prodding, they gradually began to come up with ideas. "We stopped attending the liaison meeting with linen services because we didn't think they were listening to our concerns." They also recalled being told that over $200,000 in linens had been replaced during the year because of employee theft. That money could have helped pay for a higher-capacity washing machine that would process linens more quickly. The final contributing factor that they identified was their common practice of hoarding linen and stashing it in all kinds of places so that it would be available when needed. This practice had made it impossible to get an accurate inventory count, giving linen services inaccurate figures and thus causing inadequate planning. Once the group identified these issues, it began to work more effectively on the problem.

In a radiology department, the problem was incomplete requisitions for procedures. The radiology employees themselves had contributed to the problem over the years by accepting the patient and doing the procedure in spite of incomplete or inaccurate requisition forms. As a result, there were no consequences for completing (or not completing) the forms.

The problem statement is a concise description of the problem. Novice problem-solving groups tend to put the solution into the problem statement.

One group, for example, came up with this problem statement: "The problem is inadequate staffing." This statement, however, limited problem-solving creativity because the solution was, "Get more staff." Changing the problem statement to, "There is more work than the available employees can handle," makes multiple possibilities apparent, including eliminating some of the work, changing the way it is being done, or adjusting staffing levels temporarily.

Once the group has clearly identified the problem, it next determines its level of authority in solving the problem (see Chapter Five for a discussion of levels of authority). Determining the level of authority at this point is crucial so that everyone's expectations are appropriate. The group can plan necessary communication and involvement with others in the organization. A low level of authority does not preclude a group's working on a particular issue; it simply helps them stay within their scope of authority. And clarity about authority levels will prevent misunderstandings when it is time to implement decisions.

Compare the following two groups. Both chose to work on an employee-benefits problem for which they had only level one authority, which included gathering information. The first group was very aware of its level of authority. The members spent their time investigating the problem and gathering information; they reviewed their findings and developed a strategy for sharing the information with the human resource department. Their work focused on a desired future that included the successful presentation of their information and specific steps aimed at their strategies for delivering the findings in a manner that would create movement on the issue.

The second group had not clarified its level of authority. The members proceeded with enthusiasm throughout the entire process, developing a future vision that included employee benefits, offered in a cafeteria-style approach, from which employees could select. Their action planning revolved around the implementation of the new benefits. They were excited and eager when they finished the problem-solving process—only to become frustrated and angry when the organization did not act on their work. Group members cynically observed that it was the last time they would volunteer for a problem-solving task force, never realizing that the work they had done substantially exceeded their level of authority.

Step Two: Statement of a Desired Future

A common mistake that problem-solving groups make is to focus almost exclusively on the problem and its causes rather than on what they would like to build or create for the future. Russell Ackoff, the originator of interactive planning, has demonstrated clearly that solutions are more creative if the focus remains on desired outcomes rather than on details of the current problem (Ackoff, Finnel, and Gharajedaghi, 1984).

This step requires asking, What would this look like if there were no problem, if it were solved? The group then writes a description of the ideal situation. For example, if the group's problem statement is, "Communication between hospital and home health personnel is poor, creating problems in delivery of quality patient care," a statement of a desired future might be, "Communication between hospital and home health personnel is free-flowing, timely, and accurate." In another system, a group was working on coordinating community services for seniors. Their desired future statement read: "Community services for seniors are coordinated and easily accessible to participants, with information flowing freely and fluidly between agencies for the benefit of our program participants."

Focusing exclusively on the problem statement leads to more limited solutions. A clear statement about a desirable future creates a picture for those involved and generates more imaginative and original ideas, as well as a broader scope of possibilities.

Step Three: Solution Generation and Analysis of Alternatives

This stage is both creative and analytical, and it is critical that the group separate the two phases of this step. The group first generates all possible solutions but withholds analysis, discussion, and critical thinking about the solutions until it has identified all possibilities. Nothing impairs creative flow faster than criticizing or analyzing ideas as they are presented. Being well versed in creativity techniques is important at this stage because these techniques are useful for generating ideas. Many sources explain approaches such as nominal group technique, mind mapping, list making, attribute analysis, and the use of storyboards (Manion, 1990). A particularly helpful source,

Innovation Leadership: Creating the Landscape of Health Care (Porter-O'Grady and Malloch, 2010), presents a thorough analysis of creativity techniques and offers examples.

The second phase of this step is to analyze all the solutions generated in phase one. Once the group has identified all of the possible alternatives, it can begin to converge regarding the most viable options. A series of helpful questions can help sort and categorize feasible alternatives:

- Are some alternatives very similar? Do they overlap?
- Can we combine certain solutions?
- Do we need to rearrange any alternatives?
- Can we eliminate any? (If yes, do we need to consider any worthwhile applications or characteristics of this option?)
- What is good about a solution?
- How would it solve the problem or help create the desired future?
- Are there any possible unexpected consequences of this option?
- If anything goes wrong, what would be the course of action?
- What is the group's degree of control or level of authority over this option?
- Are there key stakeholders who need to be involved to make this option a success? Are those stakeholders likely to support it?
- What resources would be needed to implement this solution, and are they obtainable?
- Do we need more data and information?

Each of these questions is important. However, the group needs to think about the answers and not hesitate to move on. There is no perfect solution for the problems in organizations today, and it is better to implement something than to be caught in a never-ending spiral of data collection. If the selected solution does not work, at least the group has more knowledge and information on which to base a new decision.

At the end of step three, the group should have identified at least two or three viable solutions. Stopping at only one solution is dangerous. If it is not accepted or cannot be implemented, group members feel demoralized and think they have wasted their time. Also, research has demonstrated that problem solvers are dominated by pressure to solve the problem and that adopting the first solution may reflect this pressure. Forcing the group to develop at least two or three viable alternatives results in more creative solutions because group members focus on the desired future as opposed to the need to find an answer.

Deciding among the alternatives requires knowledge of decision-making approaches. There are several types of decision making, including voting and reaching consensus, which this chapter considers later.

Step Four: Action Planning and Implementation

Determining specific actions to be taken, the time frame within which to complete them, and responsibility assignments for each action must be specific and realistic. Once the group has identified these elements, it prioritizes the steps to take. In some instances, actions must be sequential because some are dependent on completion of others.

Once the plan is reasonably complete, the group costs out both current practice and recommended alternatives. Spending money or time now in order to save a substantial amount of money or time later can be a compelling incentive to adopt a new practice. In some instances, an alternative can have a positive effect on quality of service without requiring more money. At this stage, the group develops a communication strategy based on who needs to know about the plan and who to include in developing additional expectations. The problem-solving group decides how and when to present its results.

During implementation, one group member must monitor the plan closely to maintain momentum. The group chooses an individual who can also reinstitute the group if further work is necessary.

Step Five: Evaluation

The final step in the problem-solving process is to establish criteria for evaluating success and determine who will be responsible for the evaluations. The implementing parties must know how they will measure success. This evaluation criterion should be as precise and objective as possible, which in some instances is fairly simple. A percentage error rate, the number of completed diagnostic tests, the number of patient falls, and figures on employee productivity are a few examples of easily obtained objective measures. Organizations that participate in the National Database of Nursing Quality Indicators (NDNQI) have access to a measurement program that gives unit-level performance reports with comparison to national averages and percentile rankings on a variety of clinical patient care measures. Other measures can be more difficult to quantify, such as improvement in relationships between teams or departments, satisfaction levels of key customers, or more subtle changes in the quality of service.

The group establishes specific review dates and makes plans to celebrate the completion of this phase of the work. Group members must monitor results and make necessary corrections. Divergence from expected outcomes will mean that the group must identify the cause and find another workable solution. The second and third solution alternatives formulated earlier in the process are helpful in this case. At this point, the leader may need to encourage and remind the group that even if the first recommendation or solution did not work exactly as planned, they are closer to a solution now than they were before.

This problem-solving process was used effectively in a hospital in the U.S. Sunbelt. An annually recurring problem of a lack of patient beds during the winter months with the influx of visitors from the northern states created conflict between employees and physicians, all scraping to come up with needed resources. Finally, during the summer, the administration put together a problem-solving team composed of employees, managers, executives, and physicians. This process took several months, but the result was a plan that increased the number of available beds during the winter and clearly identified backup contingency plans. For the first time in years, the hospital staff managed the winter season without coming to blows over beds.

Most successful quality improvement methodology in organizations use some form of this traditional problem-solving approach. Six Sigma is a data-driven quality improvement methodology that is designed to eliminate variation from a process. The five elements are define, measure, analyze, improve, and control. The Toyota Production System/Lean Management is a business philosophy and approach that seeks to improve quality and efficiency by identifying and eliminating waste. Each process is meticulously broken down to identify the value and non-value added steps with the intent reaching a zero deficit status. Transforming Care at the Bedside is a national program that was launched in 2003 by the Robert Wood Johnson Foundation and the Institute for Healthcare Improvement. This initiative engages leaders at all levels in the organization and empowers both frontline nurses and other care team members to improve the quality of care delivered on medical-surgical units. The basic process taught has four steps: plan, do, study, and act ("Transforming Care at the Bedside," 2009).

Pitfalls of the Problem-Solving Process

The most common pitfall occurs when the group does not deliberately consider whether the situation calls for a more traditional problem-solving or process improvement approach, or whether another approach, such as appreciative inquiry or polarity management, might be more appropriate. All of these approaches can be effective in dealing with challenges. Some issues are simply better tackled with an approach such as appreciative inquiry, while others are not clear-cut problems but polarities to be managed. Determining from the start which approach to use can prevent a great deal of wasted effort.

A second common pitfall occurs when the group includes a suggested solution in the problem statement. This limits the variety and creativity of alternatives the group identifies. It comes up with the same old answer one more time. Not only is the solution ineffective, but everyone involved ends up disenchanted.

A third pitfall relates to the group's level of authority. Steps for action must fit the level of authority and the problem. Too often groups develop grandiose action plans that go far beyond their authority and any reasonable parameters. A group of staff working on problems with the employee benefit package when they have no authority to influence the organization's selection or expenditure on benefits is a good example. However on this issue, gathering information about employee preferences and sharing it with the human resource department would be completely appropriate.

Hidden agendas and personal platforms make up the next pitfall. Some group members may have a strategy they want to promote, even if it has little to do with the issue at hand. This cannot be allowed to interfere with a fully explored problem-solving process.

Another common pitfall occurs when the group fails to determine time frames and people responsible for each action step. These components are critical to the implementation stage, when it is easy for the group to lose steam and neglect to carry out agreed-on steps. Monitoring and follow-through are essential.

Following the process sequentially is difficult for many groups. The process is a blend of both right- and left-brain activities, and some groups have trouble with one or the other or simply with switching between the two. Problem identification, analysis of alternatives, and selection of action steps and evaluation measures are examples of logical left-brain thinking. Establishing a desired future and generating all possible options require creativity and spontaneity and call on right-brain thinking. Groups may be facilitated in moving from one stage to the other by taking a brief break between them or actually carrying out each step in separate meetings. This creates boundaries between the two types of thinking processes and helps members make the transition. If people in the group are characteristically logical and concrete thinkers, such as clinical laboratory professionals or perioperative staff members, the group leader may need to be firm in keeping the group focused during the right-brain activities because the left-brain thinkers will exert tremendous pressure to move to analysis and left-brain logical activities.

Not respecting the problem-solving process as a methodical, sequential process leads to several common problems. The most common is called the bandage approach, often a knee-jerk reaction, when the group moves straight from problem identification to action planning without taking the time to think through a desired future or develop a full range of creative options, as illustrated in Figure 6.2.

Figure 6.2 The Bandage Approach

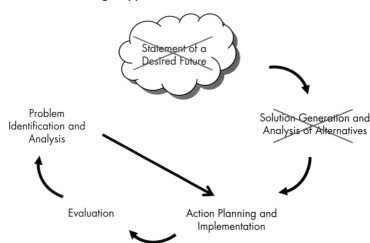

Another common problem, analysis paralysis (see Figure 6.3), occurs when the group stays in the problem identification phase so long that paralysis sets in. The group seems never to have enough data to make a decision; they may say that not all the facts have been collected or they don't have enough information for moving ahead. The goal here is to reach a happy medium between gathering information and coming to a decision. Collect enough data to provide information for adequate analysis through a specific agreed-on process and agree to an acceptable time frame for making a decision.

Some groups have an exaggerated sense of responsibility and take on too much ownership for the problem. Groups can often avoid this by asking the important question: What is our level of authority for solving this problem? They may discover that they do not have an adequate level of authority for implementing a solution to the problem and can therefore accept that doing so is not their responsibility. In some instances, they may realize that they are trying to solve a problem for a key stakeholder that is not represented in the group and as a result modify the membership of their group.

Figure 6.3 Analysis Paralysis

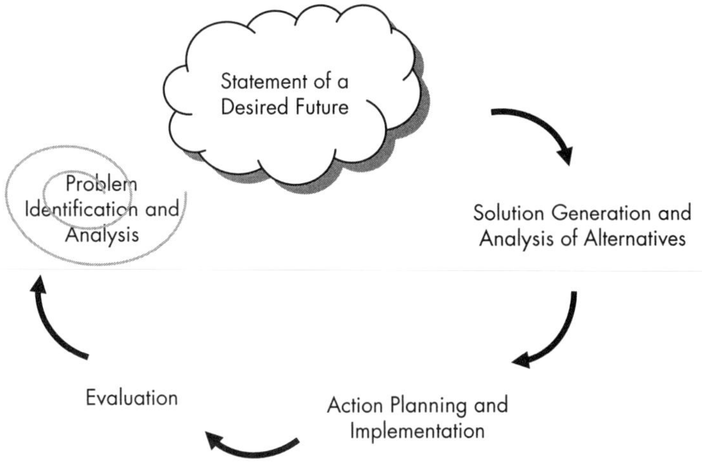

Reasons Groups Bog Down in Process

Both individuals and groups must develop effective problem-solving skills. Most groups process problems rather than solve them, continually discussing the symptoms or effects—anything but the root causes. In many instances, the problem itself escapes discussion without the group's ever having defined it. Groups engage in unproductive processing for at least three reasons:

- The group uses voting to determine plans of action, which forces members to pick sides. Once one person takes a side and another opposes it, the two opposing parties become even more adamant and continue to grow further apart.

- Groups neglect monitoring the group process. Although members may observe an unproductive process, they too often are unwilling to address it. For example, no one asks the nonparticipatory member to contribute, everyone ignores the apathetic group member, and everyone tolerates disruptive behavior.

- The group does not recognize or understand its patterns of behavior, which may include closing discussions prematurely or reaching decisions without fully analyzing the problem. Members may not recognize groupthink or their behavior is so polite and courteous that no one dares talk about the real issues. When others do not accept the group's solutions or alternatives, too often the group blames those with authority rather than reviewing its own process and truly evaluating the quality of its work.

Groupthink is a phenomenon "whereby team members become afraid of offering ideas that might conflict with the group's policies and actions. New ideas are often offered weakly and withdrawn quickly if opposed" (Chaleff, 1997, p. 4). Groupthink can destroy creative initiative and even reach the point where people with opposing views are forced out. The remedy for groupthink is continual self-evaluation of the group's patterns and outcomes.

Leaders who understand problem solving also understand its relationship to decision making. The two are closely interwoven and highly interdependent. Good problem solvers make decisions, and good decision makers often use a problem-solving approach.

Decision Making

A decision in this context is a choice among alternative courses of action that, it is hoped, will lead to a desired result. If there are no alternatives, there is no decision to make. Leaders and followers alike assume responsibility for the consequences of their decisions. This can be frightening at times because many decisions are made under conditions of uncertainty.

Decisions are evaluated based on their results or consequences, which are often unpredictable. An individual or group does not have to be right all the time, only most of the time. A sign in a printing shop provided this profound piece of wisdom: "Good decisions come from experience. Experience comes from wisdom. Wisdom comes from making bad decisions." An individual or group that has difficulty dealing with uncertainty either postpones decisions until all uncertainties are resolved or makes poor decisions to avoid coping with the uncertainties.

Types of Decisions

"As important as sound decision-making is, many executives [and groups] neglect to use any formal decision-making process" (Clancy, 2003, p. 343). Good decision makers combine a logical, systematic approach with their intuition. They sort and classify information; differentiate the valuable, worthless, and redundant; prioritize; and are able to integrate the whole into an accurate picture of reality. As the amount of information available increases, the complexity of decision making also increases (Davenport, 2009). A leader who is a good decision maker evaluates and recognizes the type of decision the situation calls for. In groups there are at least five types of decisions:

- Individual decisions
- Minority decisions
- Majority decisions
- Consensus decisions
- Unanimous decisions

Individual Decisions

These decisions are made by one person: a leader, a manager, or an individual with the responsibility and authority to decide. Others involved are expected to abide by this decision. This type of decision is used when there is no choice, the decision is not important, or the group does not want to make a decision. One example of this is called the "plop"—a suggestion that gets accepted without any discussion. Any member of the group can offer the plop.

Individual decisions are sometimes seen as an imposition or a mandated solution directed by someone with the authority to impose such a solution. Impositions are justified when the issue is truly nonnegotiable in terms of responsibility, when a group does not accept responsibility for the solution, or when the decision will have a low impact.

Minority Decisions

Minority decisions occur when a few people or a subgroup of the larger group involved in a situation meets to consider the matter and make a decision. If a group agrees to use a minority decision, the individual or group delegating the responsibility must clearly articulate the expectations for the minority or subset of the group accepting the responsibility. The decision of the minority group is considered binding for everyone.

Teams and large employee groups often use this approach. A subset of the team examines an issue and makes a decision for the team, which can be a very effective method of decision making when a larger group has difficulty taking the time to navigate the entire process together. It requires a high level of trust within the team or group. Team members with a vested interest in the decision are expected to be part of the subset and are not allowed to sabotage the decision later.

Majority Decisions

A majority decision is one in which more than half of the people involved in a situation agree on it (this is often referred to as a majority-rules vote). The resulting decision is binding on all. This type of decision is problematic because it may mean that not all members support the result.

A significant disadvantage to majority decision making is that it forces people to take one side or the other, and often the best solutions lie somewhere in the middle. The more firmly one argues for a certain side or solution, the less likely he or she will support an opposing solution if it wins. This form of decision making can be useful when the decisions involve minor issues that do not require 100 percent support to implement (such as where to hold the summer picnic) or when large numbers of people are involved and no forum or structure exists for resolving minority positions.

Consensus Decisions

A consensus decision results when the entire group or team addresses a problem with all group members, who fully present their views. Consensus exists when each group or team member can honestly make these three statements to every other member (Creative Healthcare Management, 1994):

"I believe I understand your point of view."

"I believe you understand my point of view."

"I believe the decision has been made in an open and fair manner, and I am willing to support the decision whether or not it's my first preference."

In true consensus, no majority-rules voting, bargaining, or averaging of votes is allowed. The process takes more time to achieve but results in active support and prevents later sabotage and undermining of decisions. Consensus is especially useful when full team or group commitment to the decision is essential for implementation. In an organization, for example, major decisions such as whether to embark on a major cultural change initiative or purchase another facility should require the consensus of the entire executive team. If the team makes the decision in any other manner, support may not be present during implementation, when it is required from the entire team.

Unanimous Decisions

In a unanimous decision, each group member fully agrees on the action to be taken, and the level of commitment is high. This may be needed when the decision significantly affects each member. A unanimous decision requires 100 percent agreement from group members. Consensus might be described as 70 percent agreement and 100 percent commitment. In other words, the difference between the two is that unanimity requires complete agreement, whereas consensus can be reached with a lower level of agreement. Both result in total commitment.

Group Versus Individual Decisions

Although moving up the decision-making scale from individual to unanimous decisions increases the level of commitment, it also increases the difficulty in arriving at agreement. A leader who is responsible for deciding whether to use individual or group decisions must consider at least five factors:

- *The nature of the problem or task.* Some problems are more easily solved by a group and others by an individual. In creating a new alternative or doing independent tasks, individuals often surpass groups. A project such as creating a new crossword puzzle is best completed by an individual rather than a group. When tasks are convergent or integrative and require bringing various pieces of information together to produce a solution (such as solving that crossword puzzle), a group is better. Most goal setting is also more effective in a group because it increases the diversity of contributions and level of commitment.

- *The importance of acceptance of the solution.* When people participate in the process of reaching a decision, they have more commitment to the decision. They work harder and have a greater interest in making the decision successful. When an individual solves a problem or makes a decision, two things must happen: others must be persuaded that this decision is best, and they must agree to act on the decision to carry it out. Not all decisions require widespread commitment, and these can be made appropriately by an individual.

- *The value placed on the quality of the decision.* If a leader is concerned with acceptance of a decision and with empowering others, he or she may accept a decision of somewhat lesser quality because it has widespread acceptance. Decisions that a group makes in the beginning of members' skill development may not have the same quality as the decisions an experienced individual makes. If the quality of the decision is paramount, the group might use an expert in the field. For example, if a group's members are having communication problems among themselves, they may produce and decide on the problem-solving alternatives to implement. If the outcomes are not beneficial, the group goes back to the drawing board and engages in additional problem solving. Getting it right the first time is not critical. However, if computer hardware problems with a particular application could significantly affect the organization's information systems, a decision to bring in an external expert to solve the problem or make recommendations may be the prudent choice.

- *The characteristics of individual group members.* Effective leaders consider the expertise of the various group members, the stake each has in the outcome, and the role each is likely to play in implementing the decision.

- *The operating effectiveness of the group.* Asking an individual to solve a problem or make a decision may be better than asking a group that is too new to decide or whose members cannot seem to work together. The skills of the group facilitator have an impact as well.

On the upside, group decision making represents greater total knowledge and information. Each group member brings a different perspective, resulting in a greater variety of approaches. Group decisions may have better acceptance and fewer communication problems. Implementation is likely to be smoother and to require less monitoring.

On the downside, a group setting may bring strong social pressure to conform. Groups also tend to err on the side of quick convergence, perhaps settling prematurely on a decision that seems to have support. High-quality ideas introduced late in the discussion have a limited chance of serious consideration. A dominant individual can prevail because of status, verbal skills, or persistence. Hidden agendas create problems in group decision making. Unless the leader brings these to the surface, they result in skewed and sometimes unfair or poor decisions. A significant problem for group decision making is that it simply takes longer for a group to decide.

Pitfalls of Decision Making

The most common decision-making pitfall is approaching decisions without due consideration of the various types of decision making. Without carefully analyzing the situation or giving sufficient thought to outcomes, a leader may miss opportunities for effectively engaging others in the decision. Followers can fall into the same trap. There are appropriate occasions for all types of decision making, but if followers expect to participate and reach consensus and the leader is making an individual decision, the group will not meet followers' expectations.

In one urgent care business, Ellen, the CEO, decided to reorganize and restructure the leadership and management ranks. Several managers were furious because Ellen did not include them in any discussion but simply told them what the new structure would be. Ellen elected to make an individual decision, which was within her responsibilities as CEO. Unfortunately, however, she had been preaching empowerment and employee involvement for some months, and those committed to empowerment in the company felt slapped down by her individual decision. An open discussion about how decisions would be made and which were to be individual and which were to be group decisions might have prevented some of these hard feelings.

The second common pitfall is a lack of understanding of consensus. *Consensus* has become an overused and misused buzzword in recent years.

Some people mistake participatory decision making (in which the leader gets input from members but a small group or an individual makes the decision) as consensus. Consensus is first and foremost a group decision-making process. If a decision truly needs to be made by consensus, no one should assume that the group has met the conditions of mutual belief, understanding, and support. Because reticent or disagreeing group members may not come forward or openly oppose the decision, the leader needs to ask each member of the group to state his or her commitment to the decision.

As an example, a statewide ad hoc committee, whose task was to recommend a new organizational structure for the state hospital association, spent long hours debating this hot political issue. When the group finally settled on a recommendation, the leader asked for consensus. The leader individually asked every group member the following three questions: "Do you believe you understood everyone else's point of view? Do you believe your point of view was fully expressed and understood by the others? Can you support this decision?" Each person then stated his or her agreement. At the annual meeting, however, one of the committee members had second thoughts when he realized that members from a special interest group of which he was also a member were upset about the committee's final recommendation. This member began talking with key association members, trying to engender support for an alternative and basically undermining the committee's work. During a public discussion of the issue, the leader reminded association members that they had reached the recommendation by consensus and reviewed exactly what consensus means. When reminded that he had agreed to support the committee's decision, the individual ceased his efforts to overturn the recommendations.

Not carefully considering the various factors in group versus individual decision making can be a major pitfall for a leader. A healthy combination of the two is important. In some instances, explaining why the group will use one or the other is also appropriate.

Decision making is closely related to problem solving but has its own special issues. Exemplary leaders are good decision makers, but they also are able to relinquish control and engage others in decision making when circumstances warrant. Shared decision making can strengthen any organization as long as it follows careful consideration. Understanding and applying the four key concepts of empowerment—capability, responsibility, authority, and accountability—can lead to successful shared decision making.

Appreciative Inquiry

An alternative approach to traditional problem-solving or process improvement methodology is a form of action research known as appreciative inquiry. It is based on the belief that something is already working well in the organization. Finding and studying it can lead to not only a deeper understanding but also insight into how to overcome the current difficulties and design a more desirable future.

The research world knows well that what we dwell on increases in our life. It follows that focusing on problems simply brings more problems or difficulties. To appreciate something suggests that we hold it as positive; we see the positive traits or characteristics; and this increases its value, much as property appreciates in value over the years. Appreciative inquiry is based on generative learning: "an ability to see radical possibilities beyond the boundaries of problems as they present themselves in conventional terms. High-performing organizations that engage in generative, innovative learning are competent at appreciating potential and possibility. They surpass the limitations of apparently 'reasonable' solutions and consider rich possibilities not foreseeable within conventional analysis" (Barrett, 1995, p. 2).

Comparing Traditional Problem Solving and Appreciative Inquiry

Traditional problem solving often involves looking back at our failures and trying to discover the causes. Appreciative inquiry instead inquires into our successes so that we can discover the distinctive attributes we can use to build on performance and create new strategic approaches. Traditional problem solving is a more linear or mechanized approach based on the belief that problems can be isolated, broken down into separate parts, repaired, and then restored to wholeness. As an approach, it often totally misses the systems implications.

And just as one can dissect the body and learn about it at the smallest cellular level, we have yet to discover the true essence of the person—the soul or the personality that makes each of us who we are. In the same way, problem solving often misses the essence of a situation and what really makes it work.

Problem solving can be very effective in dealing with issues that are more oriented toward process improvement such as increasing the number of accurate radiology requisitions received or decreasing extended waiting times for patients in the emergency department. Appreciative inquiry is more of a nonlinear approach and works well for issues related to less logical and methodical processes, such as changing the work culture. In some instances, a major issue might use both approaches. Reducing patients' waiting times in the emergency department is an example of an issue that has both specific process improvement opportunities and needed cultural changes.

Proponents of appreciative inquiry point out that a problem-solving approach has many consequences, including the following:

- *It limits our approach to the issue.* Often we accept the constraints of the status quo, which leads to coping with a problem rather than fixing its cause—for example, the problem of a very high patient census and the potential need for diverting patients from the emergency department to another local facility. Employees in one hospital were asked what they would do if the city's other emergency department was also diverting patients. They were stymied and could come up with no solutions. They said nothing could be done to resolve or prevent the situation. When asked about setting a limit on elective admissions to ensure that beds were available for emergency admissions, they found this inconceivable because they felt administration would never consider such an approach. Yet it is a solution, just not a popular one. And until the organization does something to create a different scenario for these people, all of their planning is based on coping with an untenable situation. At what point does it become riskier to continue to admit patients when there are not enough resources to provide for their safe care? This example illustrates the difficulties inherent in using a mechanistic problem-solving approach.

- *Problem solving creates an orientation toward finding deficiency.* The assumption is that something must be wrong somewhere. Managers develop self-worth as problem solvers, and so do executives. Thus, the more problems there are, the more important these people are. This can lead to the dysfunctional behavior of stirring the pot and creating problems in order to step in to solve them.

- *It creates a fragmented view of the world.* People in the organization become more and more expert in smaller parts of the system. Along the way it is easy to lose our ability to see the system as a whole and understand the interdependencies and their intricate connections.

Ludema, Cooperrider, and Barrett (2000, p. 8) sum up the consequences of an organizational focus on problem solving quite well: "As people in organizations inquire into their weaknesses and deficiencies, they gain an expert knowledge of what is 'wrong' with their organizations, and they may even become proficient problem-solvers, but they do not strengthen their collective capacity to imagine and build better futures."

In health care today, one of the most important organizational tasks is the creation of learning cultures (Tichy, with Cardwell, 2002). An appreciative learning culture allows employees to explore, extend their capabilities, and experiment at the very margins of their expertise and knowledge. This all serves to improve our ability to meet our mission: high-quality care for patients and exceptional client service.

The Appreciative Inquiry Process

Although there is no cookie-cutter approach to appreciative inquiry, scholars have identified several general principles and stages. One of the most important principles is to form a positive question or statement of the topic. This is the most critical part of the entire process because it serves as an intervention in and of itself (Zemke, 1999). And although it sounds easy enough to accomplish, most people who are faced with a difficult issue or challenge to deal with tend to focus on the negative and create a problem-oriented question. If the need is to improve physician and employee interpersonal relationships and communication, the tendency is to identify this issue as a "need to improve physician-employee working relationships." This statement implies that something is currently wrong, and it carries with it complex baggage such as the unequal positional power of physicians and employees or the difference between employees and independent practitioners and business owners.

The question asked determines what you will find. The challenge is to create questions that "inspire and encourage people to give . . . positive examples to use as models" (Zemke, 1999, p. 29). A leader might say: "Give me examples of positive working relationships between employees and physicians." One could further explore the characteristics of these relationships: "What makes these relationships work so well?" Another approach would be to say: "Describe what it is like when you have a good working relationship with a physician [or with an employee]." If the topic is not affirmative, the initiative will fail. So we don't ask, "Why are people leaving?" Instead we ask, "Why are people staying?" Questions such as, "How do we create a magnetic work environment?" or "How do we create upward spirals of accomplishment in the workplace?" are very powerful.

Stages of Appreciative Inquiry

The stages of appreciative inquiry are discovery, dreaming, design, and destiny (Figure 6.4).

Figure 6.4 Stages of Appreciative Inquiry

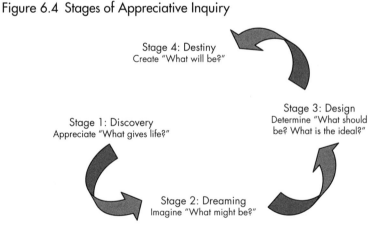

Discovery

Often referred to as the appreciating phase, discovery involves storytelling. It is a very collaborative stage. Participants think of examples and experiences that illustrate or answer the appreciative question and share them. They focus on those moments of excellence and identify the factors and characteristics that made them possible. This stage basically answers the question: What gives life? From this work, it is possible to build consensus around the strengths or basic principles inherent in the issue.

One organization was concerned about creating a more positive work environment in order to attract and better retain employees. The leader used an appreciative inquiry approach. These were questions from this first stage: "Think of a time when you felt most energized and alive at work. What was happening? Who was there? Describe the workplace environment." These are some of the answers:

"I felt valued."

"I was learning a new skill."

"My manager coached me so I could build my expertise."

"I was involved in helping make the decision."

"There was progress as a result of our actions."

"What I did made a difference."

"I liked the people I was working with."

"We had a great team."

"I was asked my opinion, and it was used in making the final decision."

"I had a high level of autonomy."

From this first step, the group developed a list of positive attributes that described these environments.

Dreaming

In the dreaming stage, also known as the envisioning phase, the basic question is, "What might be?"

This stage often starts off with an exercise such as this: "Let's assume that tonight we fall asleep and wake up five years from now. When you wake up, the hospital has become exactly the organization you would like it to be. What do you see that is different and how do you know it is different?" (Zemke, 1999, p. 30). The result of this stage is that the group coalesces around a vision of the organization and drafts a statement of what it will look like in the future. Based on the example in stage one, a vision statement might be something like: "Our workplace environment is one in which there are healthy working relationships between people, there is a high level of employee involvement in decision making, and people are treated with respect and valued for their contribution."

This stage is similar to the visioning approach presented in Chapter Three. It is not merely a dream but a vision that is grounded in history, tradition, and facts. It is based on concrete, real-life examples of what has worked.

Design

This is also referred to as the co-constructing phase because the work is to design the ideal. The questions here are: "What should be? What is the ideal? What are the principles that will help translate this vision into action? How can we make this happen?" Many successful books in the business literature use this approach. Interested individuals carefully study successful organizations or businesses to determine the principles that led to their success and then, as authors, share them with others who attempt to emulate them. Joel Barker, a futurist well regarded for his work in innovation, suggests that this is a solid start for finding new ideas. He suggests identifying two or three success stories, study the distinctive qualities that made them successful, and then put these findings to work (personal communication, June 1, 2010).

A disadvantage of trying to duplicate another organization's successes is the resistance one often encounters because "no other organization or business is exactly like ours." People often use the differences as explanations (or excuses) for why a change cannot happen. One of the advantages of using an appreciative inquiry approach within the organization is that it takes away this rationalization or excuse. If this positive environment can be created in the imaging department, why can it not be created in the laboratory department? After all, similar financial constraints exist; organizational structure and the medical staff are basically the same; the community issues are shared; and so on.

Destiny

In the destiny phase, also known as the sustaining phase, the question is: "What will be?" The participants focus on how to actualize, sustain, or create these characteristics. Zemke (1999) notes that originally this stage stood for delivery; the work was focused on developing action plans, building implementation strategies, and monitoring outcomes. Cooperrider and his colleagues (Zemke, 1999) have greatly deemphasized this concrete work in favor of more spontaneous, free-form activities. Simply preparing people in the organization with the process of the first three steps and then letting them apply them on their own in the organization has been successful in many different types of businesses around the world. This nonlinear approach is much more appropriate for the emergent nature of organizations where very little actually unfolds as predicted or planned.

The end result of an appreciative inquiry process depends on the topic that started the cycle. It may be a culture change or the development of a vision and plan to put into place.

Application

For a leader, the use of appreciative inquiry is presented here as an alternative to a traditional problem-solving approach. It has been used effectively in this manner in many organizations and projects over the past decade. Efforts to improve communication and collaboration within the organization, redefine the culture, and make process improvements have all been reported in the literature (Havens, Wood, and Leeman, 2006; Shendell-Falik, 2008; Stefaniak, 2007). Beyond health care, it has been used as a positive change methodology in businesses and more recently in cities and countries grappling with paralyzing challenges (Snyder, 2009). Cooperrider consults regularly using this technique to conduct summits (regional, national, and international) where highly energized stakeholders are prepared to implement actions that bring their dream to a reality.

However, appreciative inquiry has value beyond its action research methodology. It is also a philosophy or an attitude of approach that can function to bring the focus to the positive. One executive, during the weekly

Monday morning team huddle, starts every meeting by asking members to identify the two or three best things that happened the week before. The positivity generated by the answers helps the group to find the energy to deal with the challenges they are facing. The use of a positive question can turn the tide of an overly negative team or staff meeting. The leader can use it to emphasize what is most important and remind people of their purpose. Leebov (2005a, 2008a, 2008b) uses this approach throughout much of her work in very effective ways.

Polarity Management

There is yet another approach to dealing with challenges in getting our work accomplished. In some instances, the issue or difficulty we are dealing with is not a problem as such but rather what Barry Johnson (1996, p. xviii) calls a polarity: "Polarities are sets of opposites which can't function well independently. Because the two sides of a polarity are interdependent, you cannot choose one as a solution and neglect the other." Believing that everything we face is a problem results in trying to solve some problems that are simply unsolvable, even with all the necessary resources. By seeing polarities as problems to solve, we greatly undermine ourselves, wasting time in futile efforts. There are many examples of polarities in health care organizations today:

- Which is more important: leadership or management skills?
- When and how do we emphasize and reward individual effort versus team initiative?
- As a leader, when should I coach others to do difficult things versus doing them myself?
- How do I balance leadership accessibility and visibility versus having adequate quiet time to think and privacy?
- Should policies be implemented rigidly or with humanistic flexibility?
- Are employee needs or patient needs more important?
- When should we provide a service regardless of cost versus eliminating services that are not cost-effective and represent the wise use of our resources?

- On what issues do we need commitment, and when is it acceptable to settle for compliance?

- What's more important: the specialization of skills or employees and physicians with generalized knowledge?

- When is it better to centralize services, and when should they be decentralized?

- In the face of workforce shortages, when does urgency to produce a supply of workers override a concern for professional standards and patient safety?

If we see any of these polarities as problems to be solved, we waste our efforts. There are no clear-cut solutions to these issues. Implementing a solution just ensures that we will be dealing with the issue again at some point in the future.

Johnson's approach (1996) is to identify when the issue is actually a polarity and manage it as such rather than treating the situation as a problem to be solved. "The objective of polarity management," he writes, "is to get the best of both opposites while avoiding the limits of each" (p. xviii). In other words, the manager has the judgment to reward both individual and team effort and understands that any contemporary organizational system not only has room for both models but needs both. In some instances, an individual can best carry out the work, and in other situations, a team is much more effective. Overemphasis on either end of the polarity can result in problems. Most people would agree that policies are meant to be guidelines for action, and they must be implemented with humanistic considerations. However, there has to be some consistency or managers from different departments would choose to apply the absenteeism policy based on their own inclination and interpretation, resulting in potentially serious consequences for both employees and the organization.

Determining action in the presence of a polarity requires sound thinking, reflection, and judgment skills on the part of the leader, along with a high level of expertise in decision making. The first step is to recognize that a polarity exists. In recent years, several major consulting groups have recommended that their clients offer leadership development days on a quarterly basis in the organization. They further suggest that a council or committee of organizational managers take responsibility for this function to ensure a high level of ownership. Of course, this makes sense on the surface. However, many of these operational managers become exhausted and frustrated in handling some of the details that have long been managed by a centralized education or organizational development department. So instead of expert meeting planners handling the logistics, a continual stream of managers takes on this responsibility and have to be brought up-to-date on approaches for contacting the hotel and arranging for meeting space, contacting speakers and negotiating contracts, and dealing with the myriad details entailed in producing these events. This can lead to an enormous outpouring of energy without concomitant benefit. There is likely a middle point that could be reached that would include involving the frontline leaders in the planning and design of the program; a skilled event planner savvy in these areas could handle the meeting planning details.

The level of judgment required for leaders in dealing with polarities cannot be underestimated. Martin (2007) spent fifteen years studying how exemplary leaders think. All of the leaders he studied shared a somewhat unusual trait:

> They have the predisposition and capacity to hold in their heads two opposing ideas at once. And then, without panicking or simply set-tling for one alternative or the other, they're able to creatively solve the tension between those two ideas by generating a new one that contain elements of the others but is superior to both. This process of consideration and synthesis can be termed integrative thinking. It is this discipline—not superior strategy or faultless execution—that is a defining characteristic of most successful businesses and the peo-ple who run them [p. 3].

Understanding polarities and using Johnson's approach to mapping a polarity is the way a successful leader can become a more integrative thinker as well as assist his or her followers in thinking in a more integra-tive fashion.

Polarity Mapping

The way to manage a polarity, Johnson (1996) suggests, is through using a grid or polarity map with two poles (Figure 6.5). The left half (L in the figure) represents one side of the polarity, and the right half (R in the figure) represents the other. The upper half represents the positive outcomes that focus on the particular pole, and the lower half represents the negative outcomes that come from focusing only on that pole. Before you can effectively manage a polarity, you have to be able to see all four quadrants of this polarity grid. Johnson suggests filling out whichever quadrants are easiest first and then working from there.

Figures 6.6 and 6.7 show polarity maps that represent the four quadrants of an issue that a respiratory care department in a large tertiary medical center faced. The pediatric respiratory therapists included those who worked in general pediatrics and others in the neonatal intensive care unit. Conflict arose periodically over the years about the issue of specialization versus generalization of these practitioners. The neonatologists and pediatricians

Figure 6.5 Polarity Map

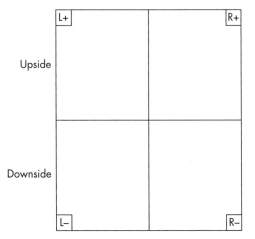

Source: Reprinted From *Polarity Management: Identifying and Managing Unsolvable Problems,* by Barry Johnson, copyright © 1992, 1996. Reprinted by permission of the publisher, HRD Press, Amherst, MA, (800) 822-2801, www.hrdpress.com.

Figure 6.6 Polarity Map: Patient Needs Versus Employee Needs

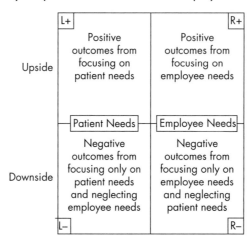

	L+	R+
Upside	Positive outcomes from focusing on patient needs	Positive outcomes from focusing on employee needs
	Patient Needs	Employee Needs
Downside	Negative outcomes from focusing only on patient needs and neglecting employee needs	Negative outcomes from focusing only on employee needs and neglecting patient needs
	L−	R−

Figure 6.7 Polarity Map: Respiratory Issue: Putting Patient or Employee Needs First?

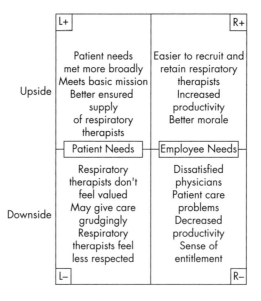

	L+	R+
Upside	Patient needs met more broadly Meets basic mission Better ensured supply of respiratory therapists	Easier to recruit and retain respiratory therapists Increased productivity Better morale
	Patient Needs	Employee Needs
Downside	Respiratory therapists don't feel valued May give care grudgingly Respiratory therapists feel less respected	Dissatisfied physicians Patient care problems Decreased productivity Sense of entitlement
	L−	R−

were often in direct conflict with each other, as well as the manager of the department about the issue. When the manager facilitated a group discussion examining this as a polarity, they identified the underlying issue as determining whether patient needs or employee needs are paramount.

Putting Patient Needs or Employee Needs First?

Mapping out this polarity enables you to see the whole picture or structure of the dilemma. To focus exclusively on patient needs may result in not meeting important employee needs, which may then result in lower morale and productivity, indirectly affecting how the respiratory therapists meet patient needs. The clearest opposites in the polarity map are the downside of one polarity and the upside of the other. Johnson (1996, p. 11) calls movement through the grid the "polarity two-step." It starts in either lower quadrant and moves across and up, down, and then repeats.

The difficulty in dealing with polarities occurs because each party is convinced that it is right in its particular conviction and basically sees only its side. Having the group work through the polarity map helps create the whole picture. Instead of the parties' disagreeing and contradicting each other's view, the task becomes to supplement each other's view in order to see the entire picture. Parties on both sides of the polarity have key pieces to the puzzle; they just need this simple structure to help identify and share them. The opposition that each side feels to the other actually becomes a key resource in dealing with the issue. No one is being challenged; instead, both parties assume the accuracy of each position. As a result, there is joint effort in combining two valid views of a situation in order to see a more complete picture.

Johnson (1996, p. 45) says that "in most organizations there are often very serious and costly confrontations that take place because a 'both/and' polarity is treated like an 'either/or' problem to solve." In working out the polarity map together, the possibility of each participant seeing the other quadrants and more fully understanding the issue occurs because the process has not contradicted their own view of reality but confirmed it. "Successful management of polarities calls for intentional interventions that support both values (poles) simultaneously" (Wesorick, 2002, p. 24).

One of the difficult challenges is knowing when there is a polarity to manage instead of a problem to solve. Johnson (1996) offers two questions to use for help in deciding which you are facing: Is the difficulty ongoing? Are there two interdependent poles?

If a solution exists that is a definite end point in a process, the problem is solvable. An example is the decision about where to have the holiday party. Once the group makes the decision, it is done. This is an either-or problem: either we go here, or we go there. Once the group makes the decision, it is carried out. Problems of choice are solved the minute the choice is made. But solving polarities is a continual process. Instead of reaching an end point, there is a never-ending change of emphasis or focus from one pole to another. For example, emphasizing and rewarding individual performance is appropriate at some times, and focusing on the team effort is appropriate at other times.

The second question is whether there are two poles that are interdependent. "The solution in problems to solve can stand alone. Unlike a polarity to be managed, the solution to a problem to solve does not have the necessary opposite that is required for the solution to work over an extended period of time" (Johnson, 1996, p. 82). Polarities instead require both poles. The issue of manager accessibility to employees is an example. On the one hand, for the manager to be available to employees is an important aspect of the job, yet the manager also needs to have quiet, uninterrupted time in order to do the work that requires concentrated thinking time. If the manager is accessible at all times, it is likely that many aspects of the leadership role are getting short shrift. And no leader who is in his or her office with the door closed the entire workday is going to be perceived as effective by his or her staff.

Once the polarity map is complete, the question is: What do we need to do to stay in the upper two quadrants? In the respiratory therapist example, the question is: How can we meet both patient and employee needs? How do we know when to shift the focus from one pole to another? The group then has identified actions to support each side of the polarity and is more likely to recognize in the future when overemphasis on either pole has occurred.

A director of education was frustrated with the seemingly constant conflict and disagreement about whether educators should be decentralized in the departments or located in the centralized education department. She used the polarity map to work her group through the issue. They identified practical strategies to manage this polarity. In a perioperative division, the director used this process to work with his staff as they explored the polarity of specialized operating room teams or emphasizing generalization of skills of staff.

Conclusion

This chapter has focused on the leader's proactivity and ability to attain results. Several key processes that effective leaders use in obtaining results, specifically the skills of problem solving and decision making, were presented. The need to think clearly about complex issues is crucial (McGinn, 2007; Vestal, 2009d). Two additional approaches, appreciative inquiry and polarity management, are included to broaden the leader's repertoire. These skills, combined with the interpersonal skills that previous chapters delineated, increase the leader's ability and credibility.

DISCUSSION QUESTIONS

1. Who are the most proactive people in your work group or department? What are the behaviors you observe that indicate to you these people have a high level of personal initiative?

2. How could you acknowledge and reinforce proactive behaviors when you see them in employees or peers?

3. What typical system, organizational, or department problems do you deal with currently? How effective are problem-solving or process improvement teams in your department or organization? Is there a specific problem-solving methodology they use? Are staff members proficient in using this process?

4. Is coaching or external facilitation available to the problem-solving groups in the organization? What is your coaching role?

5. What pitfalls in problem solving and decision making does your work group most commonly experience? What steps could be taken to prevent these?

6. What kinds of decisions are you responsible for in your leadership practice? Would any decisions that are currently being made by individuals be better made by the group or the team?

7. Think of the different types of decision making (majority vote, minority, consensus, individual, and unanimous decisions), and identify examples of each that you see in your work environment.

8. Does your team or work group deliberately determine how its decisions are going to be made?

9. Are you better with right-brain (spontaneous, creative, free-flowing) thinking or left-brain (logical, analytical, and methodical) thinking? What about your work group? What is the impact on the effectiveness of your problem-solving efforts?

10. How could you use appreciative inquiry to deal with issues you are facing?

11. How could you use appreciative questions in your leadership practice on a more frequent basis?

12. What common polarities do you see in your workplace? Have they been mistaken for problems? How could you use the polarity grid to achieve more effective results?

7

Coaching and Developing Others

CHAPTER OBJECTIVES

- Identify the most common reasons for a lack of active coaching.
- Define the term *coaching*, and differentiate it from the term *coach*.
- Identify the five basic human intrinsic motivators and their ramifications for the leader's practice.
- Explain the motivation principle of "expect the best" and why it works.
- Discuss the six steps of the coaching process.
- Use the scripting model for delivering corrective feedback.

Managers who see themselves as coaches will also
tend to see their employees as individuals of innate talent and worth.
RON ZEMKE, "THE CORPORATE COACH"

L eadership is the art of influence—the capacity to move or impel others
to a certain course of action. Each competency explored in this book
increases the leader's ability to influence others. A healthy, vibrant relationship
with followers is the foundation for transformational leadership. Shared values,
a compelling sense of purpose, and clarity of vision build commitment to a
common direction and generate energy and passion in the workplace. Free-
flowing, consistent, and accurate communication between leaders and followers
directly increases leaders' influential abilities. Skill at leading processes and
getting results are additional proactive competencies that help build momentum. A final manner in which leaders influence is by intentionally coaching
and helping followers develop their skills and abilities.

The Leader's Role

Developing others is the final leadership competency this book addresses. One
might argue that an effective leader, accomplished in the other skills already
presented, spontaneously and unconsciously helps others develop. People simply observing a leader's behaviors are influenced. Most leaders, however, are not
content with a passive role in developing others and instead choose an intentional path that actively focuses on supporting the growth and development of
employees and, in many instances, the transformation of followers into leaders.
The intentional development of others is the focus of this chapter.

The intentional development of people in the organization is a strategic focus, a future-oriented strategy that exemplifies hope and optimism.
Tichy and Cardwell (2002) believe that winning organizations are successful
precisely because they have leaders at all levels, and they have leaders at all
levels because they make the development of internal leaders a priority. They
point out that the top leaders "personally devote enormous amounts of time
and energy to teaching, and they encourage other leaders in the company to

do the same" (p. 3). Delegating the development of top performers in the organization to others is one of the most common mistakes a leader makes (Martin and Schmidt, 2010).

This chapter explores a coaching process for development of skills and performance improvement. The chapter identifies approaches that increase the leader's effectiveness and delineates a specific coaching process. All are based on the premise that the leader's influence on others increases if the leader engages actively in the process of developing followers.

Coaching

Today's leadership rhetoric is filled with references to coaching. Writers exhort leaders and managers to become coaches, articles and books on coaching in the workplace appear regularly, and seminars on the topic sell out. In recent years, national accreditation for coaches has become available, and academic programs offering in-depth preparation for the role have appeared. With this insistent and repetitive urging to become a coach, why aren't more leaders excellent coaches?

The good news is that through years of experience and learning, some leaders and managers do develop excellent coaching skills. However, they may not have a concrete framework that is easy to pass along to others because they learned their skill over years of practice, trial and error, and careful scrutiny of what worked and what did not. Excellent coaches with years of experience develop their intuition—a sense of knowing something without understanding how one knows it. Remember the specialized spindle cells in the brain that activate when we have to select the best option from a list, even for simple tasks (Goleman and Boyatzis, 2008; Veronesi, 2009). Coaching becomes a consistent and vital part of their leadership practice because they value people and have directly observed and received its many benefits. These health care leaders continually seek to further refine and define their coaching role. What exactly does *coaching* mean? What do effective coaches do for their followers?

Now the bad news: many health care managers and leaders engage in a passive form of coaching, characterized predominantly by inconsistent and sporadic coaching. On one project, they take an active coaching role, only to have followers accuse them of micromanaging; and on another project, they offer little or no guidance or advice because they are too busy. The message to followers is, "Just handle it." Perhaps the only consistent behaviors in which they engage are the annual performance appraisals and disciplinary processes meant to address and correct performance problems. This is a reactive rather than a proactive process—often something that leaders dread rather than see as an integral part of their role.

Unfortunately, the bad-news description is more common in workplaces. According to Ron Zemke (1996, pp. 26, 27), "Given the growing popularity of the coaching metaphor and the facility with which it slips from the lips of consultants and managers alike, you might expect by now that most managers would excel at listening, setting a positive example, giving praise, pointing out areas of improvement, and encouraging employees to stretch and grow—the skills of coaching. Naturally you'd be wrong." He goes on to report on recent studies, all of which conclude that "on a wide range of skills, managers were rated lowest in their ability to give employees useful feedback on job performance." A recent study found that "the biggest statistical driver of workplace satisfaction for those workers between 21–30 years of age is whether their manager recognizes and praises their accomplishments" (Murphy, Burgio-Murphy, and Young, 2007, para. 3). Only 39 percent of study participants said they did.

Why Leaders Don't Coach

If coaching is so important and popular today, why is it so rare? Why is coaching inconsistently practiced? Why is there aversion to functioning as a coach? These are reasons given by managers.

Lack of Understanding

Leaders know that coaching followers for performance improvement is important. After all, isn't everyone telling them so? Some leaders are ineffective coaches because they do not understand the principles involved; they may have received little coaching themselves and so have no role models from whom to learn. When leaders are managers and part of the organizational hierarchy, the demands of managerial responsibilities cloud the issue. Some believe that completing performance appraisals on time means their coaching responsibilities are over for the year. There is confusion over the difference between counseling and coaching. Counseling is a supportive process by a manager to help an employee define and work through problems that affect job performance. By nature, it is a reactive process. Coaching is proactively focused on development. It is defined more fully later in this chapter.

Lack of Time

Downsizing and restructuring in health care organizations in the 1990s took their toll in terms of formal leadership positions. Leaders with hierarchical positions have more responsibility and broader spans of control than ever before. The rapidly accelerating pace of change places many additional time demands on today's leaders and can result in physical, mental, and emotional exhaustion. Unfortunately, coaching is a leadership function that is easy to put off. Finding time to coach does not feel like a priority to a leader who is already facing a full and frenetically busy day crammed with meetings and unanswered e-mails. Transformational leaders understand that coaching is an investment for the future. It takes time now but later returns huge dividends.

Fear of Confrontation

Addressing performance gaps sometimes feels like confrontation, especially if the performer receives the comments less than graciously and becomes hostile or defensive. A leader's reluctance to correct or suggest alternative approaches creates a downward spiral. Afraid of offending the person or precipitating an emotionally negative response, the leader delays giving the person much-needed performance feedback. The leader becomes increasingly conscious of the performance gap and with every occurrence comes to believe more and more strongly that he or she must address it. Reluctance fuels procrastination, and when the leader and performer finally discuss it, the simple performance gap has become a major issue. When both the leader and follower clearly understand the purpose of coaching and the leader addresses the issue immediately, performance feedback is less likely to assume these horrific proportions.

Lack of Confidence

Coaching skills are learnable, but trial-and-error experience can be painful. Classroom time on coaching rarely goes beyond theory. It may teach principles and increase awareness, but it doesn't necessarily develop skill. Although being coached is one of the best ways to learn coaching, leaders who have not received coaching themselves often feel as if they are fumbling through the process. And they may be coaching followers who are more highly competent in other areas than they are, so it is no surprise that the leader's confidence may waver and weaken.

Lack of Incentive

Little in today's organization incents leaders to develop others. One department manager noted that when he worked hard to develop people within his department, they were promoted to positions elsewhere in the organization. Initially he was pleased and satisfied by this because he believed this was his role as a leader. Over time, he realized that an employee's promotion left him with a major deficit in his department and the need to start the process all over again—finding the right employee and pouring time and effort into guiding the new employee's development. As a fully mature manager leader, he continues to engage actively in this process, though he admits he is tired after several decades of this cycle. How different he would feel, he has mused, if he received a ten thousand dollar bonus for every employee promoted outside of his department. Successfully recruiting an external applicant for a position often costs far more than that, so both he and the organization would conceivably come out ahead. And if a personal bonus is not an option, an incentive in the form of money for his department with the freedom to use it as he and the employees decide would recognize their efforts.

These reasons all offer some explanation for the lack of active coaching in today's health care organizations. Admittedly the good news–bad news scenario is more likely a continuum with extremes at opposite ends. More leaders and managers are likely to fit somewhere in the middle than in the extremes. This chapter section defines coaching and proposes a concrete process that provides a structure to help make the coaching process easier to engage and apply in day-to-day work.

Coaching Defined

Coaching is another one of those buzzwords in health care leadership circles. It's used so often in an overly loose or superficial manner that it becomes virtually meaningless. Instead of frequent use increasing understanding, the opposite occurs. Distinctions become blurred. and everyone has his or her own definition.

Webster's describes *coach* as a verb, meaning "to give instruction or advice." It further defines it in terms of sports and the arts but makes no mention of the coach in the business or work world. This is a fairly narrow definition, and if the origin of the word is examined, the essence is much clearer. "The original meaning of *coach* can be traced to the concept of a horse-drawn carriage or coach and that, essentially a coach conveys 'a valued person from where he or she was to where he or she wants to be'" (McNally and Cunningham, 2010, p. 7).

This chapter defines coaching as a process of facilitating an individual's or team's development through giving advice and instruction; encouraging discovery through guided discussions and hands-on experiences; observing performance; and giving honest, direct, and immediate feedback. Coaches ask questions to stimulate discovery and thinking on the part of the follower. The goal of coaching is to improve the employee's or team's skills and abilities. Don Shula (Shula and Blanchard, 1995, p. 28), long-time coach of the Miami Dolphins, says, "A good coach provides the direction and concentration for performers' energies, helping channel all their efforts toward a single desired outcome. Without that critical influence, the best achievements of the most talented performers can lack the momentum and drive that make a group of individuals into champions."

It is helpful to distinguish between the process of coaching and the role of coach. As a process, *coaching* refers to the way outcomes are achieved. It includes the process or structure applied in order to obtain desired results. In the definition, for instance, giving advice and instruction is one way that the desired outcome—facilitating the individual's development—is realized. In this instance, *to coach* is an action—an active verb.

Coach, as a noun, describes a position or role that a person takes on. The coach is an individual who applies a process of coaching. This implies some level of formal structure, for every position or role carries responsibilities. The level of formality in the relationship can range from contractual—a legal agreement defining the role and relationship of coach to the individual receiving the coaching, with everything clearly spelled out—to a loose agreement whose details are implied by the participants involved.

In today's workplace, the structure tends to be on the loose to the nonexistent side. A leader or manager may intellectually know and accept that coaching is an important function of his or her role and yet engage in the process only sporadically and reactively, with actual coaching occurring only when the leader delegates new tasks and responsibilities or when performance shortfalls are apparent. Formalizing the coaching relationship to some degree may provide a structure that transforms an inconsistent and reactive behavior to a deliberate, consistent, and proactive process.

The Coaching Role

Comparing the coaching roles of health care leaders to athletic coaches sheds further light on the concept. There are many similarities, although also some striking differences, such as this major one: most individuals on a sports team are highly motivated to be there—not always the case in the workplace. Similarities in these different arenas, however, are striking: the coach recruits and selects players, determines the game plan, works with the team to improve performance by giving feedback, continually evaluates the team's performance, and motivates and encourages the team or the individual.

In health care organizations, as in sports, the coach does not have to be a star player—not always the best criterion for a good coach. The coach must know enough about what he or she is coaching to make suggestions that are to the point and helpful. But primarily the coach is highly skilled at helping others do better. Without the coach's objective viewpoint, a performer may repeat the same mistake over and over again. Yet often in health care settings, employees expect the leader to be the expert or star in clinical skills; indeed, many leaders expect this of themselves as well.

In sports, the coach would not dream of missing a game or not being present when the team practices or competes. Yet many leaders in health care

are so inundated with paperwork and meetings that they coach primarily by voice mail and e-mail, spending little time actually observing performers at work. And because of the demands of the work, many managers are emotionally and physically depleted of the necessary energy to engage in active coaching. "Coaching is an intensely personal business. You can't coach people from a distance, with aloofness. People need to see that you are at least as interested as they are in what's going on" (Shula and Blanchard, 1995, p. 125).

Another important point from the sports world helps health care leaders understand their coaching role. In sports, it would be ludicrous for star players not to work with a coach. As McNally and Cunningham succinctly put it, "Why does Annika Sörenstam, one of the most successful golfers in the LPGA history, need a coach? *Because she cannot see her own swing*" (2010, p. xi). Yet in a health care setting, too often the focus of the manager is on poor performers, to the neglect of exemplary performers. Because the exceptional employee is not creating any problems, the coach may believe that he or she would better spend time with low performers. Yet the future yield from investing in high-performing employees is dramatically higher than focusing all efforts on those at the lower end of the performance continuum. Many managers spend 80 percent of their time focusing on the 20 percent of their staff who fit in the low-performer category.

Sports analogies may induce visions of competition, one team winning over another. In this regard, the health care leader coach may be more like a drama or movie director, a symphony conductor, or a dance coach. These coaches function in much the same way as a sports coach, but the desired outcome is one that is mutually beneficial for all rather than victory in a win-lose competition. Coaching is about pulling the very best performance from each person.

Before presenting a process for effective coaching, two general principles or concepts that provide a grounding in the basic theory need to be explored. The first relates to the formation of a relationship between coach and performer, and the second is the application of the principles of motivation.

Building the Relationship

A prerequisite to effective application of a coaching process is the establishment of a relationship between coach and performer or player. Coaching, much like leadership, cannot exist in the absence of a relationship. The very essence of coaching is interaction between people. And without a sound relationship, the performer is less likely to be amenable to the coaching and unwilling to actively participate in the process. The presence of a relationship characterized by trust, mutual respect, support, and open communication (discussed at length in Chapters Two and Four) has a positive influence on the quality of a coaching relationship. These concepts are addressed here briefly in the context of a coaching relationship.

Trust

Trust, the foundation, comprises the three elements of competence, congruity, and constancy. A coach who knows the rules of the game and has established his or her own competency can be an excellent coach without ever having reached star status based on his or her own performance. In fact, some star players who have gone on to be coaches have failed dismally because good coaching takes far more than expert performance skills. Adequate knowledge of the game is necessary; more important are expert coaching skills.

The second element of trust, congruity, enhances faith and is heightened when the coach behaves in a manner that matches the message that the coach is sending to the performer. Successful sports coaches understand this concept. In discussing reasons for the phenomenal success of his teams, Don Shula, long-time successful coach of the Miami Dolphins, writes (Shula and Blanchard, 1995, p. 56):

> A lot of leaders want to tell people what to do, but they don't provide the example. "Do as I say, not as I do," doesn't cut it. Of course, I'm not about to show players how to run or pass or block or tackle by doing these things myself. My example is in things like my high standards of performance, my attention to detail, and, above all, how hard I work. In these respects, I never ask my players to do more than

I am willing to do. My own preparation for every game has to be exemplary. I am dedicated to success and will do whatever it takes to achieve it. I am generally the last one off the practice field.

The final element of trust, constancy, exists when the performer knows that he or she can count on the coach—that the coach is at practice sessions with the team and stays until the end of the game even through a discouraging and dismal loss. The coach does not bow out and head for the locker room early just because the team is behind. Observation of team and individual performance is not possible if the coach is not at the game. Videotaping is a wonderful way of replaying performance, but it is not the same as being there. No sports coach worth his or her salt waits until after the game to review performance and give corrective feedback.

Mutual Respect

A good relationship requires mutual respect. The coach's job is to push players to their peak performance. Players need to believe that the coach has something to offer and is focused on helping them improve. When the coach's motivation is to help the team members be their very best, players may not like what the coach asks them to do, but they respect it. "Lots of leaders want to be popular, but I've never cared about that. I want to be respected. Respect is different from popularity. You can't make it happen or demand it from people, although some leaders try that. The only way you can get respect is to earn it" (Shula and Blanchard, 1995, p. 50).

Players often resent being pushed to satisfy the coach's ego. A women's collegiate volleyball team was a good example of this. The coach had recently graduated, and this was her first coaching job. She drove the team mercilessly because she wanted a championship team in her first year out of school. Her relentless pursuit of this goal in spite of the fact that the team did not have the experience or ability necessary led to her complete ineffectiveness as a coach. By the end of the year, she did not have enough players left to take the court as a team. The players knew that she was not interested in helping them improve their performance for any reason other than her egocentric needs.

Support

Unconditional support is crucial in order for a player-performer to form a strong connection with the coach. The nature of the player role is one of continual development, honing and perfecting skills and approaches. This means there will be bungles and mistakes along the way. The coach who encourages and supports during these times wins the regard and gratitude of the players. Rather than harping on the mistake, expressing confidence that the player-performer will do better next time sets up the likelihood of future success.

Communication

Communication is the final requirement for a healthy relationship between a coach and a performer. Readers can review issues and principles of communication discussed fully in Chapter Four for their applicability to coaching. Without the ability to articulate direction, vision, and goals and to give feedback, the coaching process does not work. Good communication skills are the vehicle through which the leader carries out the coaching process. Communication that is direct, honest, and predominantly positive generates a healthy coaching relationship. If the person being coached hears mostly negative feedback, the relationship deteriorates.

Perhaps as important as the quality of the relationship between the coach and performer is the definition, or structure, of the relationship. Role definition and agreement are essential, especially in the workplace, where nebulous coaching relationships exist. Establishing the specifics of the coaching role—what it entails, what areas it includes, and what approaches the coach will use—increases clarity in an otherwise vague process. The coach and performer work out the coaching agreement together to ensure mutual understanding of the various roles. A structured coaching relationship elevates what is often a casual and sporadic process to a consistent, development-focused process.

Motivation

In addition to the underpinnings of a positive relationship, understanding and applying the principles of motivation are inherent elements of the coaching role of an effective leader. Influencing others requires comprehension of the reasons people act in certain ways. Motivation is what causes a person to act in a particular manner. A multitude of theories are related to motivation, and all have relevance for the leader who is seeking to better understand a follower's nature. These theories include need fulfillment (Maslow's hierarchy of needs), Herzberg's two-factor theory (what satisfies does not necessarily motivate), expectancy theory (a person behaves in a certain way if he or she believes the effort will yield a reward), and equity theory (one determines expected outcomes by comparing one's work and rewards to others doing a similar job). Rather than reviewing these theories, which readers can find in almost any text on organizational behavior and development (Borkowski, 2011), this section briefly looks at some common misconceptions about motivation, the factors related to intrinsic motivation, and two major principles of motivation applicable in a coaching situation. The first is the principle of expecting the best, and the second is knowing the desired outcome and then reinforcing it by reward.

Misconceptions About Motivation

Anyone seeking to influence another person needs to be skilled at motivating. McGinnis (1985) describes several of the many common misconceptions about motivation and offers examples to refute them:

- *All motivation is intrinsic.* Perhaps the most common misconception is that no one can motivate another person and that all motivation comes from within. For years managers have heard: "You cannot motivate another person; all you can do is create an environment that is motivating." Although intrinsic motivation is very powerful, it is not the only source of motivation. Everyone remembers an instance in which the presence of someone else—an inspiring teacher, a dynamic and encouraging coach, or simply the presence of loved ones—led to increased performance, even performance beyond expectation. McGinnis (1985) cites several historical examples, such as Wellington reporting that when Napoleon was on the field, it was like fighting an additional forty thousand men. Winston Churchill's leadership breathed hope into a dispirited and frightened England during the last seven months of 1940 and changed the future of the modern world.

- *Some people just are not motivated.* Everyone is motivated, though it may be by and for different things. The employee who is usually late and takes an extra half-hour to get rolling in the morning may be the first one out the door in the afternoon, full of enthusiasm. The fifteen year old who requires continual nagging to get out of bed on a school morning can get himself up and out of the house at 4:00 A.M. on Saturday for a fishing trip with friends. These two have plenty of motivation—it is just inspired by different things. The challenge for the leader is to channel that already existing energy into endeavors good for the team or organization.

Many managers and supervisors react with skepticism when introduced to the idea of shared decision-making models for employees, whether in self-directed or self-managed work teams or governance structures. From their years of observing employee behavior, these leaders simply cannot believe that employees will accept more responsibility willingly, such as participating in peer review, self-scheduling, managing inventory and supplies, or jointly interviewing applicants for an open position in the department. Unfortunately, many employees in a bureaucracy learned long ago that getting involved beyond the minimum required in a day's work simply does not pay. But when they understand that they really can, and are allowed to, make decisions that directly affect their work life, their enthusiasm returns. Most people prefer having control over their lives.

- *Motivation is manipulation.* In its negative connotation, manipulation is when a person tries to persuade another to a certain course of action that is not to the individual's benefit but to the motivator's benefit. Genuine motivation is finding mutually beneficial goals that are good for both individuals and then forming a satisfying partnership to achieve these goals.

- *Motivational people are born, not made.* Contrary to this final misconception, anyone can become an effective motivator. It simply takes an understanding of the theories and basic principles. This is good news for leaders who want to further develop their effectiveness.

Applying the principles of motivation increases the leader's ability to influence others. The following section offers a framework for understanding intrinsic motivation as well as identifying and explaining two primary principles of motivation.

Understanding Intrinsic Motivation

Intrinsic motivators are those elements within us that influence our behaviors. If motivation is what makes us do what we do, then intrinsic motivation consists of those internal factors that result in our taking a particular course of action. Although it sounds paradoxical, a good leader understands these and takes action to build on them, thus applying the added influence of external motivation.

Thomas (2000) offers a solid conceptual framework for understanding these intrinsic motivators and a compelling case for their contribution and importance in today's work world. "The new work role is more psychologically demanding in terms of its complexity and judgment, and requires a much deeper level of commitment. While economic rewards were pretty good for buying compliance, gaining commitment is a far different matter" (p. 5). He clearly believes that external motivators such as money and benefits are no longer enough to compel workers to act. Financial rewards have long been identified as a satisfier but not a motivator. When intrinsic motivators are present, an individual is more likely to feel energized and passionate about his or her work. The five intrinsic motivators, shown in Figure 7.1, are healthy relationships, meaningful purpose, competence, choice, and progress.

Recent work in the field of positive psychology has further substantiated much of the work on intrinsic motivators. Studies have found three elements important to happiness in life: pleasure, engagement, and meaning (Seligman, 2002). And to live the fullest life means that these three elements are present in all aspects of our lives: within ourselves, in our life with those we love, and in our work life. Deiner and Biswas-Deiner (2008), in examining components of a psychologically wealthy life, found many of these intrinsic motivators to be present.

Figure 7.1 The Intrinsic Motivators

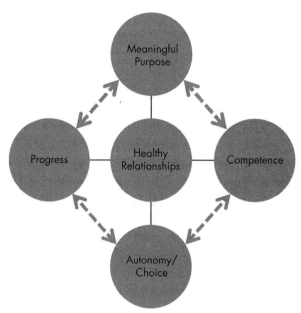

Healthy Relationships

People are clearly more highly motivated to perform in a particular way if they have a positive, healthy relationship with others in the workplace. It is very unlikely that a person goes the extra step for someone he or she actively dislikes or does not respect. Because healthy working relationships were examined more fully in Chapter Two, this discussion will not repeat these key principles. Suffice it to say that the establishment of positive relationships and a sense of connection to the people in our workplace lead to higher intrinsic motivation.

Meaningful Purpose

"People have a desire to be engaged in meaningful work—to be doing something they experience as worthwhile and fulfilling" (Thomas, 2000, p. 12). Many of us have work that is composed of tasks that serve a particular end or accomplish a specific purpose. When we are clear about what the purpose is, we can make intelligent decisions about the work. Rather than seeing work as a necessary evil or something that costs us, we find work itself to be meaningful and rewarding.

A second-career nurse who being interviewed for a research project was questioned about her experience of joy through her work in the outpatient recovery area of a diagnostic center. In the course of the interview, she mentioned casually that after almost six years, she was now nearing the salary level she had left behind to enter a nursing education program. She went on to say that she would never go back to manufacturing, even if the money was better, because her work as a nurse allowed her to see every person for whom she made a difference. In her words, our world "can live without chrome bumpers for our cars," but it could not survive without someone to care for the sick and injured (Manion, 2002a). The meaningfulness of her work far outweighed the financial considerations.

Because the very nature of health care encompasses some of the most meaningful work known to humankind, the care of others who are sick and at their most vulnerable, we might assume that health care work is inherently meaningful and think that, as leaders, we need take no specific action in this area. There are, however, several important ramifications. The first is that some individuals in the organization may do such a narrow piece of work—the volunteer who delivers patient mail, the maintenance worker who puts a fresh coat of paint on the walls, the housekeeper who circulates and empties the trash—that they may not see their connection to the contribution to the well-being of patients. Leaders can help everyone see their own contribution and the importance of the work in helping to clarify that line-of-sight concept mentioned in Chapter Three. Helping everyone see their impact on patients and the quality of health status in their community is inspiring.

Second, the leader, along with employees, must be continually alert to events or situations that indicate the organization is not living up to its stated mission and values. When organizational decisions and behaviors contradict what employees believe is the organization's mission, the resulting dissonance can severely affect the person's sense of meaning.

And finally, especially in today's health care organizations, leaders must continually seek to reduce the amount of work perceived as near meaningless that creeps into the job. Few health care workers chose their field because they wanted to spend half of their time documenting and recording what they did. The impact of increased regulation in health care has resulted in greater focus on paperwork and compliance with arbitrarily established rules—often at the cost of time spent in the delivery of actual service in the department. Add to this the amount of duplicative work and the time employees spend cleaning up the problems of other departments and the added time it takes to navigate and use the electronic medical record, and you can see that we are quickly reaching the tipping point when health care workers begin to believe that trivial concerns have overtaken the meaningful work in their day.

Competence

"You have a sense of competence on a task when you feel that you are performing your work activities well—when your performance of those activities is meeting or exceeding your own standards" (Thomas, 2000, p. 77). Most of us are more likely to enjoy work at which we are good. Seligman (2002) defines authentic happiness as knowing our signature strengths and crafting a life that uses these strengths in all aspects, personally and at work. In other words, we are more likely to be happy when we are engaged in work that taps into our abilities and reflects our competence.

Csikszentmihalyi has done extensive research on the concept of flow (1990, 1997, 2003), which he defines as an optimal experience that is the unintended side benefit of engaging in activities in which we are stretched to our limits by worthwhile challenges. It is both a sense of mastery and full engagement in an event. "Flow is the state in which people are so involved in an activity that nothing else seems to matter; the experience itself is so enjoyable that people will do it even at great cost, for the sheer sake of doing it" (1990, p. 4). Competence is an important part of this concept; the situation calls for a stretch on our part. If there is not enough challenge to our abilities, we may become bored or apathetic. And if the challenge exceeds our ability to master it, frustration results.

The ramifications of personal competence for health care leaders are far-reaching. First, this intrinsic motivator provides ample justification for the inclusion of this chapter on coaching as an important contribution to increasing the effectiveness of leaders. The role of the leader as coach is to help followers increase their level of competence, whether technical or interpersonal. Providing opportunities, learning about resources, emphasizing growth, and ensuring an organizational philosophy of continual learning are all important. Murphy (2010a) is a firm believer in the correlation between great achievements and challenging goals. In a study on goal setting, one of the areas Murphy (2010b) asked about was whether employees would have to learn new skills for their annual goals. In his words, the results were shocking. Compared to employees who do not experience new learning,

> Those who will have to learn new skills to accomplish their goals are:
>
> - Twenty-two times more likely to say, "I would like to spend my career at this organization."
> - Seventeen times more likely to say, "I recommend my boss to others as a great person to work for."
> - Twenty-one times more likely to say, "I recommend this organization to others as a great place for people to work" [p.1].

This clearly demonstrates the relationship between learning new skills and being happy and satisfied at work. Learning challenges employees to aspire to something larger than the status quo as it raises their level of expertise and makes them more valuable to the organization.

Another ramification has to do with selecting the right person for the right work or helping an individual resculpt work that does not use his or her competencies or signature strengths. Buckingham and Coffman (1999, p. 148) say that "casting is everything": "If you want to turn talent into performance, you have to position each person so that you are paying her to do what she is naturally wired to do. You have to cast her in the right role." This message was reinforced by Jim Collins's study (2001, p. 41) of why some organizations were able to make the leap from being good to exceptional performers: "The executives who ignited the transformations from good to great did not first figure out where to drive the bus and then get people to take it there. No, they first got the right people on the bus (and the wrong people off the bus) and then figured out where to drive it." Furthermore, when determining who the right people are, the greater emphasis is on character attributes rather than specific experience or education (Collins, 2001; Manion, 2004b). Having specific skills or knowledge is important, but exceptional leaders know that these are teachable, whereas character and personality traits are more ingrained.

Crafting work that fits an individual is another aspect of the leader's role. Loehr and Schwartz (2003) have extensive experience in coaching both sports athletes and corporate athletes (their term for performers in the work world). They share multiple examples of individuals who came to them for coaching because they were exhausted and nearly depleted of energy. These people had lost a sense of connection and competence in their work. Sorting through what they are extremely good at is a key aspect of redefining the work so that it engages a person's full capabilities (Loehr and Schwartz, 2003; Seligman, 2002).

Another potential role of the leader is in creating work environments that are more likely to lead to optimal experience or flow on the part of employees. Flow is also engagement; in fact, when we are in flow, we are so engaged that we do not even notice time passing. A quick examination of most health care workplaces reveals multiple barriers to the experience of flow. Workers experience countless interruptions at work—beepers and cell phones, overhead announcements, environmental noise, and e-mails—all of which interrupt or prevent flow.

An important payoff when employees work with a sense of their own competence is that they feel pride. When Byrne (2003, p. 66) interviewed Jon Katzenbach about his book, *Why Pride Matters More Than Money* (2003), Katzenbach said, "It's more important for people to be proud of what they are doing every day than it is for them to be proud of reaching a major goal. That's why it's crucial to celebrate the 'steps' as much as the 'landings.' The best pride builders are masters at spotting and recognizing the small achievements that will instill pride in their people." This is not the same as acting prideful from a sense of arrogance but is the positive emotion of feeling proud of one's accomplishments.

Autonomy/Choice

The fourth intrinsic motivator is choice. We feel a sense of choice on a task or responsibility when we see that our views, ideas, and insights matter. Choice also has to do with felt ownership—when we feel personally responsible for the outcome of our behaviors or decisions. "Choice takes on extra importance when we are committed to a meaningful purpose. Then a sense of choice means being able to do what makes sense to you to accomplish the purpose" (Thomas, 2000, p. 65).

A leader in today's workplace may not have any control over the individual's initial choice to be there, that is, whether the person must work or not. However, it was clear in the discussion on organizational commitment that people must feel they have a choice before they can feel engaged and committed to their work. A freely made choice to work in this particular organization is crucial to an employee's feelings of commitment. This has tremendous ramifications during times of severe national economic downturns. Too many people may remain in a job they don't like, increase their work hours, or change their employment status from temporary to a more stable status because of financial difficulties rather than from personal choice.

Beyond these external factors, however, leaders have a great deal of control over this intrinsic motivator. Ensuring that employees experience a sense of autonomy in their work is crucial. Models of shared decision making, operationalizing empowerment, and delegation are common ways to increase employees' exercise of choice in their work. Giving people the authority and autonomy to make decisions that are within their scope of responsibility and trusting them to do so are important transformational leadership behaviors. Creating a climate that discourages placing blame and finds positive responses to mistakes are further ways a leader encourages followers to make decisions and show initiative.

Progress

A sense of progress occurs when you feel that your activities have the impact that you intended, when you see that your work is achieving its purpose. Little is more discouraging than to feel that nothing changes as a result of our effort and hard work. When we see progress, we feel momentum and enthusiasm and the energy to continue onward. An ancient Greek legend portrayed the torture of Sisyphus, who was doomed to push a large boulder up to the top of a hill, then stand aside and let it roll back to the bottom. Then his work began again, pushing the boulder to the top. Such repetitive work with no appreciable outcome is the ultimate torture of a being who inherently seeks meaningful work.

The research on what brings people joy in their work clearly indicates that seeing results and making progress is essential (de Man, 1929; Manion, 2002a, 2003). The ramifications for health care leaders are many: we need to analyze and remove barriers to progress within our systems. For too many years, we have tolerated the same problems in our systems. Implementing an effective process improvement approach is not just the latest consulting fad or organizational culture change; instead, it is crucial if employees and leaders alike are going to have the tools to make both incremental and substantial change in our systems. Employees and leaders must share the responsibility for true process improvement. Many of the processes identified in Chapter Six (problem solving, appreciative inquiry, polarity management) are approaches for dealing with these issues.

In addition to putting into place effective processes for dealing with issues and problems, organizations must develop measurement and accountability systems so that people can track their progress and see their results. Accountability systems are notoriously weak in health care organizations. For example, with the current emphasis and focus on the leader's responsibility in recruitment and retention, few health care managers have access to department-specific measures of vacancy and turnover rates or satisfaction measurements by patients, employees, and physicians. Yet their organizations are holding these managers accountable for outcomes in areas where measurements are inadequate or so outdated as to be useless.

A final ramification for leaders to consider here is how they recognize and reward progress. If leaders do not recognize progress, they cannot acknowledge it. In recent years, a hospital in the Southeast was positioning itself to become part of a larger health care system. In order to be as financially viable as possible, the administration asked each segment of the current system to make a substantial contribution by reducing its operating expenses. In the organization's large home health agency, managers were expected to reduce their expenses by $1.5 million over the next year. These exceptional leaders worked closely with their employees in order to achieve this result. Employees were instrumental in designing and implementing a workforce reduction and work consolidation effort that was well received. In nine months, the agency reduced expenses by $1.2 million.

The system CEO and chief financial officer called the two managers to a meeting for a report on their progress. For an hour, the executives badgered, questioned, and basically harangued the two departmental leaders to determine how they would reduce the remaining $300,000 of expenses. The executives neither mentioned the progress the managers had achieved nor commended them for the exemplary way they had obtained the results. You can imagine the level of interest and motivation these two leaders felt after the meeting as they returned to their remaining task. Both left the organization within six months.

Celebrating and recognizing progress is not as easy as it sounds. We have reservations about celebrating too early. However, people pay attention to what we emphasize. A very successful leader reported that creating fun things to do was her way of emphasizing what she felt was important. For example, when new employees in her department complete their orientation period, she takes them out to breakfast, and she takes their mentors or preceptors out to dinner (Manion, 2004b).

Generational Differences and Motivation

Much has been made of the difficulties inherent in having multiple generational cohorts in the workplace. Generational diversity was "widely popularized in the early nineties when the advent of large numbers of Gen Xers into our workforce caused many Baby Boomers to shake their heads in bewilderment" (Manion, 2010, p. 8) at the seemingly different work ethic and values of the younger generation. During the past fifteen years, these differences have been the focus of many articles, books, and programs that are good reads but have not produced solid evidence-based suggestions for managers. The subject has been explored extensively in many other sources (Manion, 2009a, 2009b, 2010).

Certainly no one would deny that a sixty-two-year-old employee is likely to see things differently and have different needs from a twenty-one-year-old employee. Age diversity is a major challenge for a manager who may be trying to understand what seems incomprehensible, attempting to juggle the needs and interests of such a varied workforce. However, understanding basic human motivators is a place to begin to try to create a workplace that offers motivation to all. These principles are important to keep in mind (Manion, 2010):

- Not all motivators are equally important to everyone. One person may be more highly motivated by the presence of positive, healthy working relationships, while another may be more motivated by being able to accomplish something worthy through his or her work.

- The influence of these motivators may change over time and circumstances. A new employee or someone newly promoted to a position may be more highly motivated by his or her need to experience a high level of competence than is the long-tenured, well-experienced staff member.

- These motivators may be defined somewhat differently by members of the different generations. Meaningful work for a member of the millennial age cohort may mean community service and the ability to volunteer and make a difference in the world. A Baby Boomer may define meaningful work as making a difference for the patients under his or her care.

- Probably the most important principle is to remember that no matter the generation, we are all humans and thus tend to be motivated by at least some of the same five intrinsic factors. What may differ is the action a person will take if a key motivator is not present in the workplace. Gen Xers have been long derided for job hopping, being willing to move quickly from job to job if they aren't satisfied. On the other hand, Baby Boomers tend to hang around but if they become cynical, their dissatisfaction is evident.

Emphasizing the differences between the generational cohorts can increase divisiveness and separateness. The fact remains that we are all human beings with similar needs and motivations. It may ultimately be a more beneficial approach to focus on our similarities and the values and interests that we share. As already noted in Chapter Three, the alignment of values and beliefs can result in a shared passion for our work. The leader's role as a source of external motivation is crucial and more effective when focused on the five basic motivators.

Motivation Principles

Leaders who understand the principles of intrinsic motivation can choose behaviors that support these important principles (see Figure 7.2). The leader must also understand external motivation. Two of its most important principles are expecting the best and knowing what you want so you can reward it.

Expect the Best

In coaching, attitude is everything. To put it simply, coaches who like people and believe that people have the best of intentions often get the best performance. It is well documented that people live up to the expectations they and others have of them. Henry Ford said it best: "Whether you think you

---

Figure 7.2 The Leader's Role in Enhancing the Intrinsic Motivators

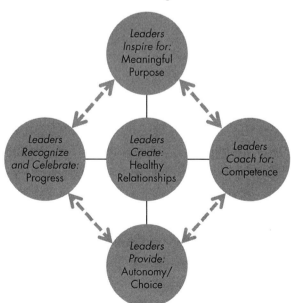

can or you think you can't, you're right!" If the coach expects the best from his or her performers, that is what the coach gets. Good coaches do not waste time looking for and exposing their performers' faults. Instead, they look for strengths and abilities that others have overlooked, and they find ways to encourage these special talents (Wiseman and McKeown, 2010). If the coach is constantly on the watch for the person's worst side, performers become defensive and self-protective, and the door to an effective coaching relationship closes.

The coach can quickly turn a person or team into what he or she expects of them. Jim, a department manager, has recently had his scope of responsibility expanded through the additional assignment of two new departments. Over the past several months, he has been grooming Susan, a long-term employee, to move into an assistant manager position in one of these departments. Although she has been gradually assuming more responsibility, Jim does not believe that Susan is yet ready to effectively make decisions that he spent years learning to make. However, he feels he has no choice because of the circumstances in which he finds himself. Jim has a short vacation planned but is concerned about what might happen in his absence. Sure enough, on his return, he learns that Susan has made a poor decision that has significant negative ramifications for the department.

Jim's reaction will greatly influence Susan's future behavior. Jim might say, exasperatedly (even if only to himself): "I should have known better than to take any time off. I didn't think she was ready, but I didn't have any choice." To reinforce this reaction, every time Susan asks for more responsibility or for less micromanaging on his part, he reminds her of the fiasco the last time she was left alone. And when he is gone for a day or longer, he makes a point to call in and check up regularly to see what's going on. Or he asks a fellow department head to check a couple of times throughout the day just to be certain nothing is amiss. What's the message to Susan? What happens the next time Susan needs to make a decision on her own? How does Susan feel about herself? Will she have the confidence to make a decision or take needed action?

Or Jim can react to the situation based on his belief that Susan can accept responsibility and make good decisions. His reaction might then be more like this: "Susan, this decision was a mistake. It isn't like you. Let's take a look at what was happening and how you can clear this up. We won't make a big deal out of this, but I want to help you figure out what you might do differently next time. We all learn from doing, and if you're not making any mistakes, you're probably not making any decisions. And I want you to make decisions, because I know you have good judgment and can make good choices." How will this affect Susan's level of confidence and willingness to accept responsibility in the future?

The leader's belief about people influences how he or she approaches these coaching situations, and these beliefs create a self-fulfilling prophecy that begins with an assumption that is not necessarily true. But by believing it is true, the leader acts as if it is and creates a cycle of behavior that results in the very behavior he or she initially expected or feared (see Figure 7.3). This concept explains how the principle of "expect the best" works. Research has documented extensively the validity of this concept and has discovered that people prefer others to behave as they expect them to (McGinnis, 1985; *Productivity and the Self-Fulfilling Prophecy*, 1997). In other words, by our assumptions (whether true or not), we create the reality that fits our expectations. If a coach has a belief about an individual and the individual does not behave in a manner to support this belief, the coach becomes uncomfortable. For example, a situation in which an individual succeeds where a coach thought the individual would fail creates dissonant feelings in the coach.

Figure 7.3 The Self-Fulfilling Prophecy

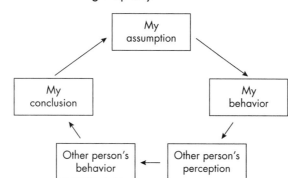

The concept of the self-fulfilling prophecy is critical for workplace coaches because they have all kinds of expectations about the people they work with, and some of these expectations are damaging. For example, executive leaders and managers who believe that employees do not want additional responsibility or involvement in decision making are less willing to share responsibility (see Figure 7.4). A manager's belief that employees without a professional education cannot manage themselves or are not as creative as employees with more education directly affects the degree of delegation that occurs. These are common beliefs operating in today's workplace, and they limit the potential of individuals and teams to achieve. Transformational leaders continually seek to understand their own behavior to determine the presence of unrecognized negative assumptions. The way to break a self-fulfilling prophecy is to question the underlying assumption and thus change behavior.

Reward the Desired Behavior

The second major motivation principle involves rewarding the behavior we want to increase. To effectively influence others, the coach must be crystal clear about the behavior he or she is seeking and then reward that behavior. If the leader does not somehow reward or recognize the desired behavior, the follower will gradually stop behaving that way. Worse, if the leader rewards and reinforces contradictory behaviors, poor outcomes may result, leaving leaders wondering what happened.

Figure 7.4 The Self-Fulfilling Prophecy in Action

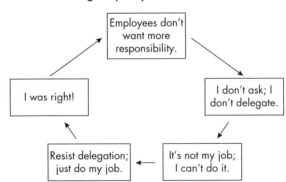

The concept of reward is far broader in scope than simply monetary rewards. Too often in the workplace, people assume that only money can be that reward. What is really needed is a variety of rewards. Money is certainly an important one, but it is often tied directly to the annual performance appraisal system. In too many organizations today, the performance appraisal system is more deflating than motivating. A large system in the Midwest implemented a new rating scheme for its annual performance appraisals. Department managers were told that roughly only one employee for every twenty should receive the highest rating. In one small department, the manager was directly advised that she could give only one of her employees this high rating.

The manager was in a dilemma because she had several exemplary performers, and she had to make a tough choice about who would receive the highest rating. One frontline employee, Jane, had led a major housewide change initiative, coauthored an article for publication in a professional journal, and given a presentation at a national conference, in addition to carrying her normal workload. Jane was devastated when her manager gave her a rating of average after a year of truly exceptional performance. The one exemplary status was given to a coworker who had coordinated the relocation of a small department. Is it any wonder that employees disengage and remove themselves psychologically from their workplace? In this instance, the difference in money was negligible, but in terms of recognition for achievement, Jane felt this rating was a slap in the face. The organization unwittingly lost the commitment of one of its best members. Coens and Jenkins explore the inadvertent destruction of motivation created by contemporary performance appraisal systems in their book *Abolishing Performance Appraisals: Why They Backfire and What to Do Instead* (2000).

Good leaders understand the difference between pleasure and gratification and use both as rewards. Pleasures bring short-term positive feelings and often create an emotional reaction. These include things such as a coupon for a free dessert in the cafeteria, a gas card, or perhaps a couple of free movie tickets. Gifts and surprises during employee recognition events also fit this category. This has been referred to as the "toys and trinkets" approach to recognition (Manion, 2009b). Gratification is a much more powerful emotion and results when something is given, but it requires involvement on the part of the recipient. Gratification is more likely to occur in relationship to one of the intrinsic motivators. Examples of gratifying rewards could include being offered increased opportunity, going to lunch with the leader, more individual time with the coach, increased flexibility in scheduling, support of attendance at a desirable continuing education program, greater freedom, and even increased responsibility. These rewards are more likely to leave an individual with something to remember and a longer-lasting effect.

Rewards are most effective when they come soon after the behavior or accomplishment the leader identifies and acknowledges. The leader must also offer the rewards sincerely. Just handing out a coupon or writing a thank-you note because the manager is required to do a certain number every month leads to a feeling of increased disconnect in the workplace.

Wells Fargo developed innovative ways of rewarding people. At year end, the organization gave every employee a fifty-dollar bill, with the stipulation that each employee must give his or her fifty-dollar to the coworker who had been the most helpful during the past year. What a wonderful way to reinforce cooperation and teamwork among coworkers. Underlying this approach was the understanding that helping others recognize people who have made a difference to them is very gratifying to both parties.

The company then gave the employees who received the most bills a choice of another holiday gift, among them two pounds of Mrs. Field's cookies every month for a year, a two-hour body massage on April 15, a puppy, a menu item named in their honor in the Wells Fargo cafeteria, a certificate for a favorite bookstore, or attending a continuing education event. These gifts made a tremendous impact and were not soon forgotten.

A good coach is careful to avoid rewarding behaviors in a way that leads to unintended negative consequences. If, for instance, the leader always gives increased responsibilities to two or three employees because they are especially willing and competent, these individuals may feel after a time that they are pulling the weight for the whole team. Not only that, the midlevel and low performers see this consequence of high performance as a good reason to avoid such a situation. Another problem occurs if the leader reinforces behaviors contradictory to what he or she wants. If the leader considers raising issues and offering different viewpoints to be positive team behavior, then the leader should recognize and remark on that behavior rather than the compliant behavior of simply going along with everyone else. An executive in one organization was known for belittling and chastising people who offered opinions differing from his, yet he constantly verbalized the importance of speaking up and being honest. He never saw that his behavior was damaging to the very behaviors he said he wanted.

A newspaper columnist some years ago gave a classic example of a punitive reward for good behavior. The nationally syndicated columnist Sandra Pesmen (1990, p. E21) received the following question: "I called my top commission salesman in another city last week and couldn't find him in the office or at any customer's offices. So I called his house at 1 P.M. and he answered the phone. When I asked what he was doing there, he answered that he'd filled his quota for the month, and if he worked any harder and made more sales, he'd just have to pay more to Uncle Sam. I'm furious but wonder what to do. He is a good rep, works well with our customers there and knows our line."

Pesmen's answer is insightful and representative of the mentality prevalent in some sectors of society: "Try and remember you're the boss. Cut his commission so he'll have to work harder to make the same personal profits. While he's doing that, he'll be increasing the company profits, which is the main goal. If he gets angry over that and quits, remember no one is indispensable" (1990, p. E21). So the bottom line here is that every time this salesman increases his sales, he will get less, not more. What is this company rewarding? And why would anyone in their right mind continue working hard for such a company?

Sometimes what we are rewarding is not quite so obvious. But it is well known that what we pay attention to and remark on is often what increases. "If you pay the most attention to your strugglers and ignore your stars, you can inadvertently alter the behaviors of your stars" (Buckingham and Coffman, 1999, p. 155). And when our best performers start slipping, it is a sign that we have been paying attention to the wrong people and the wrong behaviors. What the top performers see is that the way to receive attention is to become one of the problems. One of the key principles for any leader who is attempting to create a positive workplace is to identify the top 20 percent of performers and spend the majority of your time working with them (Manion and Muha, 2009).

These two basic concepts—building a healthy foundational relationship and applying the principles of motivation—increase the effectiveness of the leader involved in developing followers' skills and abilities. Some leaders understand these concepts inherently, but others may use this review as a reminder of their importance.

The Coaching Process

The most effective coaching process is based on a partnership relationship between coach and performer. The essence of the relationship is one of mutual benefit—an exchange of equal contribution between the two parties. Zemke (1996, p. 27) notes: "Managers who see themselves as coaches will also tend to see their employees as individuals of innate talent and worth. Managers who see themselves as coaches will strive to act as trusted advisers to help people develop those talents and use them in concert with others toward the achievement of a common and shared goal. Managers who see themselves as coaches tend not to think of their employees as vassals." Indeed, active coaches, either peer leaders or managers, see themselves in partnership with performers. The coaching process includes the following key concepts. It is not precisely a linear model because it is dynamic and continually responsive to emerging factors. However, there is some value in understanding at least a basic sequential process. Figure 7.5 delineates this process.

1. Determine your intention.

2. Assess the performer.

3. Clarify expectations and parameters.

4. Carry out the coaching intervention.

5. Observe performance.

6. Give feedback.

Figure 7.5 The Coaching Process

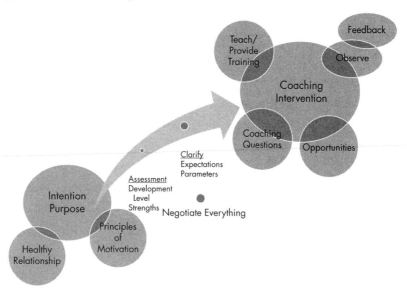

Step One: Determine Your Intention

The first step of the process is to determine the purpose of the coaching. Why is the leader coaching the individual? Is there a performance gap issue or a new expectation or process in the department? Does the individual need to improve performance simply to meet the expectations of the role or job? Is the leader trying to develop advanced skills in the performer? Is the leader evaluating the individual's strengths and capabilities to determine future promotion opportunities? Is the coaching part of a succession-planning strategy? Determining your intention actually makes the coaching much easier to approach. It both provides clarity and can serve to center the leader's positive intention. It focuses the coach on his or her positive role.

Part of this step requires setting specific performance goals. The strongest goals are those that the coach and performer develop mutually. Throughout the coaching process, negotiation contributes to the level of commitment and engagement of the performer. Goals that the leader develops for others are less likely to be embraced. The most common example occurs in disciplinary situations. Too often the manager creates a development plan and delivers it to the employee. This is often a key difference between counseling and coaching.

Without a specific goal in mind, coaching is less likely to be intentional and proactive, as I have already noted. In some instances, the coaching plan is specific and concrete enough that the leader and follower write out and agree on the goals. For instance, the CEO coaches several members of the executive team so that they are able to attend and function effectively at key meetings with the board of trustees. A manager focuses on developing an employee to lead a department action committee for solving unique or difficult problems. Department leaders implementing a shared decision-making structure often use an explicit coaching plan for each group leader and each group.

In other instances, the purpose of the coaching is more general and nonspecific: it is simply a desire to intentionally focus on others' development needs. It is comparable to the reactive form of coaching. A situation arises spontaneously, and the coach naturally intervenes in an appropriate manner (uses guiding questions, teaches, trains, or provides an opportunity) and gives feedback after observation of the performance.

A coaching session usually involves discussing intention and specific goals, which then become a frequent topic of conversation. The goals need to be brought out frequently, considered, and reconsidered. Many of us have had the experience of approaching the time for our annual performance review and suddenly realizing that we had identified goals that have been sitting in a file cabinet somewhere for the past year. This kind of goal setting has little power to influence anyone positively.

The Gallup Organization has conducted extensive research with over eighty thousand managers who excelled at turning their employees' talent into performance (Buckingham and Coffman, 1999). They found that the manager who encourages employees' development takes the time to sit down and periodically find out what the employee is interested in and what his or her job aspirations are. Research conducted to determine what health care managers actually do day-to-day to create a workplace culture of engagement found that successful managers paid a great deal of attention to their employees' growth and development (Manion, 2004b). And Murphy (2010b) advocates challenging goals that push followers well beyond their comfort zone.

Once the purpose or desired direction is clear, the coach and performer determine the latter's precise needs by completing an assessment. Although assessment of the performer's needs is the next step of the coaching process, assessment is also inherent within each step. For instance, some level of assessment occurs before the partners determine the purpose or goal. Prior to choosing an intervention, assessment of appropriate possibilities is necessary. And observing performance, the fifth step, entails assessing or appraising the results of the coaching to determine whether it was effective.

Step Two: Assess the Performer

The second step of an effective coaching process is assessment, which may be completed by the performer, the coach, or both. First, one identifies the desired skill or competency under consideration. In some instances, the performer becomes aware of a need for coaching in a specific area. It may be a new skill or job responsibility with which the individual has little or no experience, or circumstances may have changed significantly since the last time this individual accepted this responsibility. In other instances, the coach may have become aware of the need for coaching by observing a gap between actual performance and acceptable or exceptional completion of the responsibility.

Assessing Skills and Competencies

However the need for coaching is identified, the focus of assessment includes appraising the performer's level of development or accomplishment of the task or responsibility. In the classic situational leadership model (Grohar-Murray and Langan, 2011; Hersey and Blanchard, 1993), four categorized development levels (to be described in detail later in this chapter) assist both coach and performer in assessing the individual or team and determining the most effective coaching intervention. They found that the most effective leader is the one who accurately assesses what the follower needs, based on the developmental level of the particular skill, and then provides what the follower is lacking.

Patricia Benner (1984) has conducted extensive research on how clinicians, specifically nurses, learn their clinical skills. She found that nurses progress through five stages of development as they learn their practice: novice, advanced beginner, competent, proficient, and expert. The practitioner is substantially different in each of these stages in several ways. First, as a novice, the individual relies on concrete, rigid principles; as skill acquisition occurs, the person begins to rely on past experience. Let's say you are learning a new skill, such as playing racquetball. You learn exactly how to hold the racquet and to follow through with your swing. As you become more proficient, you no longer think about these details; instead, you shift your weight and handle the racquet based on what is going on in the game.

A second way we differ in these stages of development is in how we perceive the situation. A novice is often overwhelmed by all of the details in a given situation and often cannot act quickly enough. With years of experience, the person is able to quickly assess a situation, even as it unfolds, and determine the most important action to take first and what should follow. To return to the previous example, anyone who plays racquetball can remember the first time on a court and the feeling of panic and bombardment as the ball bounces from wall to ceiling to floor to ceiling again, often so quickly that it is difficult to follow. As you become skilled in the sport, you develop a sense for the ball and begin to focus on strategy.

The skill acquisition model dovetails nicely with a situational leadership model. Both respect the development of the individual and recognize the changing needs of the performer. The leader must consider the follower's skill and ability in a given situation in order to provide the appropriate leadership intervention. Two people in the same situation may need entirely different coaching.

To return to the situational leadership model, each level is based on two aspects: the performer's competence and commitment. Competence refers to the performer's knowledge, skill, and experience. Commitment includes the performer's willingness to perform or interest in accepting the responsibility or task, the performer's confidence, and the level of the performer's motivation. The following sections describe the four development levels, along with effective coaching interventions.

Development Level One: Novice

This is a new responsibility for the individual. The person may have had education and theory but no or very limited actual experience or practice with the skill or responsibility. Performers at this level are usually excited and enthusiastic about trying a new skill. Thus, their competence level is low, but their commitment is high.

Coaching interventions include sharing any information that the performer needs. This includes telling the performer what to do and how, where, and when to do it. It can include making educational opportunities available to the individual, suggesting reading resources, or even recommending practice with a specialized coach or in a simulation. However it is accomplished, the coaching intervention is to provide the competence that the performer lacks. Commitment and enthusiasm are high, so the performer needs little encouragement.

Any information that the coach provides is structured and detailed, with the coach closely controlling and monitoring the situation because the performer does not yet have well-established skills. In fact, too many explanations and examples can cause confusion because the performer needs only the basics at this stage. This level of intervention is directive in nature.

Development Level Two: Advanced Beginner

The performer now has had some experience using this skill or taking on this responsibility but is not yet accomplished. Action taken is of a more deliberative nature; it's not yet fully integrated into the person's repertoire of skills. Commitment is variable because after trying something and not having things proceed as well as expected, the performer may feel discouraged and frustrated to learn that the task is not as easy as he or she first believed. As a result, the performer lacks self-confidence and may even resist the idea of trying again.

At this level, the performer has some competence but low commitment. The coach's role is to furnish the additional technical competence the performer needs and plenty of enthusiasm and support. In addition to the how-tos of level one, the coach adds personal examples and perhaps discloses his or her own early difficulties in gaining the particular skill. The coach asks questions about the performer's experiences and previous successes and listens carefully to the answers. This provides an opportunity to redirect or reinforce behavior. Thus, the leader-coach provides what is missing: encouragement to bolster the performer's commitment and direction to support knowledge and skill.

Guided discussions are appropriate at this stage because the performer may be making progress without realizing it and may simply need someone with an objective viewpoint to recognize that and point it out. When used with praise, positive reinforcement can provide the encouragement the performer needs.

Development Level Three: Competent

The performer is now experienced in applying the skill or has the competency required to assume the responsibility but has variable commitment. He or she may have high proficiency in this skill but in a completely different setting and may lack confidence in that ability because he or she does not recognize its transferability, or the people involved may be new to the performer. This performer is high on competence but variable on commitment.

At this level, the performer is competent, and any information or knowledge the coach provides is minimal, often limited to key parameters and expectations. For example, the only structure the coach gives may be to share the final date by which the performer is to complete the task or identify key constraints, such as budget limitations or expected stakeholder involvement. The performer is fairly experienced with this responsibility and just needs a coach available to talk through ideas and possible solutions.

However, commitment is variable at this point. The performer has wavering confidence in his or her ability to achieve the desired outcomes. The current situation may be significantly different from any in his or her experience or simply more complex or difficult than usual. Whatever the case may be, at this point the coach provides much-needed encouragement and support through guided discussions, asking questions and listening carefully to answers, and reminding the performer of previous successes and lessons learned. With a highly competent performer, the focus is that little extra push of encouragement and confidence that a trusted coach can give. The coach remains available to the follower.

Development Level Four: Expert

This is the highest level of development that a performer achieves. Experience in the performance area is broad enough that the individual has not only the technical competency but a high level of judgment in applying the skills.

In addition, commitment is high. The performer is motivated, confident, and enthusiastic about the responsibility.

For the highly competent and committed performer, the coach does not need to provide much of anything. There may be a need to provide the barest of structure—perhaps clarification of a time frame or key parameters and constraints. The coach and performer often negotiate these, as would be expected in an equal partnership.

Although recognition and rewards are always important, they are less important to the performer at this level of development. Much comes simply in the form of confidence and trust that the leader has extended. The commitment and enthusiasm are generated from a profound sense of intrinsic motivation. As in development level one, the performer has plenty of zeal and is excited about the task to be accomplished.

Completing the Assessment

Ways to assess a performer's development level include observing actual performance, self-reporting by the performer, and gathering information coming from third-party sources. Yet another source of information may be demonstrated knowledge of the logical process. For example, if an individual has performed well as a leader of a department, the next step in his or her development might include leadership opportunities of cross-department or organization-wide projects or process improvement groups. If an executive leader has performed well and mastered his or her responsibilities within the organization, the next step may be systemwide opportunities.

Accurate assessment is crucial because the individual's development level determines the coaching intervention the situation requires. If the assessment is inaccurate, the resulting intervention may range from ineffective to downright harmful. For instance, if the performer is at development level one and is low on competence, the coach's role is to provide access to needed knowledge and information. If the coach erroneously assessed the individual at development level three with a high level of skill and determines that the performer needs only encouragement and support, the coach falls short. The performer then becomes frustrated and demoralized by not performing at the expected level.

A good example of this was observed in an organization undergoing massive change. A special project team of employees was identified and assigned to the project for two years. The team's purpose was to lead the organization's major change initiatives. Tom was appointed team leader. Having received his master's degree in hospital administration, Tom had recently completed his administrative residency at the hospital. A tall, imposing figure who dressed for corporate success, Tom exuded confidence and capability without being arrogant. He was a relatively young man, however, having completed his master's work immediately following his undergraduate program, and he had limited to no hands-on management experience.

Leaders erroneously believed that Tom was at a higher level of development in terms of managing the team than he was, and he certainly looked the part. Unfortunately, people overevaluated this promising young man repeatedly. Not only did he not receive the basic managerial skill development and direction he needed, but when he did not meet people's unrealistic expectations, he had to face their extreme disappointment and negative reactions. Tom was in a no-win position.

The same can happen with children. In one family, both the father and mother were very tall. Their young son grew rapidly, and at six years, he towered over all of his friends, his appearance easily that of a child twice his age. The mother reported being embarrassed and concerned by the judgmental comments and behaviors of other people who assumed that this six-year-old behavior was coming from a twelve year old. Her son's behavior was very appropriate for his age but unacceptable to others who had assessed him based on a cursory glance and had come to inaccurate conclusions.

Inaccuracies in assessment also occur in the opposite direction. When the individual or team has a higher level of competency than the leader believes and the leader provides more detail and direction than the performer needs, the performer is often irritated and concludes that the leader is micromanaging or afraid to relinquish control. When teams or individuals are at developmental level three or four, they are highly competent. If the leader closely monitors and supervises their work (appropriate behavior for levels one and two), they may become angry and resentful and refer to the overseeing manager as a micromanager.

Assessing Strengths

David McCullough, an American historian, has studied the role of American leaders for decades. In a recent interview, he notes that "spotting talent is one of the essential elements of great leadership. Washington had it to a remarkable degree. Washington was not an intellectual. He wasn't a spellbinding speaker. He wasn't a military genius. He was a natural born leader and a man of absolute integrity. And he could spot ability where it wasn't necessarily obvious" ("Timeless Leadership," 2008, p. 46).

Marcus Buckingham (2005), based on survey research of eighty thousand managers conducted by the Gallup Organization coupled with in-depth studies of selected top performers, sought to discover what the most important thing is that effective managers do. He found that extraordinary managers "know and value the unique abilities and even the eccentricities of their employees, and they learn how to best integrate them into a coordinated plan of attack" (Buckingham, 2005, p. 72). Their goal is not to try and change the individual but to release the potential and capacity from within the person. It's about continually tweaking the environment "so that the unique contribution, the unique needs, and the unique style of each employee can be given free rein" (p. 79). The success of the manager, he believes, will depend almost entirely on his or her ability to do so.

Recent years has brought about a greater appreciation for the need to focus on the performer's strengths rather than deficiencies and needs for development. The field of positive psychology brought this focus to the forefront with instruments useful for identifying an individual's strengths. It has been further emphasized by the Gallup Organization through research on strengths-based leadership (Rath and Conchie, 2008). Over ten thousand participants were asked why they follow the most influential leader in their lives. The first major conclusion drawn was that the most effective leaders are always investing in strengths. "In the workplace, when an organization's leadership fails to focus on individual's strengths, the odds of an employee being engaged are a dismal 1 in 11 (9 percent). But when an organization's leadership focuses on the strengths of its employees, the odds soar to almost 3 in 4 (73 percent)" (2008, p. 2). The leader's focus on and investment in employee strengths resulted in a startling eightfold increase in engagement.

So given these tremendous results, why wouldn't a leader focus on strengths more consistently? The answer to this question is more complex than I will explore here. However, we do know that the human brain is hardwired to deal with problems. The good things that happen to us are there, and our response, we hope, is recognition, appreciation, and gratitude. But a day going well, an employee performing in an exemplary manner, and desired outcomes being reached don't seem to require much more of a response from us. However, when relationships are problematic or the employee isn't able to handle a situation appropriately, problems occur that need to be dealt with. The focus becomes the deficiency or failure, and it can lead to what feels like an overemphasis on the negative and result in loss of self-confidence in the parties involved.

There are multiple ways to determine a person's strengths. Two of the more widely used instruments can be found on the Internet. The Values in Action Character Strengths assessment, found at www.authentichappiness.com, is free of charge and useful for determining a person's character strengths. StrengthsFinder2.0 is an instrument available on the Gallup Web site, www .strengths.gallup.com, for a fee. Both are excellent resources.

Leaders can also increase their accuracy in identifying strengths simply by being mindful and deliberately looking for the strengths they see in another individual. Using guided questions when conversing with employees helps elicit these qualities. A simple approach is to have the person think about a time when he or she was at his or her very best. This should be a time when things were going extremely well, the person was highly engaged and in flow, and was proud of his or her accomplishments. While the person describes that time, the leader listens for the strengths that are apparent. Reflecting on times when we were at peak performance often illuminates our strengths.

Behaviors can be modified and skills learned; however, if a particular job or responsibility requires a strength that the individual does not have, it is far better to determine this rather than allow the individual to continue in a situation where he or she becomes demoralized and loses confidence. When a person's strengths fit his or her particular role, performance can be dazzling. In an interview shortly before his death, Peter Drucker was asked, "What is the most important thing leaders do?" His answer: "The task of leaders is to create an alignment of strengths in ways that make a system's weaknesses irrelevant" (Cooperrider, 2009).

Step Three: Clarify Expectations and Parameters

Once the partners have clearly established the goals and direction and completed an appraisal of the performer's needs, the next step is to identify and agree on expectations and applicable parameters. Clarifying the operant expectations helps prevent misunderstandings. Expectations between coach and performer may include the role of each person, as well as the most helpful desired approaches and behaviors. The coach must clearly identify parameters, and the performer must understand them. This section examines each of these issues with examples to illustrate their relevance within a coaching situation.

Expectations: Roles and Responsibilities

Early discussions about the roles and responsibilities of each party in a coaching relationship are essential. When the coaching relationship is a legal agreement between parties, the parties make the roles particularly clear. The conductor of a symphony orchestra regularly practices with the musicians and is responsible for procuring the best possible performance from them. The athletic coach is employed for the same reason: to develop individual team members to work as a team that will achieve peak performance. But relationships in the workplace are less clearly defined. Some coaches are very effective in developing performers yet are not in management positions. And many managers today see their coaching role as additional to their other responsibilities—something they do haphazardly and only when they have time, if at all.

Thus, an increasing number of performers in today's workplace are unclear about the coaching role and may actually resent having someone else observing their performance. In fact, their experience with the manager as a coach is limited to the annual performance appraisal or the less frequent disciplinary action. And leaders often manage these processes unsatisfactorily.

A conversation about the respective roles and responsibilities of each party formalizes the relationship and moves it from incidental and accidental to intentional. This objective consideration of who does what reduces the likelihood that strong emotions will hamper the process. A coach's role is to facilitate or support the performers' development of skills by observing their performance and providing honest, direct feedback; giving advice and instruction; and encouraging discovery through guided discussions and hands-on experiences. The performer's role is to practice, perform, and use the coach's feedback, guidance, and instruction to improve performance further.

Expectations: Desired Approaches and Behaviors

Expectations concerning desired approaches and behaviors include such elements as the type of coaching required and the ways in which the coach will observe performance or deliver feedback. In discussions, coach and performer can clarify their expectations and needs related to specific behavior. This actually forms an operating agreement. For example, the coach gives the individual immediate feedback after observing performance. But what qualifies as "immediate" feedback—within a few minutes, a few hours, or several days? Is it important that the coach deliver the feedback privately? Are voice mail and e-mail messages acceptable? Is feedback kept confidential? Will there be time to discuss the feedback and ask questions? What does the coach expect of the performer who is receiving feedback? Is the performer to incorporate the suggestions and corrections in the next performance? Is the performer to receive the feedback with an open mind and a willingness to try alternatives?

Expectations and agreement on coaching interventions are determined by the performer's needs and are an important point to discuss. Ideally, in a healthy coach-performer relationship, the parties discuss the results of any assessment and reach an agreement on specific coaching interventions that the coach will provide. Even the most highly skilled performer at times has a need for direction and instruction. If the current situation is new to the performer, ways to increase his or her knowledge and competence are the focus of the coaching. No matter how capable a performer the performer is, today's workplace is continually presenting new challenges for which performers need to develop competency. The similarities of situations may accelerate the learning curve, but the need for direct instruction and advice is paramount in the rapidly changing health care environment today.

One situation in a western health care system is a classic example. Ellen, the system's CEO, knew that as the system expanded to integrate a freestanding rehabilitation facility, a large home health facility, and a physician practice clinic, she could prepare for her own role changes by selecting a chief operating officer whose focus would be primarily on hospital operations. The final candidate came from her executive staff. Don, a young man, had the necessary educational qualifications and demonstrated leadership abilities. His current responsibilities included the marketing function and physician relations in the organization. When Ellen made the appointment, she was well aware that his downside was lack of experience and knowledge of hospital operations. In making her decision, she was clear about her coaching role with Don. He would need directive interventions and learning opportunities to assist him in developing these competencies.

There can be emotional elements—both negative and positive—to consider when the coaching intervention involves providing competence and skill. Don was excited and pleased about his promotion because of Ellen's trust and confidence in his abilities. If Ellen and Don had not talked about his learning needs and the appropriate coaching interventions, he might have felt uncomfortable with the high level of direction that Ellen would provide. There is added pressure from Don's personal need to perform well after receiving such a big promotion. This was a time of increased vulnerability for Don, with others watching to judge the appropriateness of the promotion. He felt a strong need to perform capably and competently to show himself worthy of Ellen's trust.

In any department, implementing an employee team or council structure provides a multitude of examples illustrating the importance of discussing appropriate coaching interventions. When organizations implement shared decision-making models, they often underestimate the coaching needs of the new groups. Many managers and leaders make erroneous assumptions about the group's level of development. If individual department employees were at a high development level, one may wrongly assume that their group's development level is also high. Although the members' individual skills and competencies certainly influence the group's ability, the two are not the same. Cherniss and Goleman (2001) clearly report this when talking about a group's emotional intelligence. The presence of a few emotionally intelligent members does not make the team emotionally intelligent.

These false assumptions are often reinforced by highly skilled, professional, and capable team members who believe that their individual high performance automatically translates to group high performance. In early stages of group development, the group needs a manager leader who provides the competence that the collective entity lacks: how to work as a team or an effective group. Yet unless the group and manager leader discuss the role of the coach and his or her assessment, the group or team may feel that the manager is giving a mixed message: "You said we're going to be responsible for making the decisions, so why are you telling us what to do?" Everyone involved feels they have failed and been failed by their leader because the situation does not meet their expectations.

Sometimes these issues and the need to talk through and agree on expectations become clear during the process of working together. In the beginning, the parties assume many of these behaviors, but the danger of not talking through expectations is that they are much more difficult to discuss once either party has violated them. The performer may have assumed that the coach would give negative or corrective feedback privately, only to discover that the coach is giving critical feedback in the middle of an employee meeting. It is better to have a discussion prior to the occurrence of problems to avoid negative emotional reactions that can make effective resolution more difficult.

Relevant Parameters

The coach identifies any constraints, limitations, deadlines, or other parameters for the performer. If the coach does not think these through and share them with the performer, this can adversely affect outcomes; the performer's enthusiasm and commitment may spiral downward, making the performer feel as though he or she has failed. Some individuals perform acceptably without this clarification, but this is not a chance worth taking—unless, of course, the coach is trying to assess the performer's ability to sort out and determine these important boundaries (which in itself can be a useful skill).

In a major system on the eastern seaboard that was growing in both size and scope, the CEO began delegating more and more responsibility to the chief operating officer (COO). The COO took on a major project: a patient safety initiative for the acute care hospital facility. This initiative was the CEO's favorite and an important project. But this was a sink-or-swim affair in which the CEO did not actively coach the COO. The CEO covered key constraints and expectations only loosely or assumed that the COO understood them. The COO misread and reversed the importance of many of these key parameters and forced the project through in an unrealistic time frame without adequate resources. The resulting negative impact on physician and customer satisfaction—the parameters most important to the CEO and board of trustees—eventually cost the COO his job. Clarifying expectations and parameters at the beginning of the coaching process can avoid this kind of demoralizing result.

In another organization, the chief nurse executive was asked to become executive sponsor for a massive process improvement project that included the implementation of the universal room concept (where a patient is admitted to a bed and remains in that room and department for the duration of his or her hospitalization, with needed services and level of care brought to the patient rather than the patient being transferred to other departments). This was her most important large-scope project since she had assumed her role eighteen months before. Her coach told her that the most critical parameter was that the project have no negative impact on physician or employee satisfaction ratings during its implementation. Based on everything she knew about change and the organization's relationship with physicians, she knew this was an unrealistic expectation. As she accepted the responsibility, this expectation was a major discussion point. She negotiated much more realistic expectations, including an acceptable depth of decline in physician satisfaction scores over a reasonable length of time due to the change.

In another instance, a CEO told a chief nurse executive that he and his department would attain Magnet designation (which is conferred on hospitals with exemplary nursing practice) for the hospital within twelve months. The nurse executive carefully investigated and developed a plan and a list of necessary resources and returned saying to the CEO, "This is what it will take to accomplish this goal within this time frame." As a result, not only did the organization establish a more realistic time frame, but it allocated important supports and resources.

The specificity of parameters is related to the performer's development level. At level one, the performer needs more detailed information. As the performer gains in experience and skill level, parameters become fewer or less concrete. For instance, when the performer is at level three, the structure that the coach gives may be only a time deadline or budget constraint.

An employee decision-making team leading the department redecoration process in one hospital decided to purchase beautiful color-coordinated linens for the patient rooms—bedspreads, curtains, draperies, and bed linens. To everyone's dismay, they discovered that the organization's laundry equipment could not process the fabric blend they had chosen, so these decorator linens sat useless in a warehouse. It became an organizational example of why empowerment does not work and why employees cannot make decisions such as these. Granted, someone on the team could have suggested talking to the experts in linen services, but a thorough coach would have identified the important parameter that the organization's laundry equipment must be able to process the linens. Or the coach might have identified a parameter that the team involve an expert from the linen service department as a team member before making a final decision.

A major difficulty is that leaders frequently imply rather than state expectations and parameters and assume that those involved understand and agree on the important expectations. This increases the likelihood that one or the other party involved in the coaching agreement fails to meet the other's unstated expectations. No matter how highly intuitive the participating individuals may be, they probably cannot read someone else's mind. The various people involved must clearly articulate and agree on expectations, needs, and parameters.

Step Four: Carry Out the Coaching Intervention

Once the intention of the coaching is clear, an assessment is completed, and expectations and parameters have been negotiated, the actual coaching intervention occurs. The intervention can be simple and spontaneous. For example, perhaps the coach notices the performer struggling to perform a procedure and steps in to say: "Here, let me show you an easier way." Or, in response to a concern expressed about a coworker's behavior in a meeting:

"I've had that happen, and I find if I ask for ideas and make sure I give enough time for their input, people are less likely to get off track from the agenda." Coaching interventions happen as a matter of course throughout any leader's day. However, there is a need for deliberate, intentional coaching interventions, and these include the use of specific coaching questions, teaching or offering formal learning opportunities, and providing opportunities. Each is presented here.

Coaching Questions

The use of coaching questions in an interchange with the performer is likely the most common form of coaching intervention. Questioning as a communication technique was addressed in Chapter Four. Questioning is powerful because it encourages reflection and helps the performer find his or her answers. Although there are times when giving advice or counsel is appropriate, these approaches are less likely to develop the person's ability to think through and determine the best course of action.

The coach's questions have the ability to guide the performer in a proactive, positive manner. After listening carefully to the performer describing a situation, the coach can respond with these questions, in this sequence:

1. "What would it look like if this situation were fixed?"

2. "What is the first step you can take to get this result?"

3. "Which of your strengths can you use in this situation?"

Developed by Tom Muha (Manion and Muha, 2009; Muha and Manion, 2010), this sequence builds on principles from positive psychology. The first question redirects the performer to think about the future rather than focus on the past and what has happened. Any one of us who has had an employee or peer going on and on about a problem knows how easily we become mired in a downward spiral of negativity. This question redirects the person's thinking and helps him or her develop a future vision, "What would this look like if it were the way you wanted it?" The second question forces the performer to become proactive. It does not ask for the detail of all the steps that need to be taken, just the first step. This is ultimately self-empowering because most of us can commit to doing one thing to help change an unacceptable situation. And the final question focuses the interaction on the individual's strengths. It's reaffirming and increases self-confidence in the person.

Teach or Train for the Desired Skills

Another form of coaching intervention is to teach or train for desired skills. Teaching others is also a specific manner in which a coach develops others and therefore is presented more fully under its own heading in this chapter. Because it is also a step in the coaching process, it is discussed here briefly.

Once the coach and performer have determined the goals of coaching and completed the assessment, it becomes clear what specific skill development is necessary—either individual competencies or group and team skills. A good coach requires both individual and team practice. Individual practice focuses on increasing the proficiency of the individual's performance. Group or team practice is preparation aimed at the collective functioning of the group and its ability to orchestrate individual talents among them in order to deliver a fine performance.

In partnership, the coach and performer determine what needs to be taught, when, and how best to teach it. The "what" encompasses technical or professional and supportive skills. Technical or professional skills pertain to the elements of an individual's job or work, such as completing a budget analysis or preparation, counseling an employee, or preparing a collaborative strategic plan. Supportive skills are more general in nature, such as the emotional intelligence competencies of displaying empathy, communication, and coaching skills.

Selecting a teaching approach is paramount. Too often coaches rely solely on traditional methods of didactic classroom-style teaching and formal academic programs. Although these are valuable, coaches often overlook other possibilities. Audio-recording and videotaping are powerful methods of instruction that can provide immediate, objective feedback on performance. Videotaping a meeting and replaying it to learn from participants' performances provide powerful lessons in group process. In one hospital's information services department, the clinical support team decided to tape-record conversations with customers (with the customers' permission) to evaluate the team's effectiveness in handling complaints and support on the help line.

In considering how to teach or train a performer, an effective coach capitalizes on every teachable moment. It is as much an attitude as a technique. Using the day-to-day environment and continually seeking opportunities to demonstrate a point or teach a technique drives home the expectation that learning is an integral part of the workplace, not just something that happens in a classroom. The coach plans department and team meetings to include some teaching and new learning at each meeting. And teaching is not limited to what the coach provides. Exemplary performers also teach others, both formally and informally; employees are therefore expected to coach and teach one another.

When to teach is more of an issue with regard to formal learning settings such as a classroom. More formal presentations tend to be linear in approach. The most effective teaching and training are done at the time the skill or learning is needed, when the learner can apply it immediately and anchor it as a change in his or her behavior. This is a more nonlinear approach and highly appropriate in our emergent systems. However, most situations are not ideal, and the issue of when to provide training is fraught with difficulty. Formal learning sessions most often occur prior to when they are actually needed or too long after the fact, which reduces the usefulness and adversely affects learning.

Providing Opportunities

What may be one of the most powerful methods of developing others is also one of the simplest: providing opportunities. A transformational leader continually seeks opportunities to stretch and challenge followers, delighting in others' accomplishments.

The extent to which a leader makes new opportunities available to followers demonstrates the importance that he or she places on the development of new proficiencies. Furthermore, it delivers a high-impact message of trust and confidence in the follower's ability to perform well in a particular situation. Providing opportunities means seeking these occasions, presenting them to followers with enthusiasm and encouragement, removing barriers or obstacles, getting out of the way of the developing performer, and celebrating achievements.

This strategy was one that health care managers who had successfully created a workplace culture of engagement frequently identified. "I constantly seek opportunities for them." "Each employee has particular strengths and I seek to recognize those, asking them, what would they like to develop? What kinds of experiences would be beneficial to help prepare for the role they're pursuing?" (Manion, 2004b, p. 34).

Many high-performing leaders could undoubtedly look back over their own career paths and identify times when someone tapped them on the shoulder and asked them to take on a responsibility or task that they had not previously considered. Looking for ways to share the responsibility of leadership is one source of opportunities for followers. Is there a way to delegate some of the leader's responsibility? Extraordinary followers continually seek challenge. However, their path is smoother and faster if an influential leader facilitates it by working on their behalf.

Removing barriers or obstacles for the follower is an important leadership responsibility, discussed briefly in Chapter Five. In the context of follower development, it might mean introducing the follower to the right person or simply speaking highly of the follower to other leaders in the organization. Recommending a person to serve as the chair of an influential task force or committee or positioning the individual to receive appointments to boards or groups within the community or state—even promotions outside of the current position—are ways a leader can remove barriers and champion followers. Many established and highly visible leaders receive more opportunities for service than they could possibly handle. Sharing some of these opportunities with followers is a way of supporting a follower's development.

If the leader is also the performer's manager, removing obstacles may mean something as rudimentary as providing time within the normal work week for the follower to engage in these other activities. Helping arrange for coworker coverage, when necessary, and providing time away from the department to assume these new responsibilities is a way of saying to the follower: "I am serious about your development needs. They are important to me as well as to the organization."

In some instances, simply providing the opportunity is adequate, but most leaders also become involved in coaching the follower to help develop the individual's skills. If the leader is not able to provide what the follower needs, a referral or recommendation to another available coach may be effective.

A good leader is delighted, rather than threatened, when a follower's skill level surpasses the leader's own. A transformational leader treats achievement of outcomes and improvement of the performer's skills as occasions for celebration.

Step Five: Observe Performance

An active, involved coach spends a great deal of time simply watching people perform. If the coach dispenses with this necessary step of the process, the coach has no way of determining the success or effectiveness of the first four steps. Performers need to feel comfortable being observed. If the coach and performer have talked about the coach's role, the performer will perceive the need for direct observation as a gift rather than interpreting it as micromanagement. The performer should see this as an opportunity to have an objective party provide feedback that will either reinforce good performance or correct faulty technique.

Direct observation is the best and preferred method for a coach to evaluate performance. Nevertheless, third-party reporting or self-reporting is acceptable. Third-party reporting may be negatively associated with tattling, which is unfortunate. This association has developed because many people are uncomfortable sharing criticisms or negative comments directly with the person they have observed and will instead share these observations with others. To avoid this negative connotation, keep sharing of third-party reports to positive observations. Everyone enjoys and appreciates hearing positive comments about his or her performance and values the third party who takes time to give positive feedback to the coach. The coach who receives negative third-party reports can use the information as an indication that he or she needs to dig a little deeper for observing and evaluating.

In the self-reporting process, the coach and performer talk through how a scenario played out, what the performer tried, what was effective, and what did not work. Asking questions that will draw out information in a comfortable, nonthreatening manner is important for this approach to work. Another way the coach can evaluate performance is by examining actual outcomes against intended outcomes. Did the performer meet expectations? Were the outcomes acceptable or outstanding?

An advantage of observing performance directly is that the coach can evaluate the performer's ability. How long did it take the individual to learn the skill? What kind of teaching or training seemed to be most effective for this person? Did the performer demonstrate good judgment in asking for assistance during complex, difficult situations, or did he or she prefer to go it alone? Was the performer able to pace himself or herself appropriately? What workload level can this performer handle? Does this individual feel comfortable negotiating modifications of workload? By observing performance, the coach learns a tremendous amount about the performer and becomes a more effective coach for this individual.

Step Six: Give Feedback

This step closes the loop and finalizes the entire process. A coach who does not provide feedback negates the whole process, leaving the performer with no way of determining the success or effectiveness of the first five steps. Having no feedback would be like playing a baseball game without innings or a scoreboard. A score of two to one in the bottom of the first inning is quite different from a score of two to one in the ninth inning, when the game is almost over and the chances for catching up are almost gone. In the same way that the score of a baseball game lets team members know how they are doing, feedback lets performers know how they are doing.

The coach is, admittedly, only one source of feedback for good performers who are continual learners. The highest performers seek feedback from a variety of sources and are always evaluating their own performance. However, none of this other feedback can equal the value of honest, direct feedback from a trusted coach whose primary interest is in helping the performer improve.

We give feedback through body language, through our reaction to situations, and even simply in what we give our attention to. Unfortunately, this form of feedback is often overlooked. In one organization, a planning team made up of managers and executives was responsible for designing and making leadership development programs available. This team was responsible for everything: designing the content, engaging and preparing presenters, planning logistics for all meetings, sending out invitations, and creating a positive learning ambience in the room on the day of the program. On this particular day, they had worked especially hard to create a seasonal theme in decorating the room. Each table had fall centerpieces with special treats for the participants. Team members had made great efforts to create just the right atmosphere. The CEO walked in the room, took one look at the tables, and asked where the water pitchers were. His focus was on the item missing rather than all that the team had done. The entire team felt horribly let down.

The same kind of feedback is given in a department when the leader arrives at work in the morning and rather than seeing all that the night employees surmounted and the challenges they overcame instead focuses with a critical eye on work that they did not complete. Attempting to get to the bottom of the problem with third-degree questioning, the leader gives clear feedback: the night crew failed. Leaders must be aware of the feedback their behavior, whether purposeful or inadvertent, is giving to followers.

Feedback here is defined more narrowly as giving information in the present about past behavior in an effort to influence future behavior (Seashore, Seashore, and Weinberg, 1999). It is useful for leaders who want to influence the follower's behavior. "Feedback in the workplace is fundamental for helping those who wish to improve their performance, reach an objective, or avoid unpleasant reactions to their efforts" (p. 7).

To be effective, the feedback needs to be accurate. Expert coaches study the people they coach; they know them and look for strengths that others have overlooked. When small successes occur, they know how to transform them into larger successes (Buckingham and Coffman, 1999). The exemplary coach uses positive feedback, praise, and compliments, as well as redirection when necessary.

Positive Feedback and Praise

Nearly everyone wants to be appreciated and recognized for his or her performance. In fact, Smith (2003) says that the top motivator for employees is full appreciation for work well done that managers express directly, either personally or publicly. Kouzes and Posner (2003) found that 98 percent of employees said they performed better when they received encouragement. Most leaders acknowledge that they should give more positive feedback. A recent Gallup Poll "revealed that 65 percent of Americans haven't received recognition in the past year. A United States Department of Labor study found that the number one reason why people leave organizations is that they don't feel appreciated" (Wall, 2007, pp. 66–67).

However, most positive feedback is general rather than intentionally specific about the behavior that it means to reinforce. Effective praise reinforces that specific behavior. It is the difference between saying, "Thanks, you did a great job," and, "Your persistence in getting the team to explore their differences resulted in a much better decision for the department."

Tarkenton and Tuleja (1986) say that positive reinforcement for both normal behavior and exceptional performance is critical. They point out that people do a good job about four times as frequently as they do inadequate work. It makes sense, then, for anyone wanting improved results to recognize that performers do a good job at least 80 percent of the time. They say that negative feedback should be given in the same proportion. So an individual should receive praise at least four times as often as criticism. But almost the opposite is true, according to these authors: 80 percent of the typical feedback is based on the 20 percent that is poor performance.

Recent research in the field of positive psychology bears this out, finding a numerical ratio in the relationship of positive and negative feedback (Fredrickson, 2004). People need to hear good things about four to five times to every negative comment or experience in order to overcome the demoralizing effects of the negative comment.

Exemplary coaches are always seeking opportunities to give feedback, and in order to give praise, the coach must observe and catch the performer doing something right. McGinnis (1985) offers several guidelines for giving praise:

- Hand out commendations in public.
- Use every success as an excuse for celebration.
- Use some gesture to give weight to the commendation.

- Put compliments in writing.

- Be very specific in praise.

McGinnis (1985) thinks that one problem with praise is that it can be overdone. If a person has established good, consistent performance and continues to be praised for the same thing, the praise soon becomes meaningless. The coach needs to find new behaviors to praise. A second challenge is that when the performer shows signs of positive change, the coach must reinforce this new or changed behavior. It is demoralizing to go to a great deal of effort to improve a skill or change a behavior and then realize that the coach doesn't even notice.

This last principle can be tricky when the behavior is in the right direction but the outcomes are not acceptable. One manager coach was strongly urging a team to begin to take responsibility for solving problems and making decisions on team members' own initiative. The first decision they made was poor, mostly because it was limited in scope. The team had not considered the impact of their decision on other departments in the organization. The manager praised the fact that the team made a decision but then coached them through an evaluation of the outcome to help them see what key factors they had missed.

Negative Feedback

Giving negative feedback is often more difficult for coaches. "When you don't deliver critical feedback, you declare your indifference" (Clarke-Epstein, 2002, p. 79). Leaders who are reluctant to give a follower corrective feedback should ask themselves these questions:

- If I were the person in this situation, would I want to be told?

- With feedback, can the person change what's happening?

- Would the feedback be embarrassing for me to say or embarrassing for the other person to hear? (If the answer to this question is yes, spend time carefully crafting the message.)

The use of scripting the message can be very helpful if the feedback is difficult to deliver. This has been discussed extensively in other sources

(Briles, 2009; Leebov, 2010; Manion, 2009b). The basic framework contains the following steps:

1. State your positive intention.

2. Share what you observed.

3. Include the outcome or impact of the action.

4. Ask if this was the intent.

5. Add a bit of empathy.

6. Indicate what you want to change.

The conversation a manager has when giving an employee feedback about a situation in which the employee's behavior was unacceptable or likely to lead to problematic relationship issues in the workplace might go like this:

Positive intention: "I appreciate the fact that you are well experienced and very knowledgeable about your work. You're one of the most highly skilled employees in this department and I need to count on you to help your less experienced coworkers."

Your observation: "When you responded to Susan's request for help this morning, you seemed abrupt and irritated. She looked embarrassed and distressed and immediately backed away without your helping her. She probably won't come to you for help in the future."

Was this your intent? "Was that your intent?"

[Pause. Do not respond until the person answers.]

Empathy: "I understand that you have a full assignment today, and it's frustrating when you have to stop and help a coworker."

What needs to change: "However, in this department we are all expected to pitch in and help each other so our patients get the kind of care they need. In the future, I expect you to respond positively to your coworker's requests unless there is a clear reason you cannot. And I expect you to do so without complaining about your own workload."

In a coaching context, the scripting message can be shortened depending on the situation:

Positive intention: "I have a suggestion that might help you deal with a situation like you had this morning."

Your observation: "I noticed you were entering information into the medical record when Mrs. Jones asked you a question. When you responded to her, you seemed a little abrupt and distracted. She stopped asking you questions."

Empathy: "I know you were trying to get the information entered into the computer before you forgot everything; however, I think Mrs. Jones felt that the computer was more important than she is. I have found that it helps to explain briefly that I just need to get this information into the computer accurately and when I'm finished, I'll take the time to answer any questions."

A coach who is afraid to correct the performer's mistakes cannot be effective. When asked how he felt about negative feedback, one employee said, "I feel good when the feedback is positive, but I can change my behavior and improve my performance when it is negative. Hearing negative feedback may not be pleasant, but the results are more satisfying to me because it helps me more in the long run."

Coaching, then, is the primary means through which a leader can develop others. In intentional, proactive coaching, leaders use a specific process: establishing the purpose, assessing, agreeing on expectations and parameters, teaching and training, observing performance, and giving feedback.

Teaching Others

Outstanding leaders are outstanding teachers. Noel Tichy addresses this concept clearly in his work with Nancy Cardwell, *The Cycle of Leadership: How Great Leaders Teach Their Companies to Win* (2002). They believe that institutions throughout society must have the capacity to develop leaders at all levels. Tichy and Cardwell call these teaching organizations with virtuous teaching cycles "dynamic, interactive processes in which everyone teaches, everyone learns and everyone gets smarter, every day" (p. xxiv). Regardless of their hierarchical position in the organization, leaders learn from each other and from followers.

In addition to holding a philosophy of continual learning, exemplary leaders also understand the principles of adult learning and are highly skilled in their application. Their teaching is intentional, and they engage in both spontaneous and deliberate teaching, obviously delighting in a follower's learning something new as well as their own learning. Such a leader lives by the old adage: give a man a fish, and he eats for a day; teach a man to fish, and he eats for a lifetime.

Here we review the principles of adult learning that effective leaders use to reinforce their application. Some people hear the word *teaching* and think of the familiar, formal academic model. But teaching is much more than the traditional example of a teacher standing in front of a group and dispensing knowledge. The teaching-learning cycles that Tichy and Cardwell (2002) discuss occur continuously and simultaneously in the best learning organizations. It is a totally emergent, nonlinear process unfolding within the events and circumstances of the workplace.

Most leaders today have been socialized and molded by an academic setting not much different from their children's experience. After years in an educational system with a relatively traditional approach, most adults expect to listen during the learning process while the experts teach them, disseminating information and giving advice. Ironically, it is not until the role of the educator shifts from transmitter of information to facilitator and resource person for self-directed inquiry that the learner will be able to meet his or her needs.

Principles of adult learning conjure up images of participants in a learning situation who are actively participating. This means an active exchange of ideas, questioning, and perhaps hands-on practice. Active participation, however, does not necessarily mean that a person is always interacting and talking. Participation can be as simple as thoughtful, private inquiry in reaction to something the teacher has asked or presented. In fact, there is growing appreciation of the power of reflective practice as a highly effective learning tool (Freshwater, 2004; Johns, 2004).

Taking generic principles or ideas that the teacher has presented and applying them to one's own situation is also active participation. In some instances, a teacher's example may create a vivid picture in a learner's mind that helps anchor the learning. So activity does not necessarily mean flashy exercises and dynamic situations that need a skilled facilitator for guidance.

Malcolm Knowles (1970) was one of the earliest educators in this country to distinguish between methods used for teaching children in a formal academic approach and those used for teaching self-directed learners such as adults. He described adult learning as differing from childlike learning in at least four main respects. First, the orientation to learning differs. Learning for children in school is often subject centered rather than problem oriented. The chief difference is in time perspectives. A child's perspective of formal education is one of postponed application, whereas an adult usually wants to apply his or her learning immediately. Compare a child's interest in a geography lesson about a country far away to the adult who is planning a vacation to that same country in the next four months. This issue of timing is critical.

Change in a learner's self-concept is the second way that children's learning differs from adult learning. An assumption of self-directed learning is that as a person grows and matures, his or her self-concept moves from one of dependence to one of increasing self-confidence. Children are dependent on others in their earliest years, but as they grow and mature, they expect to participate more actively in decisions affecting their learning. In fact, Knowles (1970) suggests that when adults find themselves in a situation in which they are not allowed to be self-directed, they experience tension between the given situation and their self-concept, resulting in resentment and resistance. They may think, "Why is this person telling me what to do? Does he or she think I don't know?"

The third area differentiating the two types of learning is the role of experience in learning. The assumption is that as an individual matures and accumulates experiences, these serve as resources for learning and an ever-enlarging base to which to relate new learning. Teachers convey their respect for students by making use of students' past experiences as a resource for learning. The learner's readiness to learn is the last point of difference that Knowles (1970) identified. As individuals mature, their readiness to learn is more the product of what they need to know because of a change in their environment or life situation than what others believe they ought to know.

Knowles's observations (1970) are powerful for those seeking to improve their teaching skills. In the same way that individuals are at varying levels of development related to the skill they are trying to learn, each is also at varying levels of development in learning. In other words, learning is a skill that one needs to develop. If we apply the assessment model for coaching provided earlier in the chapter, the different levels of learning might look like this:

- *Development level one.* This level of learning could be likened to the learning of a young child. Enthusiasm and commitment abound. The learner lacks competence and knowledge, so the teacher provides structure by deciding on the appropriate curriculum and learning experiences required. The teacher provides required information and knowledge, guides the learning process, and evaluates outcomes.

- *Development level two.* Now the learner has some experience but variable commitment. Perhaps early attempts revealed that learning is not as easy as it seemed, and this learner requires both strong direction and lots of support and encouragement. The instructor provides the direction, determining what to teach and how to teach it. At this point, most teachers remain actively present and involved during learning situations, giving feedback and attention, as well as praise and encouragement.

- *Development level three.* The learner at this stage has fairly wide experience with learning but perhaps lacks self-confidence in the subject area. He or she needs minimal structure from the teacher, and requires mostly encouragement and support. The teacher uses guided discussions and practice or live sessions to facilitate learning.

- *Development level four.* This level represents the epitome of the self-directed learner. The learner is responsible for defining his or her own educational needs, necessary resources, and appropriate time schedules. The learner also undertakes evaluation of the learning process and works in partnership with the teacher to appropriately define the learning outcomes expected and agree on an approach to learning. The self-directed learner has the ability to evaluate educational materials and opportunities and effectively manages his or her own time.

Leaders in the workplace are often working with followers who are at levels three and four. These learners are comfortable with learning and at level three may just need more coaching. They are the most likely to fall back into the more traditional modes of learning, such as didactic classroom presentations. Most leaders are blessed with at least some followers who are self-directed learners: open, curious, organized, motivated, and highly enthusiastic. They soak up learning opportunities as the earth soaks up rain following a lengthy dry spell. They deeply appreciate anything the leader does to support their learning.

Teaching by Example

Another key principle of teaching is to teach by example. This is a way to demonstrate a skill and show how to do something. In addition, the leader demonstrates leadership behaviors that the organization expects, desires, and rewards. This person is observed for the behaviors he or she is modeling, which can create tremendous pressure for him or her. Nothing a leader does or says can escape the followers' notice. Every behavior and response, even a chance remark, gives out a signal that a follower will pick up and pass on to others. Every action of the leader either validates or negates all the messages he or she has previously sent out. Followers can tell if a leader is sincere, honest, and congruent or just for show.

Some leaders are uncomfortable with this responsibility of influence and rail against the reality, claiming not to want to be a role model, not to want the pressure of others' watching their every move. The pressure to be a person of integrity, behaving consistently in accordance with stated beliefs, feels overwhelming at times. Some leaders complain: "I'm only human. I can't be perfect." Or they think: "What I do in my private life is my own business; no one needs to know." This is not to say that leaders do not need or have a right to privacy and time offstage. They not only have this right but need to have private time to rejuvenate, relax, and not feel as if someone is watching and evaluating their every move. However, the reality is that being in a position of leadership increases the leader's visibility and vulnerability. When an individual moves out in front of the pack and picks up the reins of leadership, corresponding responsibilities appear. A primary responsibility is modeling expected behavior.

The reality of leading by example can be especially difficult if the leader is somewhat shy or reserved. Instead of focusing on the privacy that one has lost, perhaps the leader could consider this exposure as a gift. Most people perform better with a small amount of competition. When others are watching and expecting a high level of performance, we often feel the motivation to reach new heights of performance and excel at our task.

Conclusion

Transformational leaders actively and intentionally participate in and contribute to their followers' growth and development. They coach for performance improvement and exemplary performance by giving advice and instruction, encouraging discovery through guided discussions and actual experience, observing performance, and giving feedback. An involved leader positively influences followers by providing opportunities and engaging in teaching new skills. Followers grow and develop in and as a result of their relationship with an exemplary leader.

DISCUSSION QUESTIONS

1. Think about people who have been influential in your life—someone who has helped you develop new skills or served as your mentor. What were that person's special coaching skills? What was most helpful to you? What and how did you learn from him or her?

2. How do you serve as a coach for others? Who have you coached in the past? What was your relationship like? What did you do successfully? What could you have done better?

3. Do you coach others as much as you think you should? What keeps you from coaching more actively? How can you eliminate these barriers to becoming a more active coach?

4. Is your coaching deliberate and intentional? Do you have a specific coaching plan for the high performers in your workplace? Do you have a performance improvement plan for the low performers?

5. Who would be in your top 20 percent of performers? How could you use these people as a team to attain results within your scope of responsibility?

6. Identify a situation in which you are actively coaching another individual. What is that person's developmental level with the task or behavior? What is your coaching intervention?

7. Do you emphasize strengths or deficiencies in the people you coach? Is it easy for you to identify another person's strengths? What is a current example of a way you've used strengths-based coaching?

8. Think about your personal and professional life. Think of a time when you were at your very best. You were deeply engaged in and passionate about the situation and succeeded in your efforts. What were the strengths you used? What were the intrinsic motivators that seemed to be present? Rank the motivators in order of their importance to you.

9. Complete a personal strengths assessment tool. Go to www.authentichappiness .com and complete the VIA (Survey of Character Strengths), which is an assessment of character strengths. Print off a list of your top five strengths. Do any of these strengths surprise you? How do you use these in your leadership practice? Identify at least three ways you could use each of these strengths in a new and different way at work.

10. What motivates you (what's most important to you)? What internal motivators get you going in the morning and keep you coming back? How are they present in all aspects of your life: personal, work, and community?

11. What are examples of the self-fulfilling prophecy that you have seen that had positive effects? What are examples of those with negative or devastating effects? What self-fulfilling prophecies do you have of others? How can you interrupt the cycle?

12. What kinds of behaviors are you emphasizing and rewarding in others around you? Is this the behavior you want to emphasize? Are you inadvertently rewarding or recognizing any behaviors you don't want?

13. What opportunities have you have been given in the past? How have they helped you grow? What are possibilities you have for sharing opportunities with others?

14. How do you incorporate the principles of adult learning in your interchanges when you teach others? How do you demonstrate respect for the people you are coaching? In what ways are the people you are coaching self-directed learners?

15. How do you feel about being a role model for others? Does this place pressure on you in any way? What examples of negative role modeling have you observed? What positive examples of role modeling have you seen?

8

Going Forward into Our Future

Knowing is not enough, we must apply.
Willing is not enough, we must do.
GOETHE (FROM BROWN, *ON SUCCESS*)

Health care has never been in greater need of transformational leaders. It is at a major crossroads, with system integrations, new business structures emerging, mergers and acquisitions, hospital closures, downsizing and rightsizing, increased government involvement, new reimbursement models, increased regulatory constraints, accelerating consumer expectations, and intensified human relations issues, all creating a tremendous demand for extraordinary leaders. The leadership paradigm has shifted dramatically: the old command-and-control approach is no longer effective, and leaders at all levels need different skills for the future.

Some of these leadership skills or characteristics—integrity, a sense of mission, and a clear and inspiring vision—cannot be taught in traditional ways. Experiential learning is what is called for—learning in life's classroom. The wisdom that comes from thoughtful personal reflection and deep knowledge of what is most important brings a commitment to living by these values day to day, especially when we must make difficult choices that require courage and belief. Most exemplary leaders have a desire to serve, to act in the interest of future generations. They function as true servant leaders, putting the needs of others first. And they believe they are in the right place at the right time. Passionate and fully engaged, with hearts committed, they clearly understand their purpose and envision a better future. A leader's vision creates the momentum that draws people to them and to their cause, to work together despite obstacles and challenges, to forge a new reality with hope and optimism for the future.

Although values, mission, and vision are not commonly taught through traditional methods, many leadership skills are—the numerous interpersonal skills that are this book's focus. Without excellent interpersonal skills and a high level of emotional and social intelligence, tomorrow's leaders cannot be successful. Paramount to this success are communication skills and the ability to form positive relationships with followers and gain their commitment to and engagement in a shared and deeply felt purpose, as well as the ability to manage processes and develop others.

Positive, dynamic relationships with followers greatly determine the degree of a transformational leader's success. Trust, mutual respect, support, and open communication allow a leader's influence to flourish. Tomorrow's leaders collaborate and work with others in partnership. They thrive on interdependence and interconnections with other people.

Transformational leaders not only recognize the distinction between compliance and commitment; they help followers find their passion and fully engage with their hearts. These leaders are not afraid to express their deeply held values and cherished beliefs, creating a collective sense of mission and a shared vision—a powerful force for transformation.

Exceptional leaders are master communicators. They constantly reflect on and evaluate their effectiveness, seeking to expand their verbal and non-verbal skills. They use anecdotes, analogies, and metaphors and evoke powerful symbols to communicate the organization's most important and deeply held values. They work diligently to overcome barriers to effective communication, becoming versatile in interpreting differences in common language forms, gender, and style.

Outstanding leaders also understand and effectively facilitate process so that the processes they and their followers engage in are meaningful in that they achieve results and progress. They recognize and knowledgeably apply the sequential steps of a process, allowing it to unfold within its natural time frame, and they develop sound judgment that alerts them to the need to nudge a process along. As process facilitators, these leaders demonstrate by example how to empower others, resolve conflict, lead a problem-solving process, reach decisions, create teams, and lead change. They use their judgment to determine when to use appreciative inquiry or a traditional problem-solving process. Their in-depth understanding of processes enables them to avoid the most common pitfalls. They recognize when the issue before them is a polarity to manage rather than a problem to solve.

And finally, extraordinary leaders constantly seek opportunities to develop others. They do this by intentional and proactive coaching, facilitating the development of followers' skills by giving instruction and advice and encouraging discovery through guided discussions and hands-on experiences. They observe performance and provide honest, direct, and timely feedback. These leaders diligently seek to provide opportunities for followers and constantly teach and share their knowledge with them. Leaders themselves are continual learners, thriving among colleagues who are also continual learners.

Each of these competencies is essential, and without the complete package, influence is difficult to attain. No competency is easy to develop, however, and it often requires years of experience of taking risks and making mistakes, trying again and yet again. It is helpful to remember Brown's (1994, p. 78) sage advice: "Remember that overnight success usually takes about fifteen years." Malcolm Gladwell studied people who had achieved great success in life. In his book, *Outliers: The Story of Success*, he shares example after example of the importance of repeated practice and preparation for success. He found that the closer psychologists "look at the careers of the gifted, the smaller the role innate talent seems to play and the bigger the role preparation seems to play" (2008, p. 38). In other words, what often distinguishes one performer from another is not just that the top performers work harder than everyone else. They work much, *much* harder. "Practice isn't the thing you do once you're good. It's the thing you do that makes you good," Maxwell writes (2008, p. 42). He coined the term *10,000 hour rule* because when he studied these extraordinarily successful individuals, there was a striking commonality: when questioned, each said it took about 10,000 hours of repeated performance to attain the high level of accomplishment that led to success.

Society cannot afford the costs and consequences of weak leadership in health care. Health care leaders today are stewards for the future, and we will build healthier communities only through full collaboration between the health care system and its leaders, local government, civic leaders, and federal legislators.

Leadership development is an intensely personal, lifelong journey. Warren Bennis (1989, p. 112) puts it particularly well: "No leader sets out to be a leader. People set out to live their lives, expressing themselves fully. When that expression is of value, they become leaders. So the point is not to become a leader. The point is to become yourself, to use yourself completely—all your skills, gifts, and energies—in order to make your vision manifest. You must withhold nothing. You must, in sum, become the person you started out to be, and to enjoy the process of becoming."

This journey is not an easy one, and it may help to reflect on the following story about a bedridden gentleman. One day this man noticed a caterpillar crawling along the windowsill next to his bed. To his delight, it stopped in the corner and began spinning a cocoon. The man was excited because he knew that eventually he would watch a beautiful butterfly emerge. Weeks later, he noticed movement in the cocoon. Eager to behold the transformation to a new butterfly, he watched and waited, but the struggle continued. Growing impatient, the man decided to help speed the labor along. He opened the window and gently picked up the cocoon. Carefully opening it, he was enchanted to see the new butterfly emerge. It staggered a few steps and, to the man's dismay, fell over and died. What the man failed to realize is that it is in the efforts to emerge from the cocoon that a butterfly gains enough strength to fly away.

Like the difficulties of a butterfly emerging from a cocoon, the struggles of leading are precisely what help build the strength to lead and meet the challenges of today's health care organizations. Leadership is not glamorous; it is hard work. Doing the right thing even at high personal cost takes courage, and it takes a belief in something bigger than oneself. It takes the optimism and hope to dream about wonderful possibilities, although dreaming is not enough. Perseverance and dedication are needed to implement the strategies that will transform current reality into that desired future. Leadership is an opportunity, a rare privilege, and a gift to those with the courage to accept its challenges.

REFERENCES

Ackoff, R., Finnel, E., and Gharajedaghi, J. *A Guide to Controlling Your Corporation's Future*. Hoboken, N.J.: Wiley, 1984.

Adams, J. L. *The Care and Feeding of Ideas: A Guide to Encouraging Creativity*. Reading, Mass.: Addison-Wesley, 1986.

Aiken, L. H., Clarke, S. P., and Stone, D. M. "Hospital Staffing, Organization, and Quality of Care: Cross-National Findings." *Nursing Outlook*, 2002, *50*(5), 187–194.

Altuntas, S. A., and Baykal, U. "Relationship Between Nurses' Organizational Trust Levels and Their Organizational Citizenship Behaviors." *Journal of Nursing Scholarship*, 2010, *42*(2), 186–194.

Amabile, T. M., and Kramer, S. J. "Inner Work Life: Understanding the Subtext of Business Performance." *Harvard Business Review*, 2007, *85*(5), 72–83.

Ambler, M. "Social Media and the Health Care Leader: Maximizing Your Information Intake." *Voice of Nursing Leadership*, Nov. 2009, pp. 10–12.

American Hospital Association. "Staffing Watch." *Hospitals and Health Networks,* Sept. 2001, p. 22.

Anderson, P. *Great Quotes from Great Leaders*. Lombard, Ill.: Celebrating Excellence, 1990.

Annas, G. J. "Beyond the Military and Market Metaphors." *Healthcare Forum Journal*, May/June 1996, pp. 30–34.

Annison, M. "Leadership." *Westrend Letter*, June 1994, pp. 1–4.

Annison, M. Keynote address at the Florida Hospital Association annual meeting, Orlando, Fla., Nov. 13, 1997.

Aronson, E. *The Social Animal.* (7th ed.) New York: Freeman, 1995.

Baggs, J. G., and Schmitt, M. H. "Collaboration Between Nurses and Physicians." *Image: Journal of Nursing Scholarship*, 1988, *20*(3), 145–149.

Bardwick, J. M. "Emotional Leaders." *Executive Excellence*, Apr. 1996, pp. 13–14.

Barker, J. A. *The Power of Vision.* Burnsville, Minn.: Charthouse Learning Corporation, 1990. Videotape.

Barker, J. A. *Paradigms: The Business of Discovering the Future.* New York: HarperCollins, 1992.

Barney, S. M. "Radical Change: One Solution to the Nursing Shortage." *Journal of Healthcare Management*, 2002, *47*(4), 220–223.

Barrett, F. J. "Creating Appreciative Learning Cultures." *Organization Dynamics*, 1995, *24,* 36–49.

Becker, H. S. "Notes on the Concept of Commitment." *American Journal of Sociology*, 1960, *66,* 32–40.

Beckhard, R., and Pritchard, W. *Changing the Essence: The Art of Creating and Leading Fundamental Change in Organizations.* San Francisco: Jossey-Bass, 1992.

Benner, P. *From Novice to Expert.* Reading, Mass.: Addison-Wesley, 1984.

Bennis, W. *On Becoming a Leader.* Reading, Mass.: Addison-Wesley, 1989.

Bennis, W., and Nanus, B. *Leaders: The Strategies for Taking Charge.* New York: HarperCollins, 1985.

Berry, L. L. "Qualities of Leadership." *Retailing Issues Letter*, 1992, *4*(1), 1–4.

Block, P. *The Empowered Manager: Positive Political Skills at Work.* San Francisco: Jossey-Bass, 1987.

Blouin, A., and Brent, N. "Strategic Partnering: Clinical and Risk Management Concerns." *Journal of Nursing Administration,* 1997, *27*(6), 10–13.

Borkowski, N. *Organizational Behavior in Health Care.* Sudbury, Mass.: Jones and Bartlett, 2011.

Bossidy, L., and Charan, R. *Execution: The Discipline of Getting Things Done.* New York: Crown, 2002.

Bowcutt, M. "Maintaining a Balance." *Nurse Leader,* Apr. 2004, pp. 25–27.

Boyatzis, R., and McKee, A. *Resonant Leadership: Renewing Yourself and Connecting with Others Through Mindfulness, Hope, and Compassion.* Boston: Harvard Business School Press, 2005.

Breen, B. "The Clear Leader." *Fast Company,* 2005, *78*(3), 65–67.

Brickman, P., Wortman, C. B., and Sorrentino, R. (eds.). *Commitment, Conflict, and Caring.* Upper Saddle River, N.J.: Prentice Hall, 1987.

Bridges, W. *Surviving Corporate Transition.* Mill Valley, Calif.: William Bridges & Associates, 1988.

Bridges, W. *Managing Transitions: Making the Most of Change.* Mill Valley, Calif.: William Bridges & Associates, 1991.

Bridges, W. *Participant's Guide: Managing Organizational Transitions.* Mill Valley, Calif.: William Bridges & Associates, 1992.

Briles, J. *Sabatoge! How to Deal with the Pit Bulls, Skunks, Snakes, Scorpions and Slugs in the Health Care Workplace.* Aurora, Colo.: Mile High Press, 2009.

Brown, H. J. Jr. *Life's Little Treasure Book on Success.* Nashville, Tenn.: Rutledge Hill Press, 1994.

Buckingham, M. "What Great Managers Do." *Harvard Business Review,* 2005, *83*(3), 70–79.

Buckingham, M., and Coffman, C. *First, Break All the Rules: What the World's Greatest Managers Do Differently.* New York: Simon & Schuster, 1999.

Bunker, K. A. "Leading Change: A Balancing Act." *Nurse Leader*, 2006, *4*(2), 43–45.

Bürkner, H. "The Best Advice I Ever Got." *Harvard Business Review*, 2007, *85*(12), 21.

Burns, B. M. *Leadership.* New York: HarperCollins, 1978.

Bush, H. "Time to Tweet?" *Hospital & Health Networks*, June 2009. Retrieved from http://www.hhnmag.com/hhnmag_app/jsp/articledisplay. jsp?dcrpath=HHNMAG/Article/ data/06JUN2009/0906HHN_FEA_twitter&domain=HHNMAG.

Byers, J. F., and White, S. V. (eds.). *Patient Safety: Principles and Practice.* New York: Springer, 2004.

Byrne, J. A. "How to Lead Now: Getting Extraordinary Performance When You Can't Pay for It." *Fast Company*, Aug. 2003, pp. 62–70.

Campbell, R., and Inguagiato, R. "The Power of Listening." *Physician Executive*, 1994, *20*(9), 35–37.

Chaleff, I. "Effective Leadership." *Executive Excellence*, Apr. 1996, pp. 16–17.

Chaleff, I. "The Groupthink Challenge." *Team Management Briefings*, June 1997, p. 4.

Champy, J. "The Hidden Qualities of Great Leaders." *Fast Company*, Nov. 2003, p. 135.

Chawla, S., and Renesch, J. (eds.). *Learning Organizations: Developing Cultures for Tomorrow's Workplace.* Portland, Ore.: Productivity Press, 1995.

Cherniss, C., and Goleman, D. (eds.). *The Emotionally Intelligent Workplace: How to Select for, Measure, and Improve Emotional Intelligence in Individuals, Groups, and Organizations.* San Francisco: Jossey-Bass, 2001.

Ciancutti, A., and Steding, T. L. *Built on Trust: Gaining Competitive Advantage in Any Organization.* Chicago: Contemporary Books, 2001.

Clancy, T. "The Art of Decision-Making." *Journal of Nursing Administration*, 2003, *33*(6), 343–349.

Clark, M. "Metaphorically Speaking." *Healthcare Forum Journal*, May/June 1996, pp. 20–27.

Clarke-Epstein, C. "Truth in Feedback." *Training and Development*, Nov. 2002, pp. 78–80.

Coens, T., and Jenkins, M. *Abolishing Performance Appraisals: Why They Backfire and What to Do Instead*. San Francisco: Berrett-Koehler, 2000.

Coles, D. "Because We Can: Leadership Responsibility and the Moral Distress Syndrome." *Nursing Management*, Mar. 2010, pp. 26–30.

Collins, J. *Good to Great: Why Some Companies Make the Leap . . . and Others Don't*. New York: HarperCollins, 2001.

Collins, J. *Good to Great and the Social Sectors*. Boulder, Colo.: Jim Collins, 2005.

Collins, J. "The Secret of Enduring Greatness." *Fortune*, May 5, 2008, pp. 73–76.

Collins, S. *Stillpoint: The Dance of Selfcaring, Selfhealing*. Fort Worth, Tex.: TLC Productions, 1992.

Cooper, R. K. "21st Leadership: Excelling Under Pressure." Paper presented at a meeting of the American Organization of Nurse Executives, Charlotte, N.C., Mar. 1999.

Cooperrider, D. Presentation at the General Session at the First World International Positive Psychology Meeting. Philadelphia, June 20, 2009.

Covey, S. *The Seven Habits of Highly Effective People: Restoring the Character Ethic*. New York: Simon & Schuster, 1989.

Covey, S. *Principle-Centered Leadership*. New York: Simon & Schuster, 1990.

Covey, S., Merrill, A. R., and Merrill, R. R. *First Things First*. New York: Simon & Schuster, 1994.

Cox, S., Manion, J., and Miller, D. *Nature's Wisdom in the Workplace: Managing Energy in Today's Health Care Organization*. Bloomington, Minn.: Synergy Press, 2005.

Creative Healthcare Management. *Leaders Empower Staff Participant Manual*. Minneapolis: Creative Healthcare Management, 1994.

Csikszentmihalyi, M. *Flow: The Psychology of Optimal Experience.* New York: HarperCollins, 1990.

Csikszentmihalyi, M. *Finding Flow: The Psychology of Engagement with Everyday Life.* New York: Basic Books, 1997.

Csikszentmihalyi, M. *Good Business: Leadership, Flow, and the Making of Meaning.* New York: Penguin Putnam Books, 2003.

Curtin, L. "Blessed Are the Flexible." *Nursing Management,* 1995, *26*(3), 7–8.

Davenport, T. H. "Make Better Decisions." *Harvard Business Review,* 2009, *87*(11), 117–123.

Deiner, E., and Biswas-Deiner R. *Happiness: Unlocking the Mysteries of Psychological Wealth.* Malden, Mass.: Blackwell, 2008.

de Man, H. *Joy in Work.* London: Allen & Unwin, 1929.

DePree, M. *Leadership Is an Art.* New York: Doubleday, 1989.

Detert, J. R., and Edmondson, A. C. "Why Employees Are Afraid to Speak." *Harvard Business Review,* May 2007. www.harvardbusinessonline .hbsp.harvard.edu.

Drucker, P. *Managing for the Future: The 1990s and Beyond.* New York: Penguin Books, 1992.

Edmondson, A., Bohmer, R., and Pisano, G. "Speeding up Team Learning." *Harvard Business Review,* 2001, *79*(10), 125–132.

Eisler, R. *The Chalice and the Blade: Our History, Our Future.* New York: HarperCollins, 1987.

Eisler, R., and Loye, D. *The Partnership Way: New Tools for Living and Learning.* (2nd ed.). Brandon, Vt.: Holistic Education Press, 1998.

Fagiano, D. "Designating a Leader." *Management Review,* Mar. 1994, p. 4.

Fielden, J. "What Do You Mean I Can't Write?" *Journal of Nursing Administration,* 1981, *11*(3), 42–47.

Fields, M., and Zwisler, S. "Walk in Balance: Returning to the Self." *Nurse Leader,* Apr. 2004, pp. 44–45.

Flower, J. "The Chasm Between Management and Leadership." *Healthcare Forum Journal*, 1990, *33*(4), 59–62.

Flower, J. "Being Effective." *Healthcare Forum Journal*, 1991, *34*(3), 52–57.

Fredrickson, B. "What Good Are Positive Emotions?" Online presentation for the Authentic Happiness Coaching seminar, June 10, 2004.

Fredrickson, B. *Positivity: Groundbreaking Research Reveals How to Embrace the Hidden Strength of Positive Emotions, Overcome Negativity, and Thrive.* New York: Crown, 2009.

Frese, M. "Proactivity and Engagement." Presentation at the First Annual World Congress of the International Positive Psychology Meeting, Philadelphia, June 19–21, 2009.

Freshwater, D. "Reflective Practice: A Tool for Developing Clinical Leadership." *Reflections on Nursing Leadership*, 2004 (2nd qtr.), 20–26.

Frick, D., and Spears, L. (eds.). *On Becoming a Servant-Leader: The Private Writings of Robert K. Greenleaf.* San Francisco: Jossey-Bass, 1996.

Friedman, S. D. "Be a Better Leader, Have a Richer Life" *Harvard Business Review*, 2008, *86*(4), 112–118.

Gelinas, L., and Bohlen, C. *Tomorrow's Work Force: A Strategic Approach.* Irving, Tex.: Voluntary Hospitals of America, 2002.

Gentile, M. C. "Keeping Your Colleagues Honest: How to Challenge Unethical Behavior at Work—and Prevail." *Harvard Business Review*, 2010, *88*(3), 114–117.

Gibson, C. "A Concept Analysis of Empowerment." *Journal of Advanced Nursing*, 1991, *16*, 354–361.

Gilbert, J. *Strengthening Ethical Wisdom: Tools for Transforming Your Health Care Organization.* Chicago: AHA Press, 2007.

Gilbert, J. *Ethics and the Board: Pathways to Leadership Excellence in Healthcare.* San Diego, Calif.: Governance Institute, 2008.

Gladwell, M. *Outliers: The Story of Success.* New York: Little, Brown, 2008.

Goleman, D. *Emotional Intelligence: Why It Can Matter More Than IQ.* New York: Bantam Books, 1994.

Goleman, D., Boyatzis, R., and McKee, A. *Primal Leadership: Realizing the Power of Emotional Intelligence.* Boston: Harvard Business School Press, 2002.

Goleman, D., and Boyatzis, R. "Social Intelligence and the Biology of Leadership." *Harvard Business Review*, 2008, *86*(9), 74–81.

Grohar-Murray, M. E., and Langan, J. *Leadership and Management in Nursing.* Upper Saddle River, N.J.: Pearson, 2011.

Grossman, R. J. "The Looming Crisis: Health Care Organizations Are Behind Other Industries in Cultivating Tomorrow's Leaders." *Health Forum Journal*, Nov./Dec. 1999, pp. 18–25.

Guber, P. "The Four Truths of the Storyteller." *Harvard Business Review*, 2007, *85*(12), 53–59.

Gutbezahl, C. "The Benefits of Conflict." *Hospitals and Health Network Online.* March 9, 2010.

Havens, D. S., Wood, S. O., and Leeman, J. "Improving Nursing Practice and Patient Care: Building Capacity with Appreciative Inquiry." *Journal of Nursing Administration*, 2006, *36*(10), 463–470.

Heenan, D. A., and Bennis, W. *Co-Leaders: The Power of Great Partnerships.* Hoboken, N.J.: Wiley, 1999.

Heifetz, R. A., and Laurie, D. L. "The Work of Leadership." *Harvard Business Review*, Jan./Feb. 1997, pp. 124–134.

Heifetz, R. A., Grashow, A., and Linsky, M. "Leadership in a (*Permanent*) Crisis." *Harvard Business Review,* July-August 2009, 62–69.

Hemp, P. "Death by Information Overload." *Harvard Business Review*, 2009, *88*(1), p. 16.

Henry, B., and LeClair, H. "Language, Leadership, and Power." *Journal of Nursing Administration*, 1987, *17*(1), 19–24.

Hersey, P., and Blanchard, K. H. *Management of Organizational Behavior: Utilizing Human Resources.* (6th ed.) Upper Saddle River, N.J.: Prentice Hall, 1993.

Hesselbein, F., Goldsmith, M., and Beckhard, R. (eds.). *The Leader of the Future*. San Francisco: Jossey-Bass, 1996.

Hewlett, S. A., Sherbin, L., and Sumberg, K. "How Gen Y and Boomers Will Reshape Your Agenda." *Harvard Business Review,* 2009, *87*(7), 71–76.

Huey, J. "The New Post-Heroic Leadership." *Fortune*, Feb. 21, 1994, pp. 45–50.

Iverson, R., and Buttigieg, D. "Affective, Normative and Continuance Commitment: Can the 'Right Kind' of Commitment Be Managed?" *Journal of Management Studies*, 1999, *36*(3), 307–333.

Iyengar, S. S., and Lepper, M. R. "Rethinking the Value of Choice: A Cultural Perspective on Intrinsic Motivation." *Journal of Personality and Social Psychology*, 1999, *76*(3), 349–366.

Jazwiec, L. *Eat That Cookie: Make Workplace Positivity Pay Off . . . for Individuals, Teams and Organizations.* Gulf Breeze, Fla.: Fire Starter Publishing, 2009.

Johns, C. "Becoming a Transformational Leader Through Reflection." *Reflections on Nursing Leadership*, 2nd qtr. 2004, pp. 24–26.

Johnson, B. *Polarity Management: Identifying and Managing Unsolvable Problems.* Amherst, Mass.: HRD Press, 1996.

Johnson, J. A. "Warren Bennis, Chairman, The Leadership Institute." *Journal of Healthcare Management*, 1998, *43*(4), 293–296.

Joni, S. A., and Beyer, D. "How to Pick a Good Fight." *Harvard Business Review*, 2009, *87*(12), 48–57.

Kalisch, B., and Begeny, S. "Improving Nursing Unit Teamwork." *Journal of Nursing Administration*, 2005, *35*(12), 550–556.

Kalisch, B., Begeny, S., and Anderson, C. "The Effect of Consistent Nursing Shifts on Teamwork and Continuity of Care." *Journal of Nursing Administration,* 2008, *38*(3), 132–137.

Kanter, R. M. *Commitment and Community: Communes and Utopias in Sociological Perspective.* Cambridge, Mass.: Harvard University Press, 1972.

Kanter, R. M. *On the Frontiers of Management.* Middlebury, Vt.: Soundview Executive Book Summaries, 1997.

Kanter, R. M. "Transforming Giants." *Harvard Business Review*, 2008, *86*(1), 43–52.

Kanter, R. M. "What Would Peter Say?" *Harvard Business Review*, 2009, *87*(11), 650–70.

Kaplan, R. S. "Reaching Your Potential." *Harvard Business Review*, 2008, *86*(7), 45–49.

Katzenbach, J. R. *Why Pride Matters More Than Money: The Power of the World's Greatest Motivational Force.* New York: Crown Business, 2003.

Katzenbach, J. R., and Smith, D. K. *The Wisdom of Teams: Creating the High-Performance Organization.* Boston: Harvard Business School Press, 1993.

Kaye, B., and Jordan-Evans, S. "Retention in Tough Times." *Training and Development*, Jan. 2002, pp. 32–37.

Kemp, P. "Death by Information Overload." *Harvard Business Review*, 2009, *87*(9), 83–89.

Klich-Heartt, E. I., and Prion, S. "Social Networking and HIPAA: Ethical Concerns for Nurses." *Nurse Leader*, 2010, *8*(4), 56–58.

"Know How to Lead." *Tampa Tribune*, Mar. 3, 1993.

Knowles, M. *The Modern Practice of Adult Education: Andragogy Versus Pedagogy.* Chicago: Association Press, 1970.

Kostner, J. *Knights of the TeleRound Table.* New York: Warner Books, 1994.

Kotter, J. P., and Schlesinger, L. A. "Choosing Strategies for Change." *Harvard Business Review*, 2008, *86*(6), 130–139.

Kouzes, J. W., and Posner, B. Z. *The Leadership Challenge.* (2nd ed.) San Francisco: Jossey-Bass, 1987.

Kouzes, J. W., and Posner, B. Z. "The Credibility Factor." *Healthcare Forum Journal*, July/Aug. 1993a, pp. 16–24.

Kouzes, J. W., and Posner, B. Z. *The Credibility Factor.* San Francisco: Jossey-Bass, 1993b.

Kouzes, J. W., and Posner, B. Z. *The Leadership Challenge*. (3rd ed.) San Francisco: Jossey-Bass, 2002.

Kouzes, J. W., and Posner, B. Z. *Encouraging the Heart: A Leader's Guide to Rewarding and Recognizing Others*. San Francisco: Jossey-Bass, 2003.

Kowalski, K., and Yoder-Wise, P. "Five Cs of Leadership." *Nurse Leader*, Sept./Oct. 2003, pp. 26–31.

Kramer, R. M. "Rethinking Trust." *Harvard Business Review*, 2009, *87*(6), 69–77.

Kraemer, H. "Keeping It Simple." *Health Forum Journal*, summer 2003, 16–20.

Larson, C. E., and LaFasto, F. *TeamWork: What Must Go Right/What Can Go Wrong*. Thousand Oaks, Calif.: Sage, 1989.

Larson, P., and William, L. "Striving for Balance: A Thing of the Past?" *Nurse Leader*, Apr. 2004, pp. 37–39.

Leebov, W. "Inviting the Soul to Work." *H&HNOnline*. 2005a, February 15. [Online information; retrieved 2/26/2005.] www.hhnmag.com.

Leebov, W. "E-Mail Etiquette." *H&HNOnline*, 2005b, April 19. [Online information; retrieved 4/24/2005.] www.hhnmag.com.

Leebov, W. *Wendy Leebov's Essentials for Great Patient Experiences: No-Nonsense Solutions with Gratifying Results*. Chicago: Health Forum, 2008a.

Leebov, W. *Wendy Leebov's Essentials for Great Personal Leadership*. Chicago: Health Forum, 2008b.

Leebov, W. "Workplace Hostility." *Wendy Leebov's HeartBeat on the Quality Patient Experience*, 2010, *1*(7), 1–3.

Lencioni, P. *The Five Dysfunctions of a Team: A Leadership Fable*. San Francisco: Jossey-Bass, 2002.

Loehr, J., and Schwartz, T. *The Power of Full Engagement: Managing Energy, Not Time, Is the Key to High Performance and Personal Renewal*. New York: Free Press, 2003.

Lorimer, W., and Manion, J. "Team-Based Organizations: Leading the Essential Transformation." *Patient Focused Care Association Review*, summer 1996, 15–19.

Losada, M., and Heaphy, E. "The Role of Positivity and Connectivity in the Performance of Business Teams: A Nonlinear Dynamics Model." *American Behavioral Scientist*, 2004, *47*(6), 740–765.

Ludema, J. D., Cooperrider, D. L., and Barrett, F. J. "Appreciative Inquiry: The Power of the Unconditional Positive Question." In P. Reason and H. Bradbury (eds.), *Handbook of Action Research*. Thousand Oaks, Calif.: Sage, 2000.

Lydon, J. E., and Zanna, M. P. "Commitment in the Face of Adversity: A Value-Affirmation Approach." *Journal of Personality and Social Psychology*, 1990, *58*(6), 1040–1047.

Mackoff, B. L., and Triolo, P. K. "Line of Sight: The Crucible in Nurse Manager Engagement." *Nurse Leader*, 2008a, *6*(4), 21–26.

Mackoff, B. L., and Triolo, P. K. "Why Do Nurse Managers Stay? Building a Model of Engagement: Part 1, Dimensions of Engagement." *Journal of Nursing Administration*, 2008b, *38*(3), 118–124.

Mackoff, B. L., and Triolo, P. K. "Why Do Nurse Managers Stay? Building a Model of Engagement: Part 2, Cultures of Engagement." *Journal of Nursing Administration*, 2008c, *38*(4), 166–171.

Maisel, N., and Gable, S. "The Paradox of Received Social Support: The Importance of Responsiveness." *Psychological Science*, 2009, *20,* 928–932.

Makin, P. J., Cooper, C. L., and Cox, C. J. *Organizations and the Psychological Contract: Managing People at Work*. Westport, Conn.: Quorum Books, 1996.

Manion, J. "Professional Collaboration: More Than a Committee Structure." *Nursing Options*, 1989, *1*(4), 9–12.

Manion, J. *Change from Within: Nurse Intrapreneurs as Health Care Innovators*. Kansas City, Mo.: American Nurses Association, 1990.

Manion, J. "Chaos or Transformation? Managing Innovation." *Journal of Nursing Administration*, 1993, *23*(5), 41–48.

Manion, J. "Managing Change: The Leadership Challenge of the 1990s." *Seminars for Nurse Managers*, 1994, *2*(4), 203–208.

Manion, J. "Understanding the Seven Stages of Change." *American Journal of Nursing*, 1995, *95*(4), 41–43.

Manion, J. "Teams 101: The Manager's Role." *Seminars for Nurse Managers*, 1997, *5*(1), 31–38.

Manion, J. "Building Commitment in Today's Workforce." *Home Care Provider*, Aug. 2000a, pp. 130–131.

Manion, J. "Retaining Current Leaders: A Gold Mine in Your Back Yard." *Health Forum Journal*, 2000b, *43*(5), 24–27.

Manion, J. "Joy at Work: As Experience, As Expressed." Unpublished doctoral dissertation, Fielding Graduate Institute, 2002a.

Manion, J. "Emergence of the Free Agent Workforce." *Nursing Administration Quarterly*, 2002b, *26*(5), 68–78.

Manion, J. "Joy at Work: Creating a Positive Workplace." *Journal of Nursing Administration*, 2003, *33*(12), 652–659.

Manion, J. "Strengthening Organizational Commitment: Understanding the Concept as a Basis for Creating Effective Workforce Retention Strategies." *Health Care Manager*, 2004a, *23*(2), 167–176.

Manion, J. "Nurture a Culture of Retention: Front-Line Nurse Leaders Share Perceptions Regarding What Makes—or Breaks—a Flourishing Nursing Environment." *Nursing Management*, 2004b, *35*(4), 28–39.

Manion, J. *Managing the Multi-Generational Nursing Workforce: Managerial and Policy Implications.* Geneva, Switzerland: International Centre for Human Resources in Nursing, 2009a.

Manion, J. *The Engaged Workforce: Proven Strategies to Build a Positive Health Care Workforce.* San Francisco: Jossey-Bass, 2009b.

Manion, J. "The Challenges and Rewards of an Intergenerational Workforce." *Voice of Nursing Leadership*, 2010, *8*(4), 8–10.

Manion, J., and Bartholomew, K. "Community in the Workplace: A Proven Retention Strategy." *Journal of Nursing Administration*, 2004, *34*(1), 46–53.

Manion, J., Lorimer, W., and Leander, W. *Team-Based Health Care Organizations: Blueprint for Success.* Gaithersburg, Md.: Aspen, 1996.

Manion, J., and Muha, T. "Flourishing in Difficult Times." *H&HN Weekly*. December 8, 2009. [Online information; retrieved 12/20/2009]. www.hhnmag.com.

Manion, J., Sieg, M. J., and Watson, P. "Managerial Partnerships: The Wave of the Future?" *Journal of Nursing Administration*, 1998, *28*(4), 47–55.

Martin, J., and Schmidt, C. "How to Keep Your Top Talent." *Harvard Business Review*, 2010, *88*(4), 54–61.

Martin, R. "How Successful Leaders Think." *Harvard Business Review*, 2007, *85*(6), 1–9.

Maun, C. Speech for the Maryland Healthcare Institute, Baltimore, Md., June 1, 2004.

Maxwell, J. "Inspiration Point." *Nurse Leader*, 2003, *1*(5), 8.

Mayer, J. D., Salovey, P., and Caruso, D. R. "Models of Human Intelligence." In R. J. Sternberg (ed.), *Handbook of Human Intelligence*. (2nd ed.) Cambridge: Cambridge University Press, 2000.

Mayer, R., and Schoorman, D. "Differentiating Antecedents of Organizational Commitment." *Journal of Organizational Behavior*, 1998, *19*(1), 15–28.

McCarthy, D. *The Loyalty Link*. Hoboken, N.J.: Wiley, 1997.

McConnell, C. R. "Interpersonal Skills: What They Are, How to Improve Them, and How to Apply Them." *Health Care Manager*, 2004, *23*(2), 177–187.

McDonald, T. "Send Clear Messages." *Team Management Briefings*, 1997, 4.

McGinn, P. "Thinking Clearly About Complex Issues" *H&HNetworks Online*. February 27, 2007. [Online information; retrieved 2/27/2007.] www.hhnmag.com.

McGinnis, A. L. *Bringing Out the Best in People*. Minneapolis: Augsburg Fortress, 1985.

McNally, K., and Cunningham, L. *The Nurse Executive's Coaching Manual*. Indianapolis, Ind.: Sigma Theta Tau International, 2010.

McNeese-Smith, D., and Crook, M. "Nursing Values and a Changing Nursing Workforce." *Journal of Nursing Administration*, 2003, *33*(5), 260–270.

Melrose, K. "Leader as Servant." *Executive Excellence*, 1996, *13*(4), 20.

Meyer, J. P., and Allen, N. J. "Testing the 'Side-Bet Theory' of Organizational Commitment: Some Methodological Considerations." *Journal of Applied Psychology*, 1984, *69*(3), 372–378.

Meyer, J., and others. "Organizational Commitment and Job Performance: It's the Nature of the Commitment That Counts." *Journal of Applied Psychology*, 1989, *74*(1), 152–156.

Miles, R. H. "Accelerating Corporate Transformations (Don't Lose Your Nerve)." *Harvard Business Review*, 2010, *88*(1), 69–75.

Miller, D., and Manthey, M. "Empowerment Through Levels of Authority." *Journal of Nursing Administration*, 1994, *24*(7), 23.

Mintzberg, H. *The Nature of Managerial Work*. Upper Saddle River, N.J.: Prentice Hall, 1980.

Morgan, C. "Growing Our Own: A Model of Encouraging and Nurturing Aspiring Leaders." *Nursing Management,* 2005, *11*(9), 27–30.

Morris, D. *Manwatching: A Field Guide to Human Behavior*. New York: Abrams, 1979.

Morse, G. "Trust, But Verify." *Harvard Business Review*, 2005, *83*(5), 19.

Muha, T., and Manion, J. "Using Positive Psychology to Engage Your Staff During Difficult Times." *Nurse Leader*, 2010, *8*(2), 50–54.

Murphy, M. "Leadership IQ Study: Youngest Workers Are the Least Satisfied." *Leadership IQ Newsletter*. [Online information retrieved 12/15/2007.]

Murphy, M. *Hundred Percenters: Challenge Your Employees to Give It Their All and They'll Give You Even More*. New York: McGraw-Hill, 2010a.

Murphy, M. "If Your Employees Aren't Learning, You're Not Leading." *Leadership IQ*, March 2010b.

Murphy, M., Burgio-Murphy, A., and Young, J. *Building Trust in the Workplace*. 2007. Media contact: dave.overton@newmancom.com.

Mycek, S. "Leadership for a Healthy Twenty-First Century." *Healthcare Forum Journal*, 1998, *41*(4), 26–30.

Nierenberg, J., and Ross, I. *Women and the Art of Negotiating*. New York: Simon & Schuster, 1985.

Oakley, E., and Krug, D. *Enlightened Leadership*. New York: Simon & Schuster, 1993.

O'Brien, M. E. *Servant Leadership in Nursing: Spirituality and Practice in Contemporary Health Care*. Sudbury, Mass.: Jones and Bartlett, 2011.

O'Connell, A. "The Essential Bennis—A Review." *Harvard Business Review*, 2009, *87*(11), 28.

O'Dooley, P. *Flight Plan for Living: The Art of Self Encouragement*. New York: Master Media, 1992.

O'Toole, J., and Bennis, W. "What's Needed Next: A Culture of Candor." *Harvard Business Review*, 2009, *87*(6), 54–61.

Ott, W., and Abrams, M. N. "Retention and the Value of Work." *H&HN OnLine*, 2008. [Online information; retrieved 3/9/2008] www.hhnmag.com.

Parker, G. "Teamwork and Team Players." *Team Management Briefings*, 1997, *5*(5), 8.

Peck, M. S. *The Road Less Traveled*. New York: Simon & Schuster, 1978.

Perlow, L. A., and Porter, J. L. "Making Time Off Predictable—and Required." *Harvard Business Review*, 2009, *87*(10), 102–109.

Pesmen, S. *Orlando Sentinel*, May 27, 1990, p. E21.

Peters, T. *Thriving on Chaos*. New York: HarperCollins, 1987.

Peters, T., and Austin, N. *A Passion for Excellence*. New York: Random House, 1985.

Phillips, D. *Lincoln on Leadership: Executive Strategies for Tough Times*. New York: Warner Books, 1992.

Pinchot, G., and Pinchot, E. "Creating Space for Many Leaders." *Executive Excellence*, 1996a, *13*(4), 17–18.

Pinchot, G., and Pinchot, E. *The Intelligent Organization: Engaging the Talent and Initiative of Everyone in the Workplace*. San Francisco: Berrett-Koehler, 1996b.

Piper, L. E. "Trust: The Sublime Duty in Health Care Leadership." *Health Care Manager*, 2010, *29*(1), 34–40.

Porter-O'Grady, T., and Malloch, K. *Quantum Leadership: A Textbook of New Leadership*. Sudbury, Mass.: Jones and Bartlett, 2003.

Porter-O'Grady, T., and Malloch, K. (eds.). *Innovation Leadership: Creating the Landscape of Health Care*. Sudbury, Mass.: Jones and Bartlett Publishers, 2010.

Porter-O'Grady, T., Alexander, D., Blaylock, J., Minkara, N., and Surel, D. "Constructing a Team Model: Creating a Foundation for Evidence-Based Teams." *Nursing Administration Quarterly*, 2006, *30*(3), 211–220.

Post, N. *Working Balance: Energy Management for Personal and Professional Well-Being*. Philadelphia: Post Enterprises, 1989.

Productivity and the Self-Fulfilling Prophecy: The Pygmalion Effect. (2nd ed.) Carlsbad, Calif.: CRM Films, 1997.

Quotable Women: A Collection of Shared Thoughts. Philadelphia: Running Press, 1989.

Rath, T., and Conchie, B. *Strengths-Based Leadership: Great Leaders, Teams, and Why People Follow*. New York: Gallup Press, 2008.

Reina, D. S., and Reina, M. L. *Trust and Betrayal in the Workplace: Building Effective Relationships in Your Organization*. San Francisco: Berrett-Koehler, 1999.

Robinson, J. "An E-Tool Bill of Rights." *Fast Company*, 2006, *79*(12), 54.

Rogers, R. "The Psychological Contract of Trust." *Executive Excellence*, July 1994, p. 6.

Schwartz, T. "The Productivity Paradox: How Sony Pictures Gets More Out of People by Demanding Less." *Harvard Business Review*, 2010, *88*(6), 65–69.

Seashore, C., Seashore, E., and Weinberg, G. *What Did You Say? The Art of Giving and Receiving Feedback*. Columbia, Md.: Bingham House Books, 1999.

Seligman, M. E. *Authentic Happiness: Using the New Positive Psychology to Realize Your Potential for Lasting Fulfillment*. New York: Simon & Schuster, 2002.

Senge, P. M. *The Fifth Discipline: The Art and Practice of the Learning Organization*. New York: Doubleday, 1990.

Senge, P. M. "Leading Learning Organizations." *Executive Excellence*, Apr. 1996, pp. 10–11.

Shendell-Falik, N. "A Positive Approach to Safer Handoffs: Using AI to Improve Patient Outcomes." Presentation at the NRC Picker annual symposium, Palm Springs, Calif., Sept. 28, 2008.

Shula, D., and Blanchard, K. H. *Everyone's a Coach*. Grand Rapids, Mich.: Zondervan, 1995.

Smith, S. S. "The Power of Praise." *Costco Connection*, Mar. 2003, pp. 16–18.

Snyder, J. "Appreciative Inquiry Empowers a City." *Monthly Newsletter of the International Positive Psychology Association*, Aug. 2009.

Spitzer, R. "Commitment Goes Both Ways." *Nurse Leader*, 2007, *5*(10), 4.

Stacey, R. *Managing the Unknowable: Strategic Boundaries Between Order and Chaos in Organizations*. San Francisco: Jossey-Bass, 1992.

Stefaniak, K. "Discovering Nursing Excellence Through Appreciative Inquiry." *Nurse Leader*, 2007, *5*(4), 42–46.

Tarkenton, F., with Tuleja, T. *How to Motivate People*. New York: HarperCollins, 1986.

Taylor, B. J. "Improving Communication Through Practical Reflection." *Reflections on Nursing Leadership*, 2nd qtr. 2004, pp. 28–38.

Thomas, K. W. *Intrinsic Motivation at Work: Building Energy and Commitment*. San Francisco: Berrett-Koehler, 2000.

Thomas, S. P. *Transforming Nurses' Stress and Anger: Steps Toward Healing.* (2nd ed.) New York: Springer-Verlag, 2004.

Tichy, N., and Bennis, W. G. "Making Judgment Calls: The Ultimate Act of Leadership." *Harvard Business Review,* 2007, *85*(10), 94–102.

Tichy, N., with Cardwell, N. *The Cycle of Leadership: How Great Leaders Teach Their Companies to Win.* New York: HarperCollins, 2002.

"Timeless Leadership: A Conversation with David McCullough." *Harvard Business Review,* 2008, *86*(3), 45–49.

"Transforming Care at the Bedside: Paving the Way for Change." *American Journal of Nursing,* Nov. 2009.

Trigg, R. *Reason and Commitment.* Cambridge: Cambridge University Press, 1973.

Ulreich, S. "Balancing Life—in Heels and a Suit." *Nurse Leader,* Apr. 2004, pp. 32–35.

Unruh, L. "Impact of Nurse Staffing on Patient Safety." In J. F. Byers and S. White (eds.), *Patient Safety: Principles and Practice.* New York: Springer, 2004.

Van Allen, L. "Permission to Balance Work and Life." *Nurse Leader,* 2004, *2*(4), 40–43.

Veronesi, J. F., "Breaking News on Social Intelligence." *Journal of Nursing Administration,* 2009, *39*(2), 57–58.

Vestal, K. "Confidence: A Key Ingredient for Success." *Nurse Leader,* 2005, *3*(4), 12–13.

Vestal, K. "Leading in Times of Uncertainty." *Nurse Leader,* 2009a, *7*(2), 6–7.

Vestal, K. "Personal Initiative: Some Have It . . . Some Don't." *Nurse Leader,* 2009b, *7*(6), 10–11.

Vestal, K. "Control Is a Good Thing." *Nurse Leader,* 2009c, *7*(10), 6–7.

Vestal, K. "Decision-Making: The Need for Clarity from Leaders." *Nurse Leader,* 2009d, *7*(12), 8–9.

Wall, B. "Being Smart Only Takes You So Far." *Training & Development,* 2007, *61*(1), 64–68.

Waterman, R. H. *The Renewal Factor: How the Best Get and Keep the Competitive Edge.* New York: Bantam Books, 1987.

Weaver, T. E. "Enhancing Multiple-Disciplinary Teamwork." *Nursing Outlook,* 2008, *56*(3), 108–114.

Weinstock, M. "Team-Based Care." *Hospitals and Health Networks.* March, 2010. [Online information; retrieved 4/2/2010.] www.hhnmag.com.

Wesorick, B. "Twenty-First Century Leadership Challenge: Creating and Sustaining Healthy Healing Work Cultures and Integrated Service at the Point of Care." *Nursing Administration Quarterly,* 2002, *26*(5), 18–32.

Wheatley, M. J. *Leadership and the New Science.* San Francisco: Berrett-Koehler, 1992.

Wiener, Y. "Commitment in Organizations." *Academy of Management Review,* 1982, *7*(3), 418–428.

Wilson, J., George, J., and Wellins, R. *Leadership Trapeze: Strategies for Leadership in Team-Based Organizations.* San Francisco: Jossey-Bass, 1994.

Wiseman, L., and McKeown, G. "Bringing Out the Best in Your People." *Harvard Business Review,* 2010, *88*(4), 117–121.

Wolf, G., Triolo, P., and Ponte, P. R. "Magnet Recognition Program: The Next Generation." *Journal of Nursing Administration,* 2008, *38*(4), 200–204.

Zak, P. J. "The Neurobiology of Trust." *Scientific American,* June 2008, pp. 88–95.

Zemke, R. "The Corporate Coach." *Training,* 1996, *33*(12), 24–33.

Zemke, R. "Problem-Solving Is the Problem: Don't Fix That Company." *Training,* 1999, *36*(6), 26–33.

INDEX

A

Ability, 190–191, 192, 193, 208

Abolishing Performance Appraisals: Why They Backfire and What to Do Instead (Coens and Jenkins), 311

Abrams, M. N., 93

Academic programs, formal, 332, 342, 343

Accessibility and availability, 45–47, 153, 161, 163–164, 170, 280

Accommodation, in conflict resolution, 205–206, 212

Accountability: and empowerment, 192, 193, 198–199, 267; level of, questioning the leader's, 49; shared, 65–66; of teams, 217, 223–224; weak systems of, issue of, 304; for the well-being of the larger community, 93. *See also* Responsibility

Accountability systems, limited, 198

Accreditation visits, 10

Acknowledging a broken trust, 48, 49

Ackoff, R., 252

Action planning and implementation, *248*, 254, 257, *258, 259*, 273

Action research, form of, 267, 273. *See also* Appreciative inquiry

Active listening, 148, 149–150

Active participatory learning, 342–343

Actively constructive response, 54

Actively destructive response, 54

Ad hoc teams, 176, 216, 228

Adams, J. L., 249

Adult learning, principles of, 341–345

Advanced beginner level, 319–320, 344

Adversaries, communication strategies for, 171, *172*

Adversity, role of, 75

Advice giving, 289, 326, 331

Affective commitment, 79, 80, 81, 82, 83

African story, moral from an, 26

Age diversity. *See* Generational diversity

Aiken, L. H., 24

Alexander, D., 220

Alignment: with change initiatives, 232; of goals, 81; of mission, 92–93, 244; of strengths, 325; of values, 85–86, 87, 244, 307; of vision, 96, 244

Allen, N. J., 80, 81

Allies, communication strategies for, *171, 172*, 173

Alternatives: analysis of, solution generation and, in problem solving, *248*, 252–254, 257, *258, 259*; decisions as a choice among, 260; focusing on, that groups have control over, 250; identifying, in negotiation, *208*, 211, 213; returning to, after unexpected outcomes, 255

Alternatives to problem solving. *See* Appreciative inquiry; Polarity management

Altru Health System (United Health Systems), 143

Altuntas, S. A., 66

Amabile, T. M., 244

Ambiguity, accelerating levels of uncertainty and, challenge of, 19–22

Ambler, M., 166

Amends, making, 48, 50–51

American Hospital Association, x, 23, 24

American Nurses Credentialing Center (ANCC), 100, 101

Analogies. *See* Metaphors and analogies, using

Analysis paralysis, 258, *259*

Anderson, C., 226

Anderson, P., 95

Anger, 22, 57, 120–121, 122, 136, 137, 233, 237, 246, 322

Ankario, L., viii

Annas, G. J., 158

Annison, M., 14, 15

Answers, admitting to not having all the, 47

Anxiety, 22, 41, 237

Apologizing, 48, 50, 51

Appeal, as a conflict resolution strategy, 206

Appearance, nonverbal communication through, 156

Apple, 15, 63

Appreciating phase, 271

Appreciation, showing, 130, 152, 324, 337. *See also* Recognition; Rewards and benefits

Appreciative inquiry: as an alternative approach, 274; application of, 273–274; choosing to use, 256, 267; comparing traditional problem solving and, 267–269; defining, 267; general principles of, 269–270; stages of, 270–273

Appropriateness: of appearance, 156; of communication settings, *125*; of written content, 167, 168

Aronson, E., 111

Arthur Andersen, 18

Articulate communication, issue with just, 116. *See also* Clear communication

Asian culture, 158

Assessment. *See* Measurement; Outcome evaluation; Performance assessment

Assumptions: about feedback, 123; about group development, 327, 327–328; about problems, 269; about speaking up, 44; about values, 88; and behavioral expectations, 309, 310; challenging your own, 48; and communication, 118, 121, 127, 192; identifying, in written communication, 167, 168; and negotiations, 208, 210

Attention: exercising, by listening, 146; of listeners, getting the, 137; management of, 98; showing, through body language, 151; to something, giving feedback through, 336–337; in teaching, 344

Attentive listening, 149

Attitude, importance of: in coaching, 307–308, 333; in organizations, 186

Attracting talent, 24

Audiovisuals, use of, 139–140

Austin, N., 46, 142

Authority: blaming those with, 260; and coercion, 204; and commitment, 80, 108; concentrated decision-making, 226; earned, 193; and empowerment, 191–192, 193, 195–198, 267, 303; legitimate, issues with, 6, 38; problem-solving, determining, 251, 256–257, 258; and respect, 51; reversal of, 197–198; socialization involving, 44; of teams, avoiding communication that usurps the, 176. *See also* Decision making; Power

Authority levels, 191–192, 195–197, 251

Automated telephone systems, 140

Autonomy, *298*, 303, *307*. *See also* Choice

Availability. *See* Accessibility and availability

Avoidance, 201, 205, 212–213, 214

B

Baby Boomers, 23, 81–82, 131, 305, 306

Baggs, J. G., 61

Bakker, J., 18

Balance, work-life, 27, 46

Bandage approach, 257, *258*

Baptist Health, case study involving, 99–104

Bardwick, J. M., 4

Bargaining, 262

Barker, J. A., 15, 16, 94, 272

Barney, S. M., 79

Barrett, F. J., 267, 269

Barriers, process, removing, 187–188, 304, 333, 334

Bartholomew, K., 79

Baxter Healthcare, 5

Baykal, U., 66

Becker, H. S., 78

Beckhard, R., ix, 90

Bedfellows, communication strategies for, *171, 172*

Begeny, S., 216, 226

Beginning stage, in the transition process, *236*, 238

Behavior: accepting ownership for, 49; desired, rewarding, 310–314; as a factor related to constancy, 47; future, feedback influencing, 337; reactive, 246, 257, 287; redirecting or reinforcing, in coaching, 319. *See also* Modeling behavior

Behavioral expectations, 127, 222, 229, 307–310, 325, 326–328

Behavioral neuroscience, findings from, 34–35

Benner, P., 317

Bennis, W., ix, 2, 4–5, 7, 9, 11, 13, 14, 17, 18, 38, 45, 48, 49, 59, 63, 65, 66, 98, 124, 134, 181, 352–353

Berry, L. L., 97, 145

Beyer, D., 202, 203

Biswas, Deiner, R., 297

Blameless apology, 50

Blaming, 11, 56, 199, 203, 260, 303

Blanchard, K. H., 289, 291, 292, 293, 317

Blaylock, J., 220

Block, P., 128, 170, *171, 172*, 173

Blogging, 164, 165

Blouin, A., 63, 174

Board member risk aversion, 186–187

Body language, 44, 54, 127, 134, 135–136, 151, 153, 157, 336. *See also* Nonverbal communication

Body motions and posture, 157–158

Bohlen, C., 24

Bohmer, R., 219

Boredom, 77, 300

Borkowski, N., 295

Bossidy, L., 244

Bottom line versus the horizon, focusing on the, 12–13

Bowcutt, M., 27

Boyatzis, R., 32, 34, 35, 125, 244, 285

Brainstorming, 211, 249

Breen, B., 12

Brent, N., 63, 174

Brickman, P., 72, 74, 75, 76, 77, 109, 110, 111

Bridges, W., 22, 230, 236, 237, 238

Briles, J., 340

Brown, H. J., Jr., 350, 352

Buckingham, M., ix, 301, 313, 316, 323, 337

Building commitment. *See* Commitment

Built on Trust (Ciancutti and Steding), 60

Bullying, 203

Bunker, K. A., 230

Bureaucratic organizations, 2, 11, 92, 199, 296

Burgio-Murphy, A., 286

Bürkner, H., 219

Burnout, 87

Burns, B. M., 52

Bush, H., 165

Business environment, turbulent, 25–26, 189, 214. *See also* Economic downturn

Business literacy, 129

Business partnerships, 63

Business sector leadership, 6, 226

Butterfly analogy, 353

Buttigieg, D., 79, 81, 110

Buzzwords, 61, 188, 265, 289

Byers, J. F., 250

Byrne, J. A., 302

Bywords, 94

C

Caesar, J., 6

Campbell, R., 151

Capability, 190–191, 192, 193–194, 244, 267

Capacity, 2, 5, 21, 26, 27, 39, 40–41, 57, 225. *See also* Competence

Cardwell, N., 269, 284, 341–342

Career crisis point, 88

Caring, communicating, by listening, 145–146

Caruso, D. R., 32

Casting, importance of, 301–302

Celebration, 304–305, *307*, 333, 335

Cell phones, 131, 161, 164, 302

Chaleff, I., 44, 260

Chalice and the Blade, The (Eisler), 65

Challenger role, identifying the, 221–222

Championing, 334

Champy, J., 34

Change: anchoring, 234, 238; in authority levels, avoiding, 196–197; building affective commitment during times of, 83; communication during, 169–173, 233–234; cultural, 9, 228, 234, 239, 263, 268, 273; deep level of, 72; defined, 22; desired, indicating the, in corrective feedback, 340; driving force for, 201; effect of, on the demand for leadership, 14–15, 16; emotional reactions to, 200; facilitating the process of, 229–230, 230–236; and generational differences, 25; in job requirements, capability and, 193; leader accessibility and availability during times of, 46–47; in leaders, and establishing trust, issue of, 39–40; leading to uncertainty, 19, 20–21, 21–22; major, disruptions caused by, effect of, 199–200; phases in the process of, 230–236; pitfalls of leading through, 235–236, 238–240; positive, methodology for, 273; rapid pace of, vii, 14, 19, 25, 26, 72, 90, 169–170, 229–230, 287, 326; repeating messages during times of, 127–128, 170; responding to, empowerment and, 189; stabilizing and sustaining, 234, 238; structural, authority-related problems due to, 197; sustaining a pace of, considerations involved in, 21; technological, 20–21, 63; that is unnecessary, awareness of, 21; versus transition, 230; in the workforce due to economic downturn, 24; in workforce values, 214. *See also* Innovation

Change initiatives: failure of, 230, 233; major, time involved in, 104

"Chaos or Transformation" (Manion), *231*

Character, importance of, in selection, 302

Charan, R., 244

Chat rooms, 164

Chawla, S., 93, 187

Cherniss, C., 34, 117, 125, 222, 229, 327

Chief information officers, 132

Chilean trapped miners, 143

Choice: and adversity, 75; and the development continuum, 64; as essential to commitment, 109; failure to offer, 109–110; as an intrinsic motivator, 297, *298*, 303, *307*; lack of, and the economic downturn, 24, 81; in negotiation, 211

Churchill, W., 21, 295

Ciancutti, A., 58, 60

Clancy, T., 260

Clark, M., 139

Clarke, S. P., 24

Clarke-Epstein, C., 339

Classroom-style teaching, 332, 333, 342, 343, 345

Clear communication: among team members, 222; and asking the right questions, 151–152; challenges to, 169–177; common problems blocking, awareness of, 119–124, *125*; conclusion on, 177; discussion questions on, 177–178; and emotional intelligence, 117; getting results with, 244; and information sharing, 126–131; lack of, and feedback, 43; as a leader's primary responsibility, 131–169; and listening, 144–151; of mission, 108; and moving forward into the future, 351; and nonverbal communication, 132, 152–159; overview of, 116–117; responsibility for, 195; and special issues involving, 169–177; and spoken communication, 132–152; teamwork implying, 215; of values, 87, 88, 89; of vision, 96–97, 110; and written communication, 132, 159–169. *See also* Communication; Feedback

Climate: negotiation, 211, 212; organizational, 58–60, 234

Closed questions, 151

Closure, managing, 234, 235

Clustered organization, 229

Coach, defined, 289

Coaching: and comparing roles in sports and health care, 290–291; and conflict resolution, 207; counseling versus, 287, 316; defined, 289–290; and empowerment, 194, 199; and getting results, 244, 289; and increasing competence, motivation resulting from, 300–301; lack of, or aversion to, reasons for, 286–288; and motivation, 294–314; overview of, 285–286; steps in the process of, 314–341; and supporting direct problem solving, 13, 339. *See also* Employee development

Coaching interventions, carrying out, *315*, 319–320, 321, 330–335

Coach-performer relationship: basis for the, 314; building the, 292–294; clarifying expectations in the, 325–326; structure of the, 290, 294

Coalition building, as a conflict resolution strategy, 205

Co-constructing phase, 272

Coens, T., 311

Coercion, as a conflict resolution strategy, 204

Coffman, C., ix, 301, 313, 316, 337

Cognitive (task) conflict, 201, 202

Coles, D., 28

Collaboration: among competitors, 15; associations of, forming, 64; in decision making, 180; efforts to improve, 273; elements of, 61–63; in long-distance relationships, 175; Magnet recognition of, 101; meaning of, 61; in resolving conflicts, 65; and social networking sites, 164; understanding, importance of, 60. *See also* Partnership

Collective leadership. *See* Shared leadership

Collins, J., 5, 6, 112, 225–226, 301, 302

Collins, S., 26, 27

Command-and-control methodology, viii, 71, 107, 129, 180, 182, 350

Commitment: catalyst in the development of, 75; versus compliance, 70, 72; concept of, 72–75; conclusion on, 112; to decisions, in leadership teams, 225; development based on levels of competence and, 318, 319, 320, 321, 344; discussion questions on, 112–114; elements of, 74; escalating, possibility of, missing the, 111–112; getting results as a way of creating, 244; intense, of leaders, 4; level of, to decisions, 263, 264, 266; mistaking compliance for, 108–109; and motivation, 297; and moving forward into the future, 350–351; negotiation building, 315; overview of, 70–71; personal, 70, 72; romantic, 75; stages of, 75–77; and storytelling, 142; within teams, 223. *See also* Organizational commitment

Commitment and competency, developing. *See* Coaching

Commitments: dissolution of, 111; following through on, 60

Common mission: alignment essential for a, 92–93; clarity of mission essential to a, 89, 90–91; importance of, 89; influence of a, with a shared vision and shared values, 98, 110; as one component of building commitment, 84, 89

Common working approaches, establishing, 220–223, 229

Commonalities, establishing, with listeners, 137–138

Communication: in the absence of authority, 197; across geographical separation, 174–175; with adversaries and opponents, 171; barrage of, 131; during change, 169–173, 233–234; coaching and, 292, 294; common complaints about, 117; cultural differences in, 119; defining, 117–118; developing a strategy for, during action planning and implementation, 254; efforts to improve, 273; essence of, 125; as essential to the leader-follower relationship, 36, *37*, 56–58, 66, 83; failed effort at, of vision, example of, 107; and group decisions, 265; from the heart about values, 89; increased, promise for, 164; insufficient, for commitment, 110–111; investing time in, 108; lack of information and, effect of, 117; and leadership, 124–125; methods of, within teams, deciding on, 221; obtaining closure with, 60; poor, as a major problem, 126; systemwide, to explain a Magnet journey, example of, 102–103; with teams, 175–177; and trust, 59, 60, 116, 122, 123, 135, 171, 174–175; unreasonably prolonged process of, 160. *See also* Clear communication; Feedback

Communication campaigns, evaluating, 169

Communication channels, 118, 119–121, 128

Communication flow, 175

Communication loop, 118

Communication plan, defining and implementing a, 233–234

Communication relationships, simplifying, issue with, involving teams, 176–177

Community agency risk aversion, 186

Community hospital, failed vision at a, case study involving, 106–107

Community, sense of, 59, 79

Compassion, 59

Compensation mechanisms, 234

Compensation packages, competitive, issue with, 110

Competence: assessing, 317–318; choosing tenure over, issue of, 43–44; and credibility, 48; defined, 39; development based on levels of commitment and, 318, 319, 320, 321, 344; as essential for trust, 38, 39–41, 292; as an intrinsic motivator, 297, *298*, 300–302, *307*; leadership, 4–5; lost sense of, addressing, 302

Competency and commitment, developing. *See* Coaching

Competent level, 318, 320, 321, 322, 330, 344

Competition: among PowerPoint presenters, 139; coaching and, 291; as a conflict resolution strategy, 204; in contrast to cooperation, 62; as a motivator, 346; organizational environments based on, 63; shift in, 15

Competitive compensation packages, issue with, 110

Compliance, 70, 71–72, 97, 108–109, 182

Conchie, B., 323

Confidence and trust, 37–38, 39, 233, 333. *See also* Self-confidence

Confidential information, 128–129, 162, 165

Conflict: avoiding, 201, 205, 212–213, 214; common reactions to, 200; emotions in, 200, 201, 209, 213; evaluating a, 202–203; fear of, 214, 223; positive side of, 201–202, 203; preventing, within teams, 222; repressing, 214

Conflict resolution: and collaboration, 65; effective methods of, 206–212; ineffective methods of, 203–206; leadership role in, 202–203; pitfalls of, 212–214; responsibility for, 195; skill in, need for, 199–200; and the use of space, 156

Conflicting values, 85–86, 87, 88, 89

Conformity pressure, 265

Congruence: and body language, 134; during the change process, 233, 234; and communication, 132, 141, 158; and credibility, 48; as essential for trust, 38, *39*, 42–45, 292–293; in missions, 220; in modeling behavior, 345; between values, 80, 85, 87, 89

Consensus decisions, 262–263, 265–266

Consistency, 4; in coaching, issue of, 285–286; in modeling behavior, lack of, example of, 107; in policy implementation, 275; of support, 55, 66; of team membership, 219, 226

Consolidations, 174

Constancy: and credibility, 48; as essential for trust, 38, *39*, 45–47, 55, 293

Consultation, 62

Continual improvement, drive for, 12

Continual learning, 301, 333, 342

Continuance commitment, 78–79, 80, 81, 82, 110

Contrariness, 22, 48, 59

Control: managerial, 10; span of, 224, 287. *See also* Command-and-control methodology; Power

Conviction, 59

Cooper, C. L., 78, 80, 82

Cooper, R. K., 95

Cooperation, 61, 62, 63, 215, 233

Cooperrider, D., 269, 273, 325

Coordination, 61, *62*, 63, 233

"Corporate Coach, The" (Zemke), 284

Corrective feedback, 339–341. *See also* Negative feedback

Correctness, 167, 168

Corruption/scandals, 18, 142

Costs and rewards, issue of, in commitment, 78, 81

Counseling versus coaching, 287, 316

Courage, 4, 16, 19, 21, 47, 48, 59, 87, 89, 116, 180, 186, 350, 353
Covey, S., 64, 91, 95, 147, 148, 183
Cox, C. J., 21, 27, 78, 80, 82, 230, 231, 235
Crafting work, 302
Creative Healthcare Management, 262
Creative tension, 96
Creativity: pitfall involving transition and, 240; potential for, transition stage characterized by, 238; in problem solving, importance of, 252–253; team, phase of, *231*, 233–234. *See also* Innovation
Credibility, 48, 117, 244. *See also* Trust
Credibility gap, 42, 43, 86
Crises, 72, 143, 184, 238
Crisis points, 23, 88
Crook, M., 87
Csikszentmihalyi, M., 300
Cultivating relationships. *See* Leader-follower relationship
Cultural change, 9, 228, 234, 239, 263, 268, 273, 304
Cultural differences: anticipating and understanding, for effective communication, 157–158; in body language, 157; communication channels and, 119; in eye contact, 159; in terms of physical contact, 154
Cunningham, L., 289, 291
Curtin, L., 21
Cycle of Leadership: How Great Leaders Teach Their Companies to Win (Tichy and Cardwell), 341

D

Damage control, opportunity for, 188
Davenport, T. H., 261
de Man, H., 304
Decision making: and behavioral expectations, 308–309, 310; collaboration in, 180; complexity of, 261; concentrated authority for, 226; and deciding among alternatives, 254; empowerment and, 189, 265, 267, 303; evaluating and recognizing the types of decisions for, 260–263; feedback on, 339; individual, development of, weakening, 10; leadership teams and, 225; listening leading to better, 145; pitfalls in the process of, 265–267; and polarity management, 275; rational, elements of, 111; shared, 62, 130, 266–267, 303, 327; shared values and mission guiding, 89; skill in, need for, 245; structure for, providing the, in the change process, 232, 233; team, approaches to, deciding on, 221, 262; using individual versus group decisions for, factors for consideration in, 263–265, 266; vision guiding, 12. *See also* Authority; Getting results

Decisions: defined, 260; evaluation of, 260; good, source of, 260; group versus individual, consideration of, factors in, 263–265; quality of, value placed on the, considering the, 264; types of, 260–263; undermined, 197, 198
Defensiveness, 122, 152, 287, 308
Deiner, E., 297
Delegation, 199, 261, 285, 303, 310, 328–329
Delivery of care: improving, vision for, case study involving, 104–106; shifts in, 230
Delivery of messages. *See* Message delivery
Department vision, 96
Dependence, 64, 86, 130, 189, 343
DePree, M., 4, 11, 52, 65, 90, 124
Depression, 22, 237
Design stage, *270*, 272
Desired behavior, rewarding, 310–314
Desired future statement, *248*, 252, 257, *258*, *259*
Desired results/outcomes, achieving. *See* Getting results
Destiny stage, *270*
Detert, J. R., 44
Developing others. *See* Employee development
Development continuum, 64, 65
Development levels: assessing, ways of, 321; described, and coaching interventions, 318–321; and differences in skill acquisition, 317–318; inaccurately assessing, 321–322; in learning, described, 344–345; specificity of parameters related to, 330
Devil's advocates, serving as, 48
Dialogue. *See* Communication
Different, being, finding ways of, 138
Diplomacy, 167
Direct dialogue/communication. *See* Clear communication
Direction setting, 4, 231, 232
Disasters, effects of, 17, 143
Discovery, encouraging, 289
Discovery stage, *270*, 271
Discrepancies: avoiding, 43–45; common, 42–43
Dissent, respectful, 48, 134
Dissonance, 85–86, 87, 89, 299, 309
Distractions, removing, to improve listening, 147–148. *See also* Noise
Distrust, 37, 48–51, 117, 122, 126, 129, 154, 155, 177, 201, 204. *See also* Trust
Diversity, 24–25, 52, 219, 305, 306
Dominance and intimidation, as a conflict resolution strategy, 204
Dreaming stage, *270*, 271–272. *See also* Vision

Drucker, P., ix, 4, 21, 32, 42, 89–90, 94–95, 324–325
Duplication, 20, 195, 300

E
Earthquake in San Francisco (1989), 143
Eastern cultures, 159
Economic downturn, 24, 26, 42, 81, 199–200, 303
Edmondson, A., 44, 219
Educated workforce, 129
Education and training. *See* Employee development
Efficiency versus effectiveness, focusing on, 7–8
Egocentricism, 293
Eisler, R., 65
Elderly people, 131
Electronic communications, 159, 161–166.
Electronic medical record (EMR), issues with the, 20, 28, 300
E-mail: advantages of, 161; coaching via, 291; communication by, issues with, 117, 119, 120–121, 121–122, 131, 161–164, 167; as an energy drain, 27; interruptions from, 302; and long-distance relationships, 175; unnecessary, eliminating, 163; volume of, managing, 161–162. *See also* Written communication
E-mail etiquette, 161–162
Emotional intelligence, 32–34, 116, 117, 118, 161, 222–223, 229, 240, 327
Emotional ties, 79
Emotional tone, 125
Emotionally Intelligent Workplace (Cherniss and Goleman), *33*
Emotions: and change, 22, 170, 200, 237, 239–240; in coaching, 287, 325, 328; communication of, 125; in conflict, 200, 201, 209, 213; and dissolution of commitments, 111; due to mixed messages, 124; listening for, 145; manager's effect on, 244; in reactive behavior, 246, 287; and transition, 200, 237, 239–240. *See also specific emotions*
Empathic (reflective) listening, 148, 149–150
Empathy, 34, 340, 341
Employee development: conclusion on, 346; discussion questions on, 346–348; intentional, leader's role in, 284–285; investing in, issue of, 12–13, 184–185, 193, 194; and moving forward into the future, 351–352; through teaching, 284, 341–346. *See also* Coaching
Employee discretionary effort, 71
Employee empowerment. *See* Empowerment
Employee engagement: challenge of, 23, 24, 81; during the change process, 234; and common mission, 92;

current emphasis on, 70; employee development creating, 316, 323; need for, 72; negotiation building, 315; and organizational commitment, 70–71, 82, 303; and proactivity, 246–247; reflecting on times of, to identify strengths, 324; and shared values, 85; and shared vision, 110
Employee loyalty and commitment: debunking a belief about, 71; predictors of, 59–60; storytelling and, 142; trust and, 59. *See also* Commitment; Organizational commitment
Employee needs versus patient needs, polarity mapping, 278, 279–280
Employee performance: and commitment, 80, 81; and geographical distance, 175; greater, expectations requiring, 199. *See also Performance entries*
Employee selection, 301–302
Empowered Manager, The (Block), 170, *171, 172*
Empowerment: applying the process of, 192–193; and conflict resolution, 203; and decision making, 189, 265, 267, 303; definitions of, 189; described, 188–190; elements of, 190–192; failure to recognize the need for, 184–185; for group problem solving, creating, 248; pitfalls in the process of, 193–199; proactivity and, 246
Encoding messages, 128
Encouragement, providing, 54, 319, 320, 321, 333, 338, 344
Encouraging the Heart (Kouzes and Posner), 244
Ending stage, in the transition process, 236–237
Energy drain, challenge of the, 26–28
Engagement, importance of, 297, 302. *See also* Employee engagement
English culture, 159
Enron, 18
Enthusiasm, 54, 74, 75, 85, 110, 142, 151, 227, 231, 296, 304, 319, 321, 333, 344
Entitlement, environment of, 193
Environment: tweaking the, to unleash employee strengths, 323; using the, to communicate a message, 136, 144. *See also specific type of environment*
Environmental pressures, external, 72, 189, 214
Envisioning phase. *See* Dreaming stage
Equity theory, 295
Escalating commitment, 111–112
Ethical commitment, 93
Ethical concerns, of social networking sites, 165
Ethical erosion, 86
Ethical leaders, 18, 28

Evaluation: of decisions, 260; in the problem-solving process, *248*, 254–256, 257, *258*, *259*, 260; of quality measures, 234, 235. *See also* Measurement; Outcome evaluation; Performance assessment

Excuses, using challenges as, 19

Execution phase, 234

Execution: The Discipline of Getting Things Done (Bossidy and Charan), 244

Exemplary performers. *See* High performers

Expectancy theory, 295

Expectations, clarifying: in the coaching process, *315*; for desired approaches and behaviors, 325, 326–328; and identifying parameters, 325, 328–330; for roles and responsibilities, 325–326. *See also* Behavioral expectations

Experience: role of, in learning, ix, 343–344, 350; source of, 260

Expert level, 318, 320–321, 322, 344–345

Exploration stage, *75*, 76

External accountability, 198

External environmental pressures, 72, 189, 214

External motivation, added influence of, applying the, 297, 307

Eye behavior, 159

F

Facebook, 164, 165

Face-to-face communication, importance of, 117, 118, 119, 120, 128, 161, 162, 174

Facilitating processes. *See* Process facilitation

Facts, gathering, in negotiation, 210, 211

Fagiano, D., 98

Failed vision, case study involving a, 106–107

Failure: of change initiatives, 230, 233; fear of, and punitive consequences, 188; focus on, resulting in loss of confidence, 324; learning from, 186; looking back at, problem solving involving, 267

Familial differences, in terms of physical contact, 154

Family values, 85

Favoritism, avoiding, 175

Fear: of conflict, 214, 223; of confrontation, 287; of continual improvement, 12; of failure and punitive consequences, 188; of giving corrective feedback, 341; and groupthink, 260; of innovation, 186; and reactive behavior, 246; of reprisals for speaking up, 43, 44, 59; during transitions, 22, 237; and uncertainty, 260

Federal Bureau of Investigation (FBI), 135

Feedback: about performance, need for, 287; about value incongruency, 87; asking for, 170; in coaching, 289, 294, *315*, 326, 328, 332, 335, 336–341; in the communication loop, 118, 121; communication problems involving, 121–123, *125*, 150; misunderstanding, 135–136; obstacles in, 43, 44–45; promoting, 43; in questioning, 152; seeking, for message clarity, importance of, 136; in teaching, 344; using, importance of, 161. *See also* Communication

Feedback loop, 118, 121, *125*, 149

Feelings and emotions. *See* Emotions

Fence sitters, communication strategies for, *171*, *172*

Fielden, J., 160, 166, 167

Fields, M., 27

File sharing, 164

Financial performance, leading indicator of, 71

Financial rewards, intrinsic motivation and, 297, 299, 311

Financial-based commitment, issue with, 79, 110

Finnel, E., 252

First-order problem solving, 245

Flooding in North Dakota (1997), 143

Flow, 300, 302, 324. *See also* Employee engagement

Flower, J., 7, 11, 21, 38, 45

Folk wisdom, 97

Follow up, 121, 122, 148, 150, 161, 162, 169, 176

Ford, H., 307–308

Formal academic approach, 332, 333, 342, 343

Formal learning sessions, 333

Fragmentation, 269

Fraud, 18

Fredrickson, B., 56, 338

Frese, M., 246, 247

Freshwater, D., 343

Frick, D., 93

Friedman, S. D., 27

From Good to Great (Collins), 226

From Management to Leadership (Manion), 70

Frustration, 70, 152, 193, 195, 204, 237, 245, 246, 251, 300, 319, 321

Future: conflict that faces the, 203; demands of the, meeting, 70; hope for the, 94; moving forward into the, 350–353; stewards of the, 352. *See also* Desired future statement; Vision

Future behavior, feedback influencing, 337

Future organizational structure, basis of, 229

Future, unknown. *See* Uncertainty, challenge of

Future-oriented strategy, 284

Future-oriented thinking, 246, 331

G

Gable, S., 53, 55

Gallup Organization, 316, 323, 324, 338

Gap analysis, use of, 100

Gelinas, L., 24

Generation Xers, 82, 305, 306

Generational cohorts, defined, and differences among, 25

Generational differences, 81–82, 305–307

Generational diversity, 24–25, 305, 306

Generative learning, 267

Gentile, M. C., 44

Geographical separation, communicating across, 174–175

George, J., 126

Gestures and movement, using, 137, 138–139, 157

Get-it-done mentality, 180, 239–240

Getting results: with appreciative inquiry, 256, 267–274; coaching and, 244, 289; conclusion on, 281; decision making and decisions for, 245, 260–267; discussion questions on, 281–282; and moving forward into the future, 351; overview of, 244–246; and pitfalls of the problem-solving process, 256–260; with polarity management, 256, 274–280; and proactivity, 245, 246–247; problem solving for, 245, 247–256. *See also* Decision making; Problem solving

Gharajedaghi, J., 252

Gibson, C., 189

Gilbert, J., 86, 89, 93

Girl Scouts of the USA, 6

Gladwell, M., 352

Globalization, 25

Goal setting, 263, 301, 315–316

Goals: alignment of, 81; and the line-of-sight concept, 92; organizational, acceptance of, 78; superordinate, using, as a conflict resolution strategy, 207; team, 222, 223. *See also* Mission; Vision

Goethe, J., 350

Goldsmith, M., ix

Goleman, D., 32, 34, 35, 117, 125, 222, 229, 285, 327

Good to Great and the Social Sectors (Collins), 226

Grammar and punctuation, 162, 167

Grashow, A., 3

Gratification, importance of, 311–312

Greek legend, 304

Greenleaf, R., 93

Grievance procedure, 206

Grieving, 22, 57, 237, 240

Grohar-Murray, M. E., 317

Grossman, R. J., 2

Group cohesiveness, 78, 79

Group development, assumptions about, 327–328

Group members, characteristics of, considering the, 264

Group operating effectiveness, considering, 264

Group patterns, evaluating, 260

Group practice, 332

Group problem solving: approaches to, 249–256; complexity of, 247–248; pitfalls in, 256–258, *259*; unproductive, reasons for, 259–260. *See also* Problem solving

Group values, 85

Group versus individual decisions, using, factors for consideration in, 263–265, 266

Groupthink, 259–260

Guber, P., 141

Guided discussions, use of, 320, 326, 344

Guided practice, 344

Guided questions, 324

Gutbezahl, C., 201

H

Haas, R., 129

Happiness, elements important to, 297, 301

Harvard Business Review, 27

Harvard Business School, 189

Hasty conclusions, jumping to, 249

Havens, D. S., 273

Health care environment, rapidly changing, 326

Health care reform, vii, 16, 21–22, 230

Health care systems: integration within, failure of, 239; nature of, 181

Health Insurance Portability and Accountability Act (HIPAA), 165

Healthy relationships: basis for, 36, 83, 292, *315*; as an intrinsic motivator, 297, 298, *307. See also* Coach-performer relationship; Leader-follower relationship

Heaphy, E., 56

Heenan, D. A., 63

Heifetz, R. A., 2, 3, 180

Hemp, P., 131, 162–163

Henry, B., 158

Hersey, P., 317

Herzberg, F., 295

Hesselbein, F., ix, 6

Hewlett, S. A., 82

Hidden agendas, 208–209, 257, 265

Hierarchical organizations, 43, 44, 50, 71, 92, 140, 156, 199, 216, 224, 247, 286–287, 342

Hierarchy of needs, 295

High performers: coaching, 291, 312, 313–314, 324, 337, 338; success of, elements in the, 352; as teachers and coaches, 333

High-performing teams, 57

High-stakes conflict, 202–203

HIPAA (Health Insurance Portability and Accountability Act), 165

Hispanic culture, 154

Honest/direct communication. *See* Clear communication

Honesty, 59, 159, 171, 208, 345

Hoover, J. E., 135

Horizon, focusing on the bottom line versus the, 12–13

Hospital evacuation, largest, 143

Hospital risk aversion, 186

Hospital system, vision for a, case study of, 99–104

How versus what and why, focusing on, 8–9

Huey, J., 129

Hurricane Andrew, 143

Hurricane Katrina, 143

I

IBM, 63, 138

Ignoring, 148

Impactful messages, creating, 136

Impasse, reaching an, 213

Implementation: action planning and, *248*, 254, 257, *258*, *259*, 273; basic principle of innovation involving, 228; of change, enabling, 232; with compliance versus commitment, 108, 109; of a defined communication plan, 233–234; and group decisions, 265; importance of consensus for, 263; with no clear-cut solution, 275; of policies, consistency in, 275; role of information in, 129

Implementation plan, creating an, 232

Implying expectations, problem with, 330

Impositions, 261

Incentives, lack of, for developing others, 288

Incident-reporting mechanism, 11

Independence, 10, 64–65, 86, 189, 192, 195

Individual decisions: described, 261; group versus, using, factors for consideration in, 263–265, 266

Individual practice, 332

Individual-team polarity, 275

Industrial age, management in the, 8–9

Influence, art of, 284

Information: amount of, and complexity of decision making, 261; availability of, 129–130; believing that followers already know the, 127–128; confidentiality of, 128–129, 162, 165; excess, erring on the side of, 132; importance of, 126; minimal need for, in the competent level, 320; new, listening providing, 145; provided by groups, 264; rationale that followers don't need certain, 128–129; rationale that followers don't want to know, 128; relevant, gathering, in negotiation, *208*, 210–211; respecting, that is old, 170; that is not understandable to followers, belief about, 129–131; from third-party sources, use of, in assessment, 321, 335; unequal access to, 175. *See also* Sharing information

Information overload, 122, 131, 162

Inguagiato, R., 151

Initiative, personal, 246–247

Innovation: basic principle of, involving implementation, 228; creating conflict to increase, 202; fear of, 186; focusing on the status quo versus, 11–12, 185; potential for, transition stage characterized by, 238

Innovation Leadership: Creating the Landscape of Health Care (Porter-O'Grady and Malloch), 181

Instant messaging, 164

Institute for Healthcare Improvement, 256

Instruction, giving and receiving, 326. *See also* Teaching others

Integrated systems, failure of, 239

Integration (integral) stage, of commitment, *75*, 77

Integration phase, in the change process, *231*, 234–235

Integrative thinking, 276

Integrity, 4, 18, 37, 42, 85, 86, 87, 93, 116, 350. *See also* Trust

Intelligences. *See* Emotional intelligence; Social intelligence

Intelligent Organization, The (Pinchot and Pinchot), 2

Intention, 56, 315–317, 340, 341

Interaction distances, 155

Interdependence, 36, 63, 64, 65, 189, 238, 260, 269, 279, 280

Internal accountability, 198

Internal adaptation, 237, 238–239

Internet, information on the, 129–130

Interpersonal development, stages of, 64. *See also* Dependence; Independence; Interdependence

Interpersonal skills, importance of, xi, 350. *See also* *specific skills*

Interruptions, 302

Intimate zone, 155

Intimidation and dominance, as a conflict resolution strategy, 204

Intrinsic crisis, 77

Intrinsic motivation: at the expert level, 321; misconception involving, 295; principles of, 307–314; understanding, 297–305, *307*

Intuition, 35, 87, 95, 261

Investment: in commitment, 74, 79; in employee strengths, 323. *See also* Resource allocation; Time investment

Irritability, 237, 322

Israeli culture, 159

Issues, defining, in negotiation, 208–209

Iverson, R., 79, 81, 110

Iyengar, S. S., 109

J

Jacobson, R., 143

Japanese culture, 119, 157

Jazwiec, L., 24

Jenkins, M., 311

Job descriptions, clearly articulating, 194–195

Job expertise, 8, 40

Job performance. *See* Employee performance

Job requirements, changing, 193

Job satisfaction, 87, 304

Job vacancies, 23, 24, 81, 304

Johns, C., 343

Johnson, B., 274, 275, 277, 279, 280

Johnson, C., 99, 103

Johnson, J. A., 4

Joni, S. A., 202, 203

Jordan-Evans, S., 23

Judgment calls, making good, importance of, 181, 182, 276

Just cultures, 11, 199

K

Kalisch, B., 216, 226

Kanter, R. M., 73, 78, 79, 90, 186, 189–190

Kaplan, R. S., 28

Katzenbach, J. R., 215, 216, 302

Kaye, B., 23

Kemp, P., 27

Kennedy, J. F., 95

King, M. L., Jr., 95, 97, 104

Klich-Heartt, E. I., 164, 165

Knee-jerk reactions, 257

Knights of the TeleRound Table (Kostner), 174

"Know How to Lead," viii

Knowledge: demonstrating, in performance assessment, 321; as an element of empowerment, 190, 192; as a factor related to competence, 39, *41*; minimal need for, in the competent level, 320; provided by groups, 264. *See also* Competence; Information

Knowles, M., 343, 344

Kostner, J., 174, 175

Kotter, J. P., 240

Kouzes, J. W., 4, 13, 48, 185, 244, 337

Kowalski, K., 116

Kraemer, H., 5

Kramer, R. M., 38

Kramer, S. J., 244

Krug, D., 151

L

LaFasto, F., 223

Langan, J., 317

Larson, C. E., 223

Larson, P., 27

Laughter, eliciting, 34–35

Laurie, D. L., 2, 180

Laws, 162, 183

Leader-follower relationship: and affective commitment, 83; and appearance, 156; collective responsibility and accountability in the, 65–66; conclusion on, 66; creating a trust-based organizational climate for, 58–60; discussion questions on, 66–67; emotional intelligence needed for the, 32–34; essential elements of the, 36–58, 66, 83, 184; and moving forward into the future, 350–351; nature of the, 60–65; overview of, 35–36; partnership in, viii, 63–65, 93, 184; rushing the formation of, 184; and sharing personal or leadership mission statements, 91; social intelligence needed for the, 34–35

Leaders: characteristics of, 5–6; most important role of, 181; multiple, encouraging, 96; new, establishing trust in, difficulty of, 39–40

Leadership: as the art of influence, 284; business versus social sector, 6, 226; challenges facing today's, 18–28; change in, and transition, 236; communication and, 124–125; competencies needed for, 4–5; conclusion on, 28–29; defining, 3–6, 32; demand for, reasons for the, 14–18, 350; in developing others, 284–285; discussion questions on, 29; distinguishing between management and, 3, 6–13; importance of, 2; increasing need for, 13; moving forward into the future, 350–353; overview of, 2–3; shared, 224, 225–226, 227, 334. *See also specific leadership roles and responsibilities*

Leadership and the New Science (Wheatley), 126

Leadership development, viii; importance of, 2; as a lifelong process, 352–353; meeting the challenge of, ways of, viii; methods of, 5; as a priority, 284–285. *See also* Coaching; Employee development

Leadership gap, research on the, x

Leadership interventions, for strengthening commitment: common pitfalls of, 108–112; focus of, and approaches, 82–107

Leadership IQ, 59

Leadership mission statements, 91–92

Leadership teams, 216, 224–226, 227, 228

Leadership values, 85, 91

Lean management, 256

Leander, W., 130, 220, 223, 224, 228, 230, 234, 235

Learning: continual, 301, 333, 342; experiential, ix, 343–344, 350; readiness for, 344; team, success of, influencing, 219, 229

Learning cultures, creating, importance of, 269

Learning opportunities, 186, 202, 267, 301, 309, 315, 319, 333. *See also* Employee development

Learning organizations, 71, 132, 342

LeClair, H., 158

Leebov, W., 162, 274, 340

Leeman, J., 273

Left brain thinking, 257

Legislative leadership, 226

Lencioni, P., 223

Lepper, M. R., 109

Life's Little Treasure Book on Success (Brown), 350

Lincoln, A., 6, 97, 141, 145, 160

Lincoln on Leadership (Phillips), 141

Line-of-sight concept, 92, 299

LinkedIn, 164

Linksky, M., 3

Listeners: attention of, getting the, 137; commonalities with, establishing, 137–138

Listening: continually, 184; importance of, 144–146, 150–151; levels of, 148–150; skill of, increasing, 146–148

Listening span, 146

Litigation, 154, 160

Loehr, J., 21, 27, 89, 302

Long-distance relationships, communication and trust in, 174–175

Lorimer, W., 42, 130, 220, 223, 224, 228, 230, 234, 235

Losada, M., 56

Low performers, coaching, 291, 312, 313

Low-performing teams, 57

Loye, D., 65

Ludema, J. D., 269

Lydon, J. E., 75

M

Mackoff, B. L., 92

Magnet recognition program, 3, 329; case study involving the, 99–104

Maisel, N., 53, 55

Majority decisions, 262

Makin, P. J., 78, 80, 82

Making amends, 48, 50–51

Malloch, K., 161, 181, 230, 253

Management: of attention, 98; and conflict resolution, 203, 204, 205; distinguishing between leadership and, 3, 6–13; focus on, periods calling for, 15, 16; misconception about, 6; origins of, 8–9; promoting people with job expertise to, 8; reduced need for, 13

Management by walking around (MBWA), 46

Management positions, decimation of, 2–3

Manager empowerment, 189–190

Managerial control, 10

Managerial partnerships, 63

Managing for the Future (Drucker), 32

Manion, J., 21, 23, 24, 27, 42, 46, 61, 63, 70, 79, 130, 215, 220, 223, 224, 225, 228, 230, 231, 234, 235, 237, 244, 252, 299, 302, 304, 305, 306, 311, 314, 316, 331, 334, 340

Manipulation versus motivation, 296

Manthey, M., 191

Martin, J., 70, 71, 285

Martin, R., 276

Maslow, A., 295

Mastercard and Visa, 15

Matrix organization, 229

Maun, C., 25

Maxwell, J., 77, 352

Mayer, J. D., 32

Mayer, R., 79

McCarthy, D., 190

McConnell, C. R., 117

McCullough, D., 323

McDonald, T., 135

McGinn, P., 281

McGinnis, A. L., 295, 309, 338, 339

McKee, A., 32, 244

McKeown, G., 308

McNally, K., 289, 291

McNeese-Smith, D., 87

Meaning, 124–125, 145, 220, 297

Meaningful purpose, as an intrinsic motivator, 297, 298–300, 303, *307*

Measurement: emphasis on, issue with, 12; inadequate or outdated systems of, issue of, 304; of success, following implementation, 255. *See also* Outcome evaluation; Performance assessment

Mediation, as a conflict resolution strategy, 206–207

Medicare fraud, 18

Meetings: followers arriving late to, addressing, 144; seating arrangements at, 155, 156; teaching and learning in, 333; team, 219, 221, 222; with team representatives, 176

Melrose, K., 38

Mergers/acquisitions, 111, 174, 230, 235, 236

Merrill, A. R., 91, 95

Merrill, R. R., 91, 95

Message content, listening in spite of, 147

Message delivery, 133–136, 147

Messages: mixed, 124, 134–135, 149, 170, 328; repeating, importance of, 127–128, 152, 170; restating, 148. *See also* Communication

Metaphors and analogies, using, 136, 140–141, 158, 170, 286, 291, 353

Meyer, J., 79, 80, 81

Micromanaging, 286, 322, 335

Miles, R. H., 232, 234

Military metaphors, use of, in health care, 158

Millennials, 81–82, 306

Miller, D., 21, 27, 191, 230, 231, 235

Minkara, N., 220

Minority decisions, 261–262

Mintzberg, H., 159

Mirror neurons, 34–35

Miscommunication, 117, 123, 124, 135, 150, 159, 175

Miscues, serious, involving e-mail, 161

Misinformation, 117, 129–130

Mission: alignment of, 92–93, 244; clarity of, 89, 90–91, 92, 95; defining the, responsibility for, 90; investing time in dialogue about, 108; and motivation, 299; noble purpose expressed in the, 89, 93; personal, evolution of, and statements of, 91; team, 220, 228. *See also* Common mission

Mission statements, 11, 91–92, 220

Mistakes: acknowledging, 49; admitting, 50; correcting, and accountability, 198–199; expecting and planning for, 188; learning from, 186, 309; providing corrective feedback about, 339–341; punitive response to, 11, 55–56, 188, 199; support during times of making, 294

Mistrust. *See* Distrust

Mixed messages, 124, 134–135, 149, 170, 328

Mixed-performing teams, 57

Modeling behavior: consistency in, lack of, example of, 107; lack of, for coaching, 286, 288; teaching by, 345–346; that accepts mistakes, 188; that avoids conflict, problem with, 212–213

Monitoring, 38, 255, 259, 265, 273

Mood, importance of, 34–35, 47

Moral commitment, 80

Moral distress, 28

Morgan, C., 85

Morris, D., 154, 155

Morse, G., 38

Motivation: during change, 234; of coaches, 293; coaching and, 294–314, *315*; and competition, 346; defining, 294–295; different factors inspiring, 296; external, added influence of, applying, 297, 307; generational differences and, 305–307; and getting results, 244; inspiring, 4; intrinsic, 295, 297–305, 307–314, 321; misconceptions about, 295–297; principles of, 307–314, *315*; in sports versus health care, 290; and teams, 220, 223, 227–228; theories related to, 295; top form of, 337

Movement phase, *231*, 232–233

Muha, T., 314, 331

Multiple descriptions, providing, 170

Multiple leaders, encouraging, 96

Multiple visions, need for, recognizing the, 96

Murphy, M., 59, 286, 301, 316

Mutual respect: coaching and, 292, 293; as essential, to the leader-follower relationship, 36, *37*, 51–53, 66, 83, 184; in open conflict, 201

Mutual work, sharing, 61, 62, 63

Mycek, S., 90

MySpace, 164

N

Nanotechnology, 20

Nanus, B., 2, 13, 98, 124

Napoleon, 295

National Database of Nursing Quality Indicators (NDNQI), 255

Need fulfillment, 295

Negative element of commitment, 74, 75, 76, 77, 109

Negative event support, 53, 55–56

Negative feedback, 122–123, 294, 335, 338, 339–341

Negative interactions, ratio of, to positive interactions, as an indicator, 56–58

Negative nonverbal communication, impact of, 135–136

Negative stories, 142

Negativity, downward spiral of, 57, 331

Negotiation: in coaching, 315; as a conflict resolution
strategy, 207–212

Negotiation climate, 211, 212

Negotiation map, 208–212

Network organization, 229

Neuroscience, findings from, 34–35, 37, 125

Neutral zone, in the transition process, *236*, 237–238

New beginning, differentiating between the start of
something and the, 238

New information, listening providing, 145

New leaders, establishing trust in, difficulty of, 39–40

New reality phase, *231*, 234

Nierenberg, J., 208, 211

9/11 terrorist attacks, 17, 118, 143

Noah principle, 97

Noble purpose, having a, 89, 203. *See also* Mission

Noise, 119, 127, 147, 170, 302

Noncontact cultures, 154

Nonverbal communication, 132, 134–135, 135–136,
152–159. *See also* Body language

Normative commitment: building, approaches for,
83–107; described, 80; focusing on, benefit of, 82; and
generational differences, 81–82

North American culture, 109, 119, 154, 155, 159

North Dakota flooding (1997)

Northern European culture, 154

Novice level, 318–319, 321, 330, 344

No-win situation, 194, 240, 322

Nuances, consideration of, in e-mail, 162

Nurses: professional practice of, magnet recognition of,
case study involving, 99–104; respect for, issue of,
52–53; turnover of nurses aides and, 23

Nursing function, responsibility for the, 197

Nursing skill acquisition, 317–318

O

Oakley, E., 151

Objective measures, use of, 255

Objectives, clarifying, in negotiation, *208*, 209–210

O'Brien, M. E., 93

O'Connell, A., 4

O'Dooley, P., 138

Oklahoma City bombing, 143

On Becoming a Leader (Bennis), ix

On Becoming a Servant-Leader (Greenleaf), 93

Online social networking. *See* Social networking sites

Open conflict, benefits of, 201–202

Open dialogue/communication. *See* Clear
communication

Open systems, 180–181, 229

Open-ended compliance, *108*, 109

Open-ended questions, 151

Openness, 43, 116, 165

Opinions, asking for, 152

Opponents, communication strategies for, 171, *172*, 173

Opportunities, providing. *See* Learning opportunities;
Stretch opportunities

Organizational climate, 58–60, 234

Organizational commitment: and common pitfalls
of leadership interventions, 108–112; defined, 78;
differentiating between personal commitment and,
70; elements of, 78, 303; leadership interventions for
strengthening, 82–107; and mission, 83, 84, 89–93;
partnership in, 71; types of, 78–82; understanding,
importance of, 72; and values, 83, 84, 85–89; and
vision, 83, 84, 94–107. *See also* Commitment

Organizational culture: based on learning, importance of,
269, 301; changing, 9, 228, 234, 239, 263, 268, 273,
304; that is a just culture, 11, 199; that views conflict
only negatively, 214

Organizational environment, based on competition, 63

Organizational integrity, 18

Organizational mission, 90, 92. *See also* Common
mission

Organizational structure, future, basis of, 229

Organizational support and affiliation, 80

Organizational values, 85, 87, 89. *See also* Shared values

Organizational vision, 96, 98. *See also* Shared vision

O'Toole, J., 48, 49, 59

Ott, W., 93

Outcome attachment, avoiding, 213

Outcome evaluation, 185, 188, 198, 223, 234, 235, 255,
260, 335, 339, 344

Outcome monitoring, 273

Outcome-oriented approaches, 180

Outcomes/results desired, achieving. *See* Getting results

Outliers: The Story of Success (Gladwell), 352

Outsourcing, 174

Overload, 41, 122, 131, 162

Overwhelmed feeling, 246, 345

Ownership, 12, 49, 64, 121, 176, 191, 195, 217, 220,
228, 250, 258, 303. *See also* Responsibility

P

Paradigm shifts, 15–17, 22, 350

Parameters, relevant, identifying, in coaching, 325, 328–330

Parker, G., 221

Participant's Guide to Managing Organizational Transitions (Bridges), *236*

Participatory decision making, 266

Participatory learning, 342–343

Partnership: in coaching, 314; and the leader-follower relationship, viii, 63–65, 93, 184; in organizational commitment, 71; understanding, importance of, 60

Passion stage, *75*, 76, 77

Passive coaching, 285–286

Passive constructive response, *54*, 55

Passive destructive response, *54*, 55

Patience, 5, 120, 182, 184, 187, 190, 234

Patient needs versus employee needs, polarity mapping, 278, 279–280

Patient safety and quality: and conflicting values, 86; impact of the electronic medical record on, 20; recent emphasis on, effect of, on problem solving, 11; valuing, 80, 142–143

Patton, G., 6

Peaceful coexistence, as a conflict resolution strategy, 207

Peck, M. S., 146

Peer coercion, 204

People, focusing on structure versus, 9–10

Performance: employee, and commitment, 80, 81; financial, leading indicator of, 71; repeated, role of, in success, 352

Performance appraisals, 287, 311, 325

Performance assessment, *315*, 317–325

Performance gaps, addressing, 287, 317

Performance goals. *See* Goal setting; Goals

Performance improvement, importance of, 286. *See also* Coaching

Performance observation, 289, 291, 293, *315*, 317, 321, 325, 326, 335–336, 338, 340, 341

Performance-based respect, 52

Perlow, L. A., 27

Persistence, 74, 75, 78, 246

Personal commitment: differentiating between organizational commitment and, 70; understanding, importance of, 72. *See also* Commitment

Personal initiative, 246–247

Personal mission, 89, 91, 92. *See also* Common mission

Personal space, respecting other's, 155–156

Personal values, 85, 87, 98. *See also* Shared values

Personal vision, 96, 97, 98. *See also* Shared vision

Personal zone, 155, 156

Personality traits, importance of, in selection, 302

Persuasion, as a conflict resolution strategy, 205

Pesmen, S., 313

Peters, T., 13, 46, 142

Phillips, D., 97, 141, 142, 160

Physical appearance, issue of, 156

Physical contact, issue of, 154

Physicians: and aversion to risk, 186; and coalition building, 205; and coercion, 204; ethical behavior of, 86; as key stakeholders, communicating with, 173; valuing, over patients, issue of, 80, 86

Pickford, M., 186

Pinchot, E., 2, 17, 174

Pinchot, G., 2, 17, 174

Piper, L. E., 38

Pisano, G., 219

Pitfalls: administrative, x; blocking clear communication, 119–124, *125*; of conflict resolution, 212–214; of decision making, 265–267; in the empowerment process, 193–199; in leading change and transition, 238–240; of problem solving, 256–258, *259*; in strengthening commitment, 108–112

Pleasure, importance of, 244, 297, 311

Plop decisions, 261

Polarities, defined, and examples of, 274–275

Polarity management: benefits and challenges of, 279–280; choosing to use, 256; described, 275–276; method of, described and example of, 277–280

Polarity mapping, 277–278, 279–280

Policy implementation, 275

Ponte, P. R., 3, 70

Poor performers. *See* Low performers, coaching

Porter, J. L., 27

Porter-O'Grady, T., 161, 181, 220, 230, 253

Positive change methodology, 273

Positive conflict, 201–202, 203

Positive element of commitment, 74, 75, 76, 77, 109

Positive energy, effect of, 125

Positive event support, 53–55

Positive feedback, 335, 337–339

Positive psychology, 56–57, 331, 338

Positive reinforcement, 338, 339

Positive statements or questions, forming, 269–270, 273–274

Positive stories, 142

Positive work environment, 46, 70, 215, 271, 302

Positive-to-negative interactions, ratio of, as an indicator, 56–58

Posner, B. Z., 4, 13, 48, 185, 244, 337

Post, N., 230

Posture and body motions, 157–158

Power: change in, and transition, 236; conflict resolution strategy based on, 204; and corruption, 18; defined, 189; followers giving up, 128; legitimate, 43; managers with, 190; and meeting space, 156; personal and social, 65; structural, 6; unwillingness to disseminate, 224. *See also* Authority; Control

Power map, complex, 226

Power of Vision, The (Barker), 94

Power relationships, reconfigured, 161

Powerlessness, effect of, 190

PowerPoint, issue with, 138, 139

Practice: guided, 344; importance of, 4, 352; individual and group, described, 332; role of, in success, 352

Praise, 337–339, 344

Pre-commitments, 76

Preoccupation, with the organization, 78

Preparation periods, 100–101, 108

Preparation phase, 231–232

Preparation, role of, in success, 352

Presumptive trust, 38, 129

Pretend listening, 148

Pride, building, 302

Primary work teams, 216, 228

Principle-Centered Leadership (Covey), 183

Prion, S., 164, 165

Prioritizing values, 86–88

Priority setting, during the change process, 233

Pritchard, W., 90

Privacy, 165, 345–346

Privileged information, 128–129

Proactivity, 245, 246–247, 246–247, 331

Problem identification and analysis, *248*, 249–251, 257, 258, *259*

Problem solving: consequences of, as an approach, 268–269; creative, move toward, 11; direct, coaching and supporting, 13, 339; individual and group, described, 247–248; leaders helping employees with, benefit of, 244; pitfalls in the process of, 256–258, *259*; reasons groups bog down in the process of, 259–260; shared, 62; skill in, need for, 245; steps in the process of, 248–256; team, approaches to, deciding on, 221; traditional, comparing, and appreciative inquiry, 267–269. *See also* Getting results

Problem solving alternatives. *See* Appreciative inquiry; Polarity management

Problem statement, 249, 250–251, 252, 256

Problem-centered learning, 343

Problems: coping with versus fixing, 268; creating, dysfunctional behavior of, 269; determining the solvability of, 279–280; nature of, considering the, in decision making, 263; overemphasis on dealing with, effect of, 324

Process barriers, removing, 187–188, 304, 333, 334

Process facilitation: for change and transition, 229–240; conclusion on, 240–241; for creating teams, 214–229; discussion questions on, 241–242; for empowering others, 188–199; key tenets of, 181–188; and moving forward into the future, 351; overview of, 180–181; for resolving conflicts, 199–214

Process improvement, 268, 273, 304, 329

Process improvement groups, 248

Process steps, skipping or eliminating, 182

Processes: continually challenging, 185–187; facilitating the flow of, 183, 187–188; natural flow of, 183; understanding and respecting, 182–185; work, teams deciding on approaches to, 221

Procrastination, as a conflict resolution strategy, 205. *See also* Avoidance

Productivity and the Self-Fulfilling Prophecy, 309

Productivity levels, regaining, 234

Professional associations, 73, 165

Professional practice, Magnet recognition of, case study involving, 99–104

Professional skills, teaching, 332

Proficient level, 318

Progress, as an intrinsic motivator, 297, *298*, 303–305, *307*

Promotions: past, basis for, 226; transition of, 236–237

Psychology, 56–57, 111, 249, 331, 338

Public zone, 155

Punctuation and grammar, 162, 167

Punitive consequences, 11, 55–56, 188, 199

Punitive rewards, 312–313

Purpose: of change, examining the, 232; of coaching, determining intention and, 315–317; having a noble, 89, 203; meaningful, as an intrinsic motivator, 297, *298*, 298–300, 303, *307*. *See also* Mission

Q

Qualification, as a factor related to competence, *39*, 40, *41*

Quality decisions, value placed on, considering the, 264

Quality improvement groups, 248

Quality improvement initiatives, 228

Quality improvement methodology, 246, 255–256

Quality improvement programs, techniques taught through, 249–250

Quality measures, evaluating, 234, 235

Questioning: continually, 12; the leader's level of accountability, 49; of solutions, 205; the status quo, 185

Questions: asking, techniques for, 151–152; in coaching, 315, 319, 320, 324, 331–332, 335; for defining the problem, 249; positive, forming, 269–270, 274

Quick fixes, 227

Quiet stage, 75, 77

Quotable Women, 186

R

Raines, D., 99, 100, 101, 103

Rapport (resonance), 35, 134, 156

Rath, T., 323

Rationality, importance of, 111

Reactions, feedback through, 336

Reactive behavior, 246, 257, 287. *See also* Emotions

Reactive body language, 127

Reactive coaching, 316

Readability, 166, 168

Reality, new, dealing with the, *231*, 234

Reciprocal listening, 150–151

Recognition, 234, 304–305, *307*, 311, 324, 337, 338. *See also* Rewarding desired behavior; Rewards and benefits

Reflection, 91, 145, 331, 343, 350

Reflective (empathic) listening, 148, 149–150

Regulatory environment, 25–26, 230, 300

Reimbursement changes, 26

Reina, D. S., 58

Reina, M. L., 58

Reinforcement, positive, 338, 339

Relationship conflict, 201, 203

Relationship management, 32, 33, 194–195

Relationships: communication, 176–177; complex, balancing, 64; damaging, fear of, 214; ending, 236, 237; impact of technology on, 20; leadership existing only within the context of, 10, 32; long-distance, communication and, 174–175; power, reconfigured, 161; reporting, 176–177, 197; solid, building, through empathic listening, 149–150. *See also* Coach-performer relationship; Healthy relationships; Leader-follower relationship

Renesch, J., 93, 187

Repeated performance, role of, in success, 352

Repeating messages, importance of, 127–128, 152, 170

Reporting mechanism, incident, 11

Reporting relationships, 176–177, 197

Reporting, third-party, 335

Resentment, 204, 206, 237, 322, 343

Resilience, 4, 21

Resistance, 22, 109, 151, 170, 233, 237, 272, 343

Resource allocation: for empowering employees, 184, 190, 194; inadequate, avoiding, 329; in preparing for change, 231, 232

Respect: displaying a lack of, by not telling followers the truth, 128; expectations about, 127; listening as a means of communicating, 145–146; loss of, by not admitting mistakes, 50; for old information, 170; for processes, 182–185; for students, in adult learning, 343–344; for work and personal spaces, 155. *See also* Mutual respect

Respectful dissent, 48

Responsibility: for action steps, failing to determine, 257; and authority, 176, 192, 193, 195, 196, 197, 261, 303; and behavioral expectations, 308–309, 310; clarifying expectations about, 325–326; coaching, 339; for communication, issue of, 121, 125, 131–169; for conflict resolution, 203; for defining the mission, 90; defining the, of each team member role, 221–222; delegating, 199, 261, 285, 303, 310, 328–329; earned, 193; and empowerment, 191, 193–194, 194–195, 203, 267; exaggerated sense of, 258; inspiring, 4; shared, 62, 65–66, 195, 334. *See also* Accountability; Ownership

Results, achieving. *See* Getting results

Results, measuring and assessing. *See* Outcome evaluation

Retention, 23, 24, 81

Retirement issues, 2–3, 23, 24, 81

Rewarding desired behavior, 310–314

Rewards and benefits: for both individuals and teams, 275; and commitment, 78, 81, 110; and intrinsic motivation, 297, 299, 311, 312; for making progress, importance of, 304–305; systems for, modifying, 234

Right-brain thinking, 257

Risk taking, encouraging, 186

Road Less Traveled, The (Peck), 146

Robert Wood Johnson Foundation, 256

Robinson, J., 164

Rogers, R., 48

Role expectations, clarifying, 325–326

Role models: lack of, for coaching, 286, 288; pressure felt by, 345. *See also* Modeling behavior

Romantic commitment, 75

Ross, I., 208, 211

Rumors, 126

S

Sacrifice, 74, 75, 78

Salovey, P., 32

San Francisco earthquake (1989), 143

Scandals/corruption, 18

Schlesinger, L. A., 240

Schmidt, C., 70, 71, 285

Schmitt, M. H., 61

Schoorman, D., 79

Schwartz, T., 21, 27, 89, 302

Seashore, C., 337

Seashore, E., 337

Second-order problem solving, need for, 245

Selective listening, 149

Self-awareness, 32, *33*, 38, 56

Self-care, importance of, 26–27

Self-confidence, 288, 319, 320, 321, 324, 332, 344

Self-directed learning, 343, 344, 345

Self-disclosure, selected, 137

Self-empowerment, 331–332

Self-fulfilling prophecy, creating a, 309–310

Self-justification, need for, 111

Self-management, 32–33, 130

Self-reporting, 321, 335

Seligman, M. E., 297, 300, 302

Semantic differences, awareness of, 123

Senge, P. M., 71, 95–96, 97, 110

September 11, 2001, terrorist attacks, 17, 118, 143

Servant-leadership, 93, 350

Service delivery changes, 230

Settings, inappropriate, for communication, *125*

Seven Habits of Highly Effective People, The (Covey), 64, 148

Sexual harassment, 154

Shared accountability, 65–66

Shared decision making, 62, 130, 266–267, 296, 303, 327

Shared leadership, 224, 225–226, 227, 334

Shared meaning, 124–125, 145, 220

Shared mission. *See* Common mission

Shared responsibility, 62, 65–66, 195, 334

Shared values: alignment essential for, 85–86, 87; and clarity of mission, 90; described, 85; influence of, with a common mission and shared vision, 98, 110; investing time in exploring, 108; as one component of building commitment, 84, 85; and prioritizing, 86–88; result of, 88–89

Shared vision: as a component in building commitment, 84, 94; development of a, steps in, 94–98; influence of, with a common mission and shared values, 98, 110;

investing time in development of a, 108; lack of a, example of, 107.

Sharing information, 61, 108, 116, 126–131, 175, 208, 319, 344

Sharing mutual work, 61, 62, 63

Shaw, G. B., 116

Shendall-Falik, N., 273

Sherbin, L., 82

Shotgun approach, 70

Shula, D., 289, 291, 292–293

Side bets, 78–79

Sieg, M. J., 63

Silence, issue with, 44–45

Simon Says game, 153

Simplifying, 170

Sisyphus (Greek legend), 304

Situational leadership model, 317, 318

Six Sigma, 255–256

Skill: assessing, 317–318; desired, teaching or training for a, 332–333; differentiating between talent and, ix; as a factor related to competence, 39, *41*; learning a new, and motivation, 301. *See also* Competence

Skill acquisition model, 317–318

Skill potential, selection based on, 218

Skits, using, 138

Smith, D. K., 215, 216

Smith, S. S., 337

Snyder, J., 273

Social awareness, 32, 33, 34

Social intelligence, 34–35, 116, 118

Social networking sites, 161, 164–166

Social neuroscience, findings from, 34

Social psychology, 111, 249

Social sector leadership, 6, 226

Social support. *See* Support

Social zone, 155, 156

Socialization messages, early, 44, 200

Societal dangers, top three, 17

Societal models, 65

Societal values, 85

Socrates, 6

Solution acceptance, importance of, considering the, 264

Solution generation: and analysis of alternatives, *248*, 252–254, 257, *258*, *259*; limiting, 250–251, 256. *See also* Problem solving

Sörenstam, A., 291

Sorrentino, R., 72, 74, 75, 76, 77, 109, 110, 111

Space, use of, nonverbal communication through the, 154–156

Spears, L., 93

Specialization versus generalization, 277–278

Speedy resolutions, insisting on, 60

Spitzer, R., 71

Spoken communication. *See* Verbal communication

Sports coaching, 290–291, 292–293

Stacey, R., 181

Stagnating, 186

Stakeholder agreement, 170, 171, 173

Stakeholder matrix, 171, 173

Stakeholder trust, 170, 171, 173

Stakeholders, key, specific communication approaches for, developing, 170–173, 233–234

Status: change in, and transition, 236; connotation of, through the use of space, 154–155. *See also* Authority; Power

Status quo: aspiring to something larger than the, 301; challenging, comfortable with, 247; constraints of the, accepting the, 268; forcing the examination of the, 201; versus innovation, focusing on the, 11–12, 185

Steding, T. L., 58, 60

Stefaniak, K., 273

Stone, D. M., 24

Storming, 201. *See also* Brainstorming

Storytelling, use of, 136, 141–143, 170, 271

Strengthening Ethical Wisdom: Tools for Transforming Your Health Care Organization (Gilbert), 86

Strengths, assessing, 323–325

StrengthsFinder2.0, 324

Stretch opportunities, 223, 286, 333

Stretch vision, 95–96, 100, 232

Structure versus people, focusing on, 9–10

Subject-centered learning, 343

Successes: duplicating, resistance to, 272; inquiry into, 267, 272. *See also* Appreciative inquiry

Successful individuals, commonality among, 352

Succession plans, 225

Sumberg, K., 82

Superordinate goals, using, as a conflict resolution strategy, 207

Support: coaching and, 292, 294; communication and, 116; as essential to the leader-follower relationship, 36, *37*, 53–56, 66, 83; organizational, 80; in teaching, 344; team, 222, 226

Supportive skills, teaching, 332

Surel, D., 220

Survival: organizational, and talent, 23; societal, and the demand for leadership, 17–18

Sustaining phase, 273

Swaggart, J., 18

Symbols and graphics, using, 136, 139–140, 175

Synergy, 61, 65, 88

System vision, 96

Systems integration, failure of, 239

Systems theory, 180–181

Systems thinking, importance of, xi

T

Talent: challenge of, 23, 24; differentiating between skill and, ix; spotting, 323

Tarkenton, F., 338

Task (cognitive) conflict, 201, 202

Tasks, nature of, considering the, in decision making, 263

Taylor, B. J., 91

Teaching organizations, 342

Teaching others: as a coaching intervention, *315*, 326, 344; by example, 345–346; and the principles of adult learning, 341–345. *See also* Employee development

Team creativity phase, *231*, 233–234

Team decision making, 262

Team, defined, 215

Team development, 201, 229, 327–328

Team environment, 225

Team goals, 222, 223

Team meetings, 219, 221, 222

Team members: roles and responsibilities of, discussing and defining, 221–222; selecting, 218–219

Team practice, 332

Team purpose, defining the, 220

Team recorder role, 222

Team representative role, 176

Team support, 222, 226

Team vision, 96

Team work: common approaches to, establishing, 220–223, 229; defining the, 218, 228

Team-Based Health Care Organizations: Blueprint for Success (Manion, Lorimer, and Leander), 228

Team-individual polarity, 275

Teams: accepting responsibility, 191, 195; accountability of, 217, 223–224; authority of, 196; communicating with, 175–177; and conflict resolution, 203; converting to, and capability, issue of, 194; creating, 214, 217–226; distinguishing between work groups and, 216–217, 223–224; emotional intelligence of, 222–223, 229; importance of, 214–215; performance of, 57; pitfalls of creating, 226–229; reasons for initiating, being clear about, 218; types of, 215–216

Teamwork, defined, 215

Technical skills, teaching, 332

Technological change, 20–21, 63, 230

Teleconferencing, 175

Telephone systems, automated, 140

Tempered trust, 38

Temporary workers, 24

10,000 hour rule, 352

Tenure, 43–44, 204

Terminations, announcement of, 140

Territoriality, 155

Testing stage, *75*, 76

Texting, 131, 161

Third degree, giving followers the, 152, 337

Third parties, use of, 206, 321, 335

Thomas, K. W., 297, 298, 300, 303

Thomas, S. P., 120

Thought content, 167–168

Tichy, N., 181, 269, 284, 341–342

Time: demands on, 287, 300; island, being on, 158; providing, to pursue opportunities, 334; use of, nonverbal communication through the, 153–154

Time frames, 222, 237, 239, 257, 258, 265, 329, 352

Time investment: in coaching, issue of, 287; comparing compliance and commitment in terms of, 108–109; in developing teams, minimizing, problem of, 229; in empowering employees, 184, 190, 194; in listening, importance of a, 146–147; in major change initiatives, 104; in practice, 352; in processes, 182, 187

Time lost, problems resulting in, 245

Time off, taking, 27

"Timeless Leadership," 323

Tipping point, 300

Top performers. *See* High performers

Toshiba, 15

Touch, nonverbal communication through, 154

Toyota Production System/Lean Management, 256

"Toys and trinkets" approach, 311

Training and education. *See* Employee development

Transformational leadership, defined, 3

"Transforming Care at the Bedside: Paving the Way for Change," 256

Transforming Care at the Bedside program, 256

Transition: challenge of, 22; change versus, 230; defined, 22; emotional reactions to, 200; facilitating the process of, 229–230, 236–238; pitfalls of leading through, 238–240; stages of, 22, 235–238

Transparency, 59, 116. *See also* Clear communication

Trial periods, use of, 188, 234

Trigg, R., 73

Triolo, P., 3, 70, 92

Trust: broken, repairing, 48–51; climate of, creating a, 58–60; coaching and, 292–293, 321, 333; communication and, 59, 60, 116, 122, 123, 135, 170, 171, 173, 174–175; in conflict resolution, 208–209; damaging, 56, 204, 233; defined, 37; empowerment and, 190; as essential to the leader-follower relationship, 36, 37–51, 55, 66, 83, 184; forms of, 38; gift of, self-disclosure as a, 137; giving oneself in, to the issue or solution, 72; innovation and, 11; inspiring, 4; key elements of, 38–47; and long-distance relationships, 174–175; neurobiology of, 37; presumptive, 38, 129; in the process, 183; relationships of, 10; within teams, 222; and the use of space, 155–156. *See also* Distrust

Truth, 73, 86, 128, 130

Tuleja, T., 338

Turbulent environment, challenge of a, 25–26, 90

Turnover, 23, 24, 79, 81, 87, 304, 338

Twitter/tweeting, 131, 164, 165–166

Two-factor theory, 295

U

Ulreich, S., 27

Ultimatums, 211, 213

Unanimous decisions, 263

Uncertainty, challenge of, 17, 19–22, 26, 46, 47, 55, 181, 186, 203, 230, 237, 260

Unconditional respect, extending, 51–52

Undermined decisions, 197, 198, 263

Understanding, listening for, 147

Unemployment rates, 24, 81

United Health Systems (Altru Health System), 143

U.S. Department of Labor, 338

Universal room concept, 8, 329

University of Michigan, 17

Unruh, L., 24

Utopian communities, 73

V

Vacancy measures, lack of, 304. *See also* Job vacancies

Values: alignment of, 85–86, 87, 244, 307; conflicting, 85–86, 87, 88, 89; defined, and types of, 85; and motivation, 299; noble purpose expressed in the, 89, 93; prioritizing, 86–88; workforce, changing, 214. *See also* Shared values

Values in Action Character Strengths assessment, 324

Van Allen, L., 27

Verbal communication, 132–152, 159.

Veronesi, J. F., 285

Vestal, K., 10, 19, 38, 246, 247, 281

Videotaping, 293, 332

Vietnam War, 143

Virtual office, 174

Visibility, 46, 170, 346

Vision: alignment of, 96, 244; compelling, importance of a, case studies involving the, 98–107; defining and describing the, 94–96; developing the, in the change process, 232; dialogue about the, engaging in, 94, 96–97; leaders understanding, 94; long-term, importance of, 90; noble purpose expressed in the, 89, 93; power of, 94, 98; redirecting to developing a, 331; structure for the, creating a, 94, 97–98; team, 220; that is grounded, 272. *See also* Shared vision

Vision statement, 107, 272

Visions, cascade of, 96

Voice mail, 27, 162, 291

Voice tone and word choice, 158, 161

Voting, 259, 262

W

Wall, B., 338

Wall Street, 18

Washington, G., 323

Waterman, R. H., 109–110

Watson, P., 63

Weaver, T. E., 218

Weinberg, G., 337

Weinstock, M., 215

Wellins, R., 126

Wells Fargo, 312

Wesorick, B., 279

What and why, focusing on how versus, 8–9

Wheatley, M. J., 126, 132

White, S. V., 250

Why Pride Matters More Than Money (Katzenbach), 302

Wiener, Y., 78

William, L., 27

Willingness, 190, 191, 192, 208

Wilson, J., 126

Win-lose situation, problem with, 204, 207

Win-win situation, 204, 207, *208*, 210, 212

Wisdom of Teams, The (Katzenbach and Smith), 215

Wisdom, source of, 260, 350

Wiseman, L., 308 ·

Wolf, G., 3, 70

Wolfson Children's Hospital, 99

Wood, S. O., 273

Word choice and voice tone, 158, 161

Work: crafting, 302; increasing complexity of, 214; mutual, sharing, 61, 62, 63. *See also* Team work

Work environment, 46, 70, 215, 271, 302

Work groups, distinguishing between teams and, 216–217, 223–224

Work hours, 27

"Work of Leadership, The" (Heifetz and Laurie), 2, 180

Work overload, 41

Work productivity, 87

Work space, respecting other's, 155

Workforce: as better educated, 129; changing values of the, 214; issues involving the, challenge of, 23–24, 81; nature of the, and compliance versus commitment, 72; shrinking, effect of, 199–200

Workforce shortages, 23, 72, 82

Working approaches, common, establishing, 220–223

Work-life balance, 27, 46

Workload, reducing, that is perceived as near meaningless, 299–300

Workplace diversity, 24–25, 305

WorldCom, 18

Wortman, C. B., 72, 74, 75, 76, 77, 109, 110, 111

Writing skills, improving, 166–169

Written communication, 132, 159–169. *See also* E-mail

Y

Yoder-Wise, P., 116

Young, J., 286

Z

Zak, P. J., 37

Zanna, M. P., 75

Zemke, R., 269, 270, 272, 273, 284, 286, 314

Zwisler, S., 27